Psychological Interventions in Sport, Exercise & Injury Rehabilitation

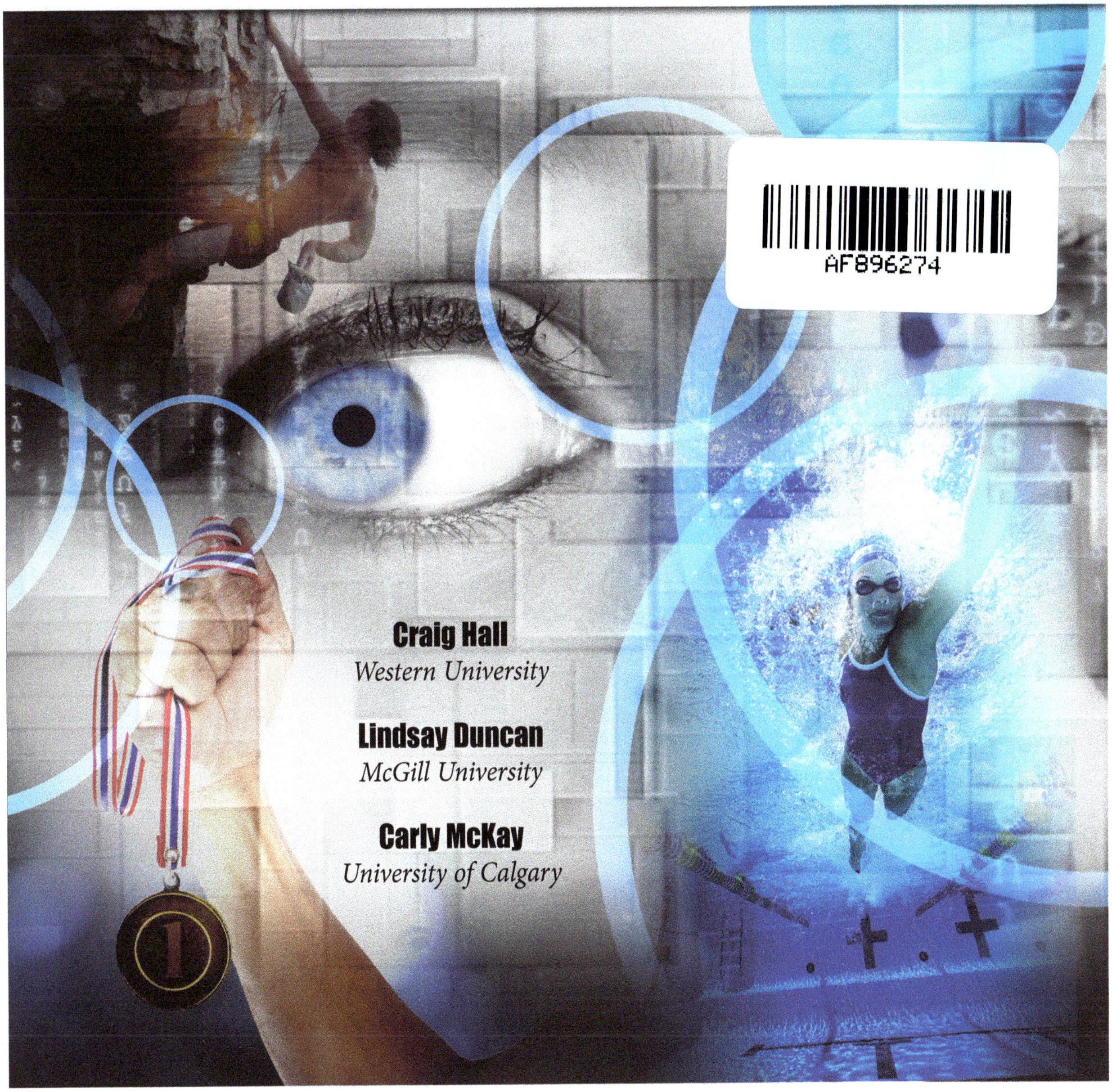

Craig Hall
Western University

Lindsay Duncan
McGill University

Carly McKay
University of Calgary

Kendall Hunt
publishing company

Kendall Hunt
publishing company
www.kendallhunt.com
Send all inquiries to:
4050 Westmark Drive
Dubuque, IA 52004-1840

ISBN 978-1-4652-6895-2

Printed in the United States of America

Contents

Chapter 4

Chapter 5

Preface

This book is written for individuals interested in psychological interventions in physical activity settings and is especially applicable to senior students in kinesiology, physical education, health sciences, or related disciplines. This book is designed to expand on the theories and concepts that are typically learned during introductory courses in sport and exercise psychology, and provide the reader with a set of techniques and tangible skills that can be practically applied in sports, exercise, and injury rehabilitation.

The book begins with three introductory chapters that discuss why and how psychological interventions can play a role in sport, exercise, and injury rehabilitation. We focus on the benefits and limitations of psychological interventions across these settings, as well as who is best placed for delivering such interventions and in what settings psychological interventions have the most success. We finish our series of introductory chapters with a discussion about expertise and the potential to optimize the use of psychological skills through the deliberate practice of these skills.

The second section of the book discusses the common interventions employed in all three of the physical activity settings and includes modeling, goal setting, imagery, self-talk, biofeedback, and coping with self-presentational concerns. Each chapter begins with an overview of the intervention technique and then discusses its application in each physical activity setting. We also present some general recommendations for the application of the intervention technique under consideration, as well as some suggested readings on the topic.

The final section of the book is comprised of three chapters that each focuses on a topic that is somewhat unique to only one of the intervention settings. In chapter 10 we discuss coping with emotions in sport, in chapter 11 we discuss the importance of the group within the context of exercise, and in chapter 12 we address fear of re-injury. As in the chapters in the second part of the book, these final three chapters also present practical recommendations and recommended readings.

Our hope is that after reading this book, individuals will feel prepared to identify the psychological intervention strategies that could be used to optimize cognitions and performance within sport, exercise, and injury rehabilitation. They also should be equipped with practical strategies for implementing these interventions. Although it takes considerable practice to become a skilled interventionist, we believe this text provides its readers the necessary information to set them on such a path.

PowerPoint slides for each chapter and a test bank are available to instructors upon adoption of this text. We welcome your comments regarding this book and your suggestions for future editions. Please contact us at 519-661-2111 (x88388) or chall@uwo.ca.

Chapter 1

Introduction

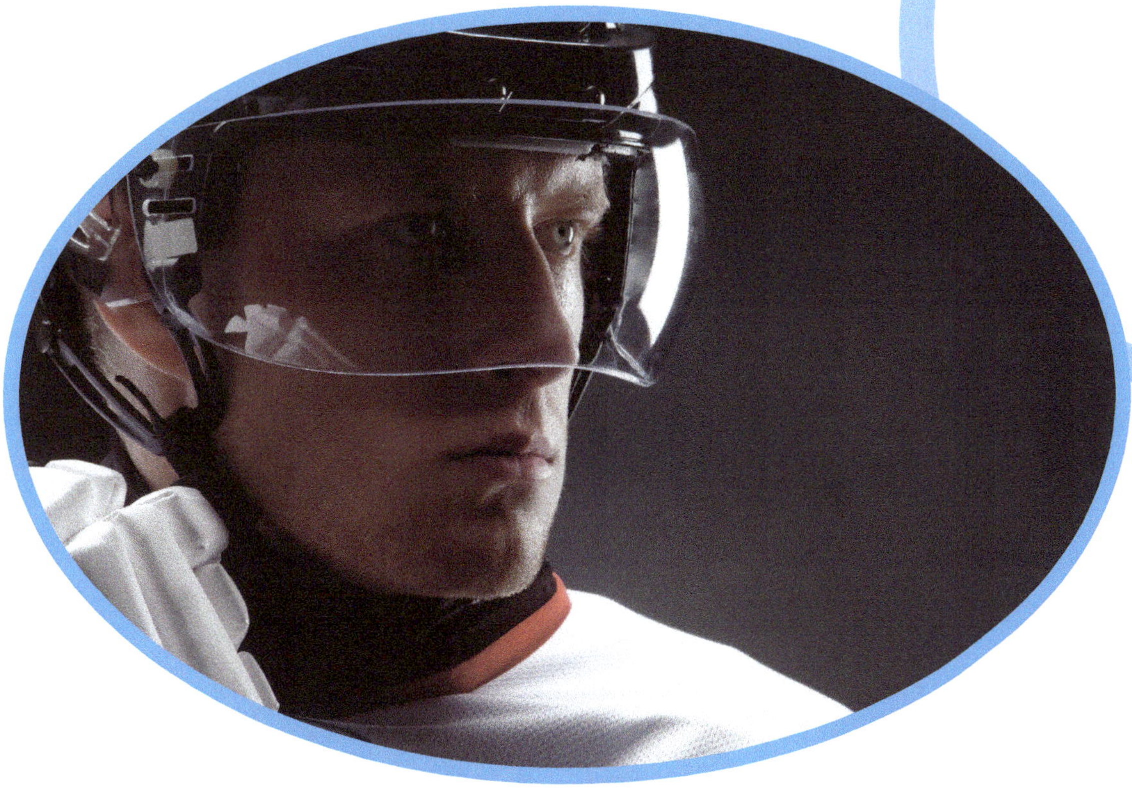

"Being strong mentally, we have to see as a skill. It's huge. We talk a lot about the technical things on the ice, but definitely your attitude and mental toughness are a huge factor."

—Antoine Vermette, National Hockey League player (Naylor, 2009)

When coaches and athletes talk about the mental side of sport, they often make comments like, "we need to have our heads in the game," "he tightened up under pressure, "or "I just try to give 110% out there." In an indirect way, these clichés are acknowledging that psychological preparation is an important part of success, but you will rarely hear a quote about how this is accomplished. What does it mean to be "mentally tough"? We hear athletes talk about it, but it is challenging to define exactly which characteristics make someone "tougher" than someone else. It is also clear that elite athletes are not the only people who can benefit from these characteristics; they can be helpful in recreational sports, exercise, performing arts, and even our everyday work and personal lives. So, what are these characteristics, and how can we develop them?

Using the jargon of sport and exercise psychology, when we talk about the "mental side" of performance we are referring to ***psychological skills***. These are defined as psychological qualities or attributes that need to be acquired and/or developed to help an individual achieve desired personal or performance outcomes. Just like physical skills, some people seem to have more inherent psychological skills than others. Luckily, these skills can be learned, and dedicated practice can yield measurable benefits for performance and personal achievement.

Psychological skills training (PST) refers to the systematic practice of mental skills to achieve specific outcomes beyond what would be attainable through physical and technical training alone. PST is used to enhance performance, increase enjoyment, or achieve greater self-satisfaction from sport or physical activity participation (Weinberg & Gould, 2003). A PST program typically includes a combination of interventions, such as goal setting, mental imagery, relaxation training, and more. These techniques have been used successfully in a number of sport contexts (Birrer & Morgan, 2010; Cohen, Tenenbaum, & English, 2006; Fournier, Calmels, Durand-Bush, & Salmela, 2005; Gucciardi, Gordon, & Dimmock, 2009; Sheard & Golby, 2006). Weinberg and Comar (1994) conducted a review of 45 published research articles that examined the use of psychological interventions with competitive athletes, and found that 38 (85%) of these studies demonstrated positive effects on performance.

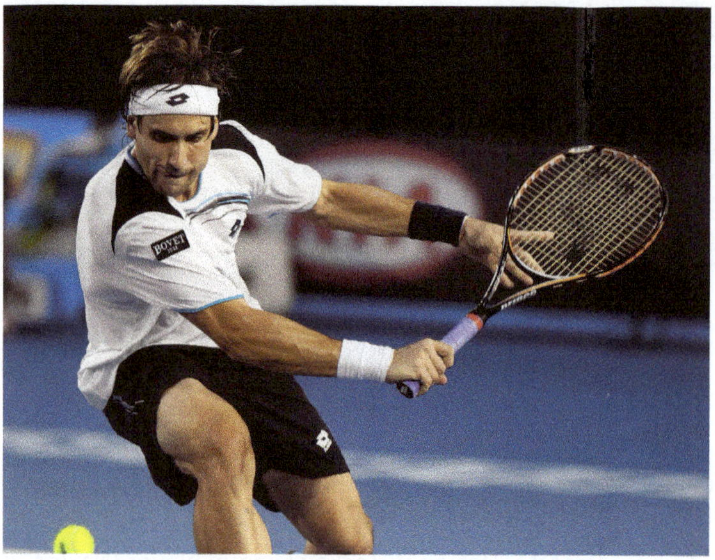

Image © Neale Cousland, 2014. Used under license from Shutterstock, Inc.

Why Are Psychological Interventions Important?

When we think about the importance of psychological skills, the first thing that usually comes to mind is sport performance. To illustrate, consider the case of an Olympic gymnastics competition. At this elite level, all of the athletes have similar technical abilities and exhibit only marginal differences in strength, endurance, and speed. What is it, then, that gives one athlete an advantage over another? As Hall of Fame baseball player Yogi Berra said, "sport is 50% physical and 90% mental." Now, it is difficult to argue that physical capabilities only account for a fraction of sport performance, but this does highlight an important concept: when athletes have similar physical abilities, psychological skills may be what determine the outcome of a competition. In fact, much of the variability in day-to-day performance can be attributed to psychological factors (Weinberg & Gould, 2003).

Consider the 2010 Olympic Winter Games held in Vancouver, Canada. In the final game of the women's curling tournament, skip Cheryl Bernard of Canada was favored to win against Anette Norberg and the Swedish team. The Canadians were counting on a gold medal in this event, and it received significant national and international media attention as one of the marquis events of the Olympics. The score was tied, sending the game into an extra end in front of a boisterous, partisan home crowd. Bernard was set to throw the second last rock of the end, and she needed to take out two Swedish rocks to assure her team of the victory. As soon as the rock left her hand, it was clear that it did not have sufficient strength or accuracy to make the shot. She managed to clear one Swedish rock, but missed the second, and Sweden won the gold medal. In this scenario, Cheryl Bernard's problem was not related to her technique. She had made this type of shot countless times before and could easily execute one with proper form. On this particular day, however, she was unable to deal with the pressure of the situation and as a result performed poorly. More physical practice would not have overcome this issue. Instead, better psychological preparation was needed to help her relax under the stressful circumstances.

Of course, psychological skills are not only useful in competitive situations. Perhaps their most important function is to facilitate skill acquisition and development. Although there is no substitute for physical practice, psychological techniques can enhance ongoing training activities by supporting the cognitive, emotional, and physiological processes underlying performance. In this way, athletes can use psychological strategies to make greater gains in shorter amounts of training time. For example, golfers may practice putting for several hours on the green, then use mental imagery to rehearse their technique to get additional practice time in while they are at home or traveling. Football teams sometimes train with recorded stadium noise to simulate the conditions of a loud arena, to get used to performing under difficult conditions. Novice rowers might use biofeedback to improve their stroke rhythm and to attune their bodies to different stroke rates. These types of strategies can be used alone or in tandem, and can lead to marked skill improvements when incorporated into a structured training regime.

Psychological skills can also be key factors in helping individuals to maintain motivation and regulate negative affect. In an athlete's career, there will inevitably be times when training becomes difficult and he or she feels as though development has hit a plateau. Some athletes will experience an injury that requires extensive rehabilitation and will keep them away from training for some time. Persevering through these challenges is just as much a question of motivation as physical tolerance. Overcoming these situations, and effectively coping with the negative emotions that often accompany them, is a function of an individual's psychological skills. Using a PST program to build these skills can ensure that the athlete is able to succeed and continue deriving enjoyment from their sport.

What Can Psychological Interventions Be Used For?

One often-overlooked aspect of psychological interventions is their usefulness in settings outside of high performance sport. Although we most often hear about sport psychologists and consultants working with professional, Olympic, or varsity athletes, they may also be helpful to novice athletes, exercisers, and those recovering from injury. Although the needs of individuals in each of these domains may be different, similar psychological techniques can be used to facilitate positive outcomes in multiple situations. Let's examine three common scenarios where PST might be useful.

In the first example, we consider a 14-year-old novice volleyball player who is just learning proper blocking technique. Although he has seen more experienced players block in competition, the timing is much more difficult than he anticipated and he needs to improve his footwork to make sure he is in the correct position to be successful. The player is getting frustrated at his lack of progress, and his coach wonders if this is something that a sport psychologist might be able to help with.

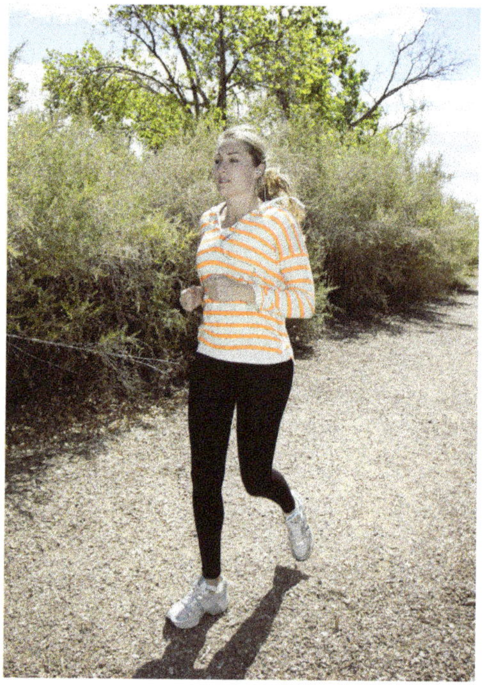

Image © Brocreative, 2014. Used under license from Shutterstock, Inc.

In the second scenario we encounter a middle-aged woman who has been sedentary for most of her adult life, but wants to begin exercising to improve her health. After beginning a routine of jogging twice per week, she decides that she would like to add one session of resistance training to her program. She has never lifted weights, however, and is unsure of the proper technique. She feels out of place at the gym because she is not very fit, and she is too intimidated by the other exercisers to ask for help with the weights. Is this a situation where a PST consultant could help?

The final example is the case of a university student who plays intramural flag football. He enjoys recreational sports, but is not particularly competitive. In his game last weekend, he sprained his ankle and his doctor has referred him for physiotherapy treatment. He has never experienced a significant injury before, and the pain and loss of mobility has become a significant source of anxiety for him. On top of that, he is nervous about having to perform difficult and uncomfortable exercises during rehabilitation. His therapist believes that he is physically capable of recovery, but worries that he will not be psychologically able to endure treatment and may actually fear returning to sport.

In each of these situations, a PST intervention could be the difference between a positive and a negative outcome. Each of these individuals is faced with having to acquire a new set of physical skills, and there is a role for psychological intervention in speeding up this process. For example, the use of peer modeling could help the volleyball player with his timing, show the woman how to correctly use the weights, or demonstrate physiotherapy exercises to the injured football player. Perhaps mental imagery would also be useful for skill rehearsal. Considering the negative affective and cognitive responses seen in these scenarios, these individuals may also benefit from positive self-talk, guided relaxation, or goal setting. These types of interventions, along with many others, can help people maximize their potential in numerous settings including exercise and rehabilitation. The key is to design PST programs to address the needs of the individual, and to match each intervention technique with the desired outcome.

The basic aim of any PST program is to provide individuals with the self-regulation skills necessary to function without constant input from a coach or psychology consultant (Weinberg & Gould, 2003). Self-regulation is the ability to work toward one's goals by effectively monitoring and managing one's thoughts, feelings, and behaviors (Gould & Chung, 2004). Essentially, PST programs help individuals develop the skills necessary to accomplish this. By teaching athletes and exercisers how to interpret situations appropriately and apply their psychological resources in adaptive ways, we can help them achieve greater levels of performance, enjoyment, and satisfaction. This is not to say that those who receive PST will not encounter difficulties or become negatively impacted by challenges. Here it is important to distinguish between ***psychological skills*** and ***psychological states***. While psychological skills are tools that can help an individual manage a given situation, psychological states refer to transient behaviors or feelings that depend on a person's current situation or motives. To illustrate, emotional states such as anger or disappointment are often brief and quickly changing, and their expression may depend on the specific situation (e.g., at home compared to at work). It is the role of PST to prepare the individual to manage these states and adapt to the changing physical and social environment in a way that facilitates performance, instead of impeding it.

What Are the Limits of Psychological Interventions?

Although sport and exercise psychology is becoming more widely accepted and understood, there are still misconceptions about its potential benefits and limitations. There are many erroneous beliefs surrounding the use of PST, causing confusion about what psychological techniques can and cannot do to help individuals improve their performance or achieve their goals.

❍ Only Athletes Can Benefit from PST

Many people think that PST is only useful for elite athletes, or those who are highly competitive. In reality, athletes at any level (including youth or those who are new to sport) can benefit from learning psychological techniques. They can even be helpful to those with physical or mental disabilities. Many sport psychology consultants are also expanding their practices to include performers from other domains (e.g., dancers, musicians, actors) (Noh, Morris, & Andersen, 2007), as well as professionals from business and medical fields, first responders (e.g., police, fire, paramedic personnel) (Brown, Mulhern, & Joseph, 2002), and the military (McCrory, Cobley, & Marchant, 2013). Anyone can utilize PST to increase their abilities to develop new physical and mental skills, perform under pressure, or gain enjoyment from achieving personal objectives.

There is also a prevailing notion that PST is for "problem athletes." It is true that clinical sport psychologists are licensed to treat various psychological problems that arise in the sporting environment, such as substance abuse, eating disorders, or severe cases of anxiety or depression. Yet, only a small proportion of athletes struggle with these types of issues. The needs of most athletes and exercisers relate to the development of psychological skills that will enhance performance. The majority of educational sport psychologists and consultants, therefore, work with individuals who fall within the normal range of psychological functioning, with the purpose of helping those individuals move toward self-regulation.

PST Is a Magic Bullet Solution

Sometimes people will ask for help performing under pressure, but will wait until a few weeks or days before a major competition to seek help. Not surprisingly, this approach usually does not work, leaving the athlete frustrated and disappointed. As tempting as it is to call in a sport psychology consultant to address problems as they arise, coaches and athletes need to have realistic expectations. Psychological skills take time and effort to develop, and one or two PST sessions are not sufficient to radically change performance.

Moreover, PST cannot turn an average athlete into a superstar, nor can it help a novice runner complete a marathon without sufficient physical training. Psychological skills can help an individual maximize his or her potential, but they cannot guarantee a performance well beyond the individual's abilities.

Consultants Are Only Needed When There Is a Problem

The need for a sport psychology consultant becomes readily apparent when an athlete or exerciser is having difficulty with a particular aspect of performance, but this is not the only time when PST can be helpful. In fact, including PST as part of a regular training routine can help an athlete avoid problems by building a foundation of psychological skills that he or she can use to enhance performance. The regular inclusion of PST during practice can help the individual improve his or her physical skills, and should be viewed as one of the fundamental elements of athlete development.

PST Is Not Going to Help Me

Despite broad acceptance of sport psychology in the athletic community, there are still those who do not believe that PST has any measurable benefit. Particularly in the exercise and sport injury domains, where the consideration of psychological skills is still relatively new, there can be resistance from individuals who are unwilling to try something "outside the box." Nonetheless, there are countless anecdotal reports and a large body of scientific literature that suggests PST is not only effective, but also rewarding for those pursuing personal improvement. PST may not always be the solution that people want it to be for performance-related problems, but when applied in a systematic, individualized way, it can have significant positive impact on desired outcomes.

There are many reasons why athletes and exercisers do not engage in PST, and the propagation of these types of misconceptions is one of them. Lack of understanding about the benefits and limitations is a major barrier to undertaking PST, but knowledge about how to implement a PST program is an even larger hurdle. Many coaches and athletes simply do not know how to teach or practice psychological skills. Because they are internal and entirely personal, there is no way to demonstrate them in the way we have grown accustomed to learning physical skills. It is also insufficient to simply give instructions. Yelling, "relax out there" is not an effective way to teach relaxation, and even though an athlete may know that he needs to reduce his anxiety, he may not know how to do it. Herein lies the difficulty in practicing PST when coaches and participants do not have access to proper training in psychological techniques.

Until recently, researchers in the sport and exercise psychology field have not been particularly effective at making evidence easily accessible to coaches and athletes (Gould, Medbery, Damarjian, & Lauer, 1999b). So, unless they have been exposed to a consultant who is well versed in PST programming, many individuals have had to rely on their own personal experiences to guide the way they teach psychological skills. Many coaches also believe that they know just as much, if not more, about sport psychology than researchers, based on a lifetime of participation in their sport (Gould, Medbery, Damarjian, & Lauer, 1999; Gould, Giannini, Krane, & Hodge, 1990).

Although experiential learning is an important source of information, it can lead to misconceptions about what psychological skills are and how they are acquired. Contrary to what many people believe, psychological skills are not simply a component of someone's personality. Just because one athlete seems to be mentally stronger or more competitive than another, does not mean that these athletes are necessarily destined to perform at more elite levels. Psychological skills are not innate characteristics, but instead can be taught directly or developed through life experiences.

Another barrier preventing the use of PST is a perceived lack of time to practice psychological skills. Coaches often feel that their players hardly have enough time to practice physical skills, and they are reluctant to devote training time to anything else. Yet, one of the most common reasons cited for poor performance is the mental state of the athlete. We often hear coaches and players attributing a loss to a lack of concentration or a "choke." It therefore seems that additional training time devoted to PST would be just as beneficial as practicing physical skills, although this is contrary to the doctrine of many coaching styles. Convincing coaches and athletes to make PST a priority is one of the greatest challenges in the field of sport and exercise psychology.

All of these barriers to PST use are compounded for individuals in non-sport domains. For example, exercisers do not typically have the coaches or other resources that sport participants have, and are often left to undertake PST on their own. If information is not easily accessible to these individuals, they may not even be aware that psychological skill development could be beneficial to them. Others who recognize the need for PST may become discouraged if they have no guidance in designing a program, and decide to give up before achieving any positive results. Similar challenges face those undergoing injury rehabilitation, where medical practitioners may be unaware of the need for psychological intervention or may simply not have the expertise or time to help the patient in this capacity.

Why Do We Study Psychological Interventions?

Even though we know that developing psychological skills is important, we cannot take for granted that the same strategies will work for everyone, or in every situation. Determining the most appropriate interventions for teaching these skills is a challenge that faces all sport psychology consultants. Researchers and practitioners must continually seek knowledge regarding the best PST techniques, as well as the most effective timing, dosage, and evaluation methods to ensure that athletes and exercisers are able to gain the greatest advantage possible from their PST programs.

Many questions about PST have still not been adequately answered. We do not yet know how best to structure PST programs for optimal performance, particularly for non-elite and youth populations. There has also been very little consideration of using PST to improve coaching performance, which is a promising area of future research (Vealey, 2007). Further investigation into the interaction between personal characteristics and the training or competitive environment will also be crucial for informing intervention design (Danish & Hale, 1981). Moreover, understanding how to apply the lessons learned in sport to other domains, including exercise and injury rehabilitation, is an important goal in PST research and practice.

We also do not yet know the most appropriate way to measure the outcomes of PST. Although a number of performance metrics are currently used, such as skill execution, race times, or shooting percentages, we may need to identify more holistic measures of success. Including psychological evaluations alongside performance outcomes could give a better overall picture of the way athletes are using psychological skills, and might speak to the effect of PST on mental well-being and self-satisfaction. Unfortunately, very little research has been conducted in this area to date.

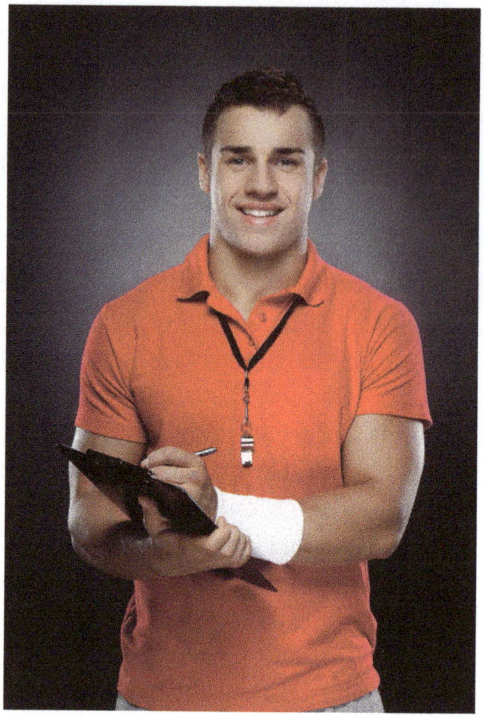

Image © BlueSkyImage, 2014. Used under license from Shutterstock, Inc.

There is an expressed need for specific guidance about how to implement PST programs. It is often ideal for these programs to be delivered by qualified sport psychologists or consultants, but this is not always feasible or even desirable. For those who wish to use PST for their own personal improvement, or for coaches or therapists who would benefit from using basic techniques with their athletes, the development of standardized programming may prove to be useful. There have also been suggestions that a focus on competition plans, or defined step-by-step mental preparation routines for individuals to go through before a performance or game, may be a successful strategy (Orlick, 1986; Vealey, 2007). Much more research is needed, however, to evaluate the effectiveness of these approaches.

CHAPTER SUMMARY

Psychological skills are important factors in achieving maximum performance in sport and related domains. These skills can be trained, and using a structured, individualized PST program can facilitate the development of mental strategies to enhance performance. Although there are a number of barriers to using PST, increasing our understanding of the most effective timing, dosage, and outcome evaluation methods will help us overcome these challenges.

In the following chapters we provide an overview of psychological strategies that can be used as part of a PST program, with emphasis on their use in sport, exercise, and injury rehabilitation. We highlight the current gaps in our knowledge, and provide suggestions for those wishing to implement these techniques in their own PST practice.

REVIEW QUESTIONS

1. How are ***psychological skills*** different from ***psychological states***?
2. What are the three main goals of PST programs?
3. Identify the four major myths surrounding PST.
4. What are the limits of our knowledge about PST, and what research questions still remain to be asked in this field?

SUGGESTED READINGS

Birrer, D., & Morgan, G. (2010). Psychological skills training as a way to enhance an athlete's performance in high-intensity sports. *Scandinavian Journal of Medicine & Science in Sports, 20*(.s2), 78–87.

Weinberg, R. S., & Gould, D. (2003). Foundations of Sport & Exercise Psychology (3rd ed.) Champaign, Ill: Human Kinetics.

REFERENCES

Birrer, D., & Morgan, G. (2010). Psychological skills training as a way to enhance an athlete's performance in high-intensity sports. *Scandinavian Journal of Medicine & Science in Sports, 20*(.s2), 78–87.

Brown, J., Mulhern, G., & Joseph, S. (2002). Incident-related stressors, locus of control, coping, and psychological distress among firefighters in Northern Ireland. *Journal of Traumatic Stress, 15*(2), 161–168.

Cohen, A. B., Tenenbaum, G., & English, R. W. (2006). Emotions and Golf Performance: An IZOF-Based Applied Sport Psychology Case Study. *Behavior Modification, 30*(3), 259–280.

Danish, S. J., & Hale, B. D. (1981). Towards an understanding of the practice of sport psychology. *Journal of Sport Psychology, 3*(2), 90–99.

Fournier, J. F., Calmels, C., Durand-Bush, N., & Salmela, J. H. (2005). Effects of a season-long PST program on gymnastic performance and on psychological skill development. *International Journal of Sport and Exercise Psychology, 3*(1), 59–78.

Gould, D., & Chung, Y. (2004). Self-regulation skills for children and adolescents. In M. Weiss (Ed.), *Developmental sport and exercise psychology: A lifespan perspective* (pp. 383–402). Morgantown, WV: Fitness Information Technology.

Gould, D., Giannini, J., Krane, V., & Hodge, K. (1990). Educational needs of elite US national team, Pan American, and Olympic coaches. *Journal of Teaching Physical Education, 9,* 332–344.

Gould, D., Medbery, R., Damarjian, N., & Lauer, L. (1999). A survey assessment of mental skills training knowledge, opinions, and practices of a national sample of junior tennis coaches. *Journal of Applied Sport Psychology, 11*(1): 28–50.

Gould, D., Medbery, R., Damarjian, N., & Lauer, L. (1999b). An examination of mental skills training in junior tennis coaches. *Sport Psychologist, 13*(2): 127–143.

Gucciardi, D. F., Gordon, S., & Dimmock, J. A. (2009). Evaluation of a mental toughness training program for youth-aged Australian footballers: A quantitative analysis. *Journal of Applied Sport Psychology, 21*(3), 307–323.

McCrory, P., Cobley, S., & Marchant, P. (2013). The effect of psychological skills training (PST) on self-regulation behavior, self-efficacy, and psychological skill use in military pilot-trainees. *Military Psychology, 25*(2), 136–147.

Naylor, Dave. "Senators looking for closure." *The Globe and Mail,* 18 May 2007.

Noh, Y. E., Morris, T., & Andersen, M. B. (2007). Psychological intervention programs for reduction of injury in ballet dancers. *Research in Sports Medicine, 15*(1), 13–32.

Orlick, T. (1986). *Psyching for Sport: Mental training for athletes.* Champaign, Ill: Human Kinetics.

Sheard, M., & Golby, J. (2006). Effect of a psychological skills training program on swimming performance and positive psychological development. *International Journal of Sport and Exercise Psychology, 4*(2), 149–169.

Vealey, R. S. (2007). Future directions in psychological skills training. In D. Smith & M. Bar-Eli (Eds.), *Essential readings in sport and exercise psychology* (pp. 295–304). Champaign, Ill: Human Kinetics.

Weinberg, R. S., & Comar, W. (1994). The effectiveness of psychological interventions in competitive sport. *Sports Medicine, 18,* 406–418.

Weinberg, R. S., & Gould, D. (2003). Foundations of Sport & Exercise Psychology (3rd ed.) Champaign, Ill: Human Kinetics.

Chapter 2

Delivering Psychological Interventions

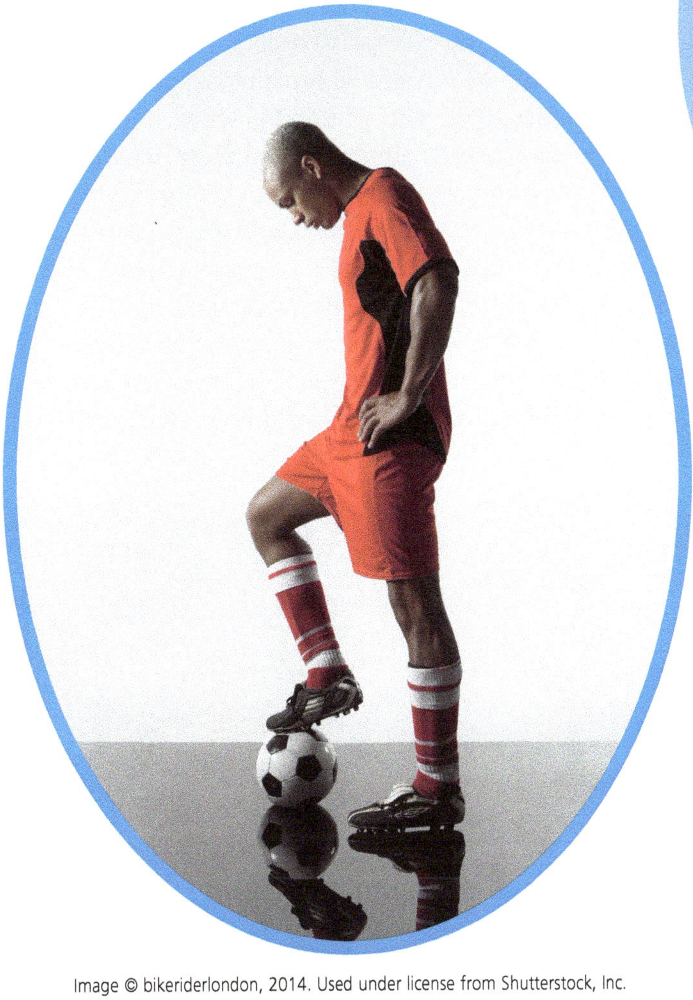

Introduction

If you stopped to think about it, you could likely remember a time that you used self-talk to help you overcome a challenge. Maybe you were feeling tired at the end of a workout and you gave yourself a little pep talk saying, "Come on, you can finish this!" Maybe you were playing a doubles tennis match and you had to remind yourself to be patient with your partner who was slightly less skilled than you. Maybe to get you through a late-night study session you took a pause to remind yourself how important it was to you to get a good grade on your upcoming exam. You can also likely think of a time that you've set your mind on accomplishing something (i.e., set a goal) or imagined what it might be like if you accomplished that goal (i.e., used mental imagery). Without thinking much about it, we all use psychological skills naturally in our day-to-day lives. As we will see in upcoming chapters, athletes and exercisers have a natural set of mental strategies that they use, for example, to help them learn and perfect skills or strategies, stay motivated to train and compete, and overcome physical pain during injury rehabilitation. You've likely seen an Olympic gold medalist during a post medal ceremony interview reflecting on the years that they spent imagining themselves winning the gold. You also may have come across popular Internet blogs showcasing pictures, videos, and descriptions of different exercise routines and fitness tips for exercisers looking to learn from the example of others. These are just two examples of how common psychological skills (imagery and observational learning, respectively) are naturally applied in the contexts of sports and exercise. Indeed, our state of mind plays an important role in helping us master the many challenges of sport, exercise, and rehabilitation and these mental strategies can help to regulate our state of mind. Although it is common for athletes and exercisers to employ some of these mental strategies naturally, the greatest success can come from developing, practicing, and utilizing a full arsenal of psychological skills. To learn and practice these psychological skills and to determine which skills to use and when to use them, psychological interventions can be helpful.

In the previous chapter you learned why and how psychological interventions can be helpful. In this chapter we will discuss the delivery of psychological interventions in sports, exercise, and injury rehabilitation. Specifically, we will discuss the interventionists—the individuals who typically deliver

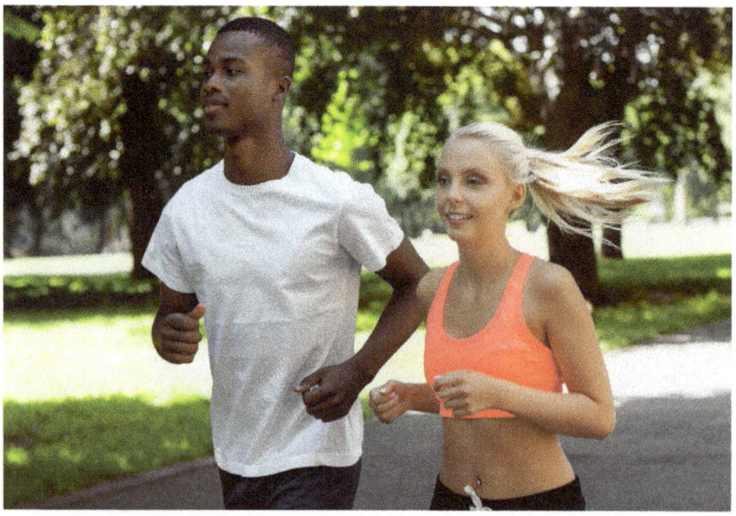

psychological interventions in each of these settings. We also will discuss the settings in which these interventions typically take place. There isn't a perfect formula for the delivery of psychological interventions, but we will describe the ways in which these interventions are most commonly delivered and discuss some of the advantages and disadvantages of current practice.

Who Delivers Psychological Interventions?

Although many of us have a natural tendency to use some psychological skills in our sport, exercise, and rehabilitative pursuits, developing a full repertoire of psychological skills and implementing those skills into a psychological skills training program may require the help of an expert. There are currently three groups of experts who are likely to deliver psychological interventions in sports, exercise, and rehabilitation: (a) sport and exercise psychology consultants, (b) coaches, trainers, or therapists, and (c) researchers. The role of each group of experts in delivering psychological interventions in sports, exercise, and rehabilitation is discussed below.

Sport and Exercise Psychology Consultants

This type of expert is most common in a sport setting, although they are becoming increasingly common in the exercise domain as well. The role of a sport psychologist or sport psychology consultant is to work with individuals or teams to teach the psychological skills that can be useful during training and in competition (both inside and outside the athletic arena). It is important to note the distinction between a ***sport psychologist (SP)*** and a sport psychology consultant. Whereas a sport psychologist is trained and certified as a clinical psychologist with expertise in sports-related issues and strategies, ***sports psychology consultants (SPC)*** may have considerable expertise in sports-related issues and strategies but do not have formal clinical training and certification. Both SPs and SPCs have the expertise necessary to help athletes develop psychological skills and implement them into training and competition; however, SPCs are not qualified to diagnose and treat clinical issues that can occur in the domain of sports psychology such as eating disorders and anxiety disorders.

The role of a SP or SPC in working with an athlete or a team can vary greatly. In certain cases, a SP or SPC is invited only to deliver a lecture or a workshop on a given psychological skill. In these cases, the SP or SPC does not develop relationships with the individual athletes but rather provides information and strategies that the athlete, team, or coach can implement at their discretion. In other cases, a SP or SPC works closely with an athlete or team throughout an entire season. These cases may involve regular, individual meetings between the SP/SPC and the athletes and frequent collaboration between a SP/SPC and the coach in order to teach and integrate psychological skills into practices and competitions. The degree to which a SP/SPC is involved with an athlete or team depends on many factors, including the coach's individual preferences and areas of expertise, availability of a SP/SPC, and the time and money available for psychological skills training.

A recent qualitative study conducted by Zakrajsek, Steinfeldt, Bodey, Martin, and Zizzi (2013) described the way in which coaches prefer to include a SP or SPC into their training program. Some of the main findings from this study indicated that coaches prefer for SPs and SPCs to work one-on-one with athletes as well as with the whole team together, and they prefer SPs or SPCs who can be flexible with their schedule and work with the athletes or the team when the general training program allows.

Whereas coaches like SPs and SPCs who can blend into the team culture and become a part of the regular support staff, they also like to use psychological skills training as a 'special event' to break up the usual practice routine. Finally, coaches report that it is critical for the coach and the SP/SPC to be 'on the same page' with regard to all facets of the training program and to the role of the SP/SPC. Building an effective relationship between a coach and a SP/SPC could be challenging given the degree of trust that a coach must place in the SP/SPC; however, once an effective relationship is established, the inclusion of a SP/SPC in the coaching/training staff could have highly-beneficial effects on the performance of the athletes or team.

Although consultants appear most frequently in the sport domain, there is growing recognition that integrating consultants into the realm of exercise and rehabilitation could help to increase adherence to physical activity and rehabilitation programs. Primary health care settings may be ideal for delivering physical activity recommendations and prescriptions because of the potential to reach a large number of individuals; however, primary care physicians are often limited by time (Abramson, Stein, Schaufele, Frates, & Rogan, 2000; Petrella & Wright, 2000; Yarnell, Pollak, Ostbye, Krause, & Michener, 2003) or by a lack of specific knowledge required for prescribing physical activity or counseling behavior change (Nupponen, 1998; Ritchie, Stetson, Bass, & Adams, 2002; Walsh, Swangard, Davis, & McPhee, 1999). Thus, physical activity counselors—individuals with specialized knowledge in the areas of physical activity assessment and prescription, theories of health behavior change, and counseling strategies (Tulloch, Fortier, & Hogg, 2006) are beginning to be integrated into primary health care settings (Fortier, Tulloch, & Hogg, 2006). Because of their specific training in counseling strategies, physical activity counselors can assist exercisers or individuals undergoing a rehabilitation program in developing the psychological skills that will assist them in persisting with exercises over the long-term. To date, physical activity counseling in primary care settings has typically occurred one-on-one; however, as the demand for physical activity counselors grows, there may be some potential for developing group-based sessions in which one counselor can aide a group of individuals in learning and practicing important psychological skills.

Coaches, Trainers, and Therapists

Coaches, trainers, and therapists are ideally positioned to deliver psychological interventions because they are the individuals who work with the athletes and exercisers most frequently. If a coach, trainer, or therapist is trained in delivering psychological interventions, there is great potential for the interventions to be well integrated into the larger training program. Because the effectiveness of psychological interventions is increased when the psychological skills are practiced, integrating psychological skills training into regular practice may allow the athletes and exercisers to develop optimal proficiency with these skills. One limitation to coaches, trainers, and therapists as psychological interventionists is that they may not be specifically trained in implementing these interventions.

Instances of coaches acting as psychological interventionists occur primarily in the sport domain because most athletes and teams work directly with a coach. There is widespread understanding among coaches that becoming versed in sport psychology is important to an athlete or a team's success (Gould, Damarjian, & Medbery, 1999; Martens, 2004; Orlick & Partington, 1988). A basketball coach who is proficient in sport psychology techniques may begin a season by working with her team to establish short- and long-term goals and follow up on the progress toward those goals throughout the season. A figure skating coach who understands the anxiety-arousing nature of his performance sport may prompt his athletes to use imagery during their training sessions to mentally rehearse the experience of performing in an arena packed with fans, judges, media, and other competitors. A moguls skiing coach may use videos of expert skiers to demonstrate to his more novice athletes the techniques they can aspire to develop. Because coaches are deeply familiar with the unique culture and terminology of their sport, they are in an advantaged position with regard to delivering highly-relevant psychological interventions. For this reason, a coach may be better able to tailor psychological interventions to the unique needs of his or her athletes compared to a SP or SPC who may be less familiar with the sport.

The degree to which coaches implement psychological skills training, however, depends on the degree to which they are comfortable with and trained to deliver such interventions. Although coaches endorse the importance of psychological skills training (Gould, Murphy, Tammen, & May, 1989; Ottley, 2000; Sullivan & Hodge, 1991), it often is excluded from practice sessions (Gould et al., 1999; Grobbelaar, 2007) because coaches feel they lack the necessary education and training to deliver these interventions (Gould & Eklund, 1991; Gould, Medbery, Damarjian, & Lauer, 1999). In fact, Reade and his colleagues (2008) reported that up to 98.4% of coaches of elite athletes recognized a need for additional training and support in delivering psychological interventions. Thus, to capitalize on the vast potential for coaches to deliver psychological interventions, it seems that more thorough training is required.

Trainers and therapists are well-positioned to deliver psychological interventions in the contexts of sport, exercise, and injury rehabilitation. Although trainers and therapists typically do not interact with athletes and exercisers as frequently as do coaches, they tend to work with them on a consistent schedule and on specific tasks. Therefore, although trainers and therapists may not be in a position to integrate psychological skills training into everyday practice, their regular interaction with athletes and exercisers would allow them to assist in development and practice of psychological skills over time. For example, consider a flexibility specialist who works with elite gymnasts. The specialist understands that extreme flexibility is advantageous in gymnastics but that stretching too much may leave an athlete susceptible to injury. In addition, this specialist understands that elite-level gymnasts may feel under pressure to push themselves to the limits when it comes to stretching. Knowing all of this, the flexibility specialist may help the athlete learn to use biofeedback techniques to determine the optimal amount of stretching that can be done safely and to develop a progressive flexibility training regimen. In the context of exercise, personal trainers at a gym are in a good position to deliver psychological interventions. Consider a 60-year-old man who is healthy and active but has noticed that as he ages, physical exercise is becoming increasingly difficult and frustrating. Although he does not work with a personal trainer each time he visits the gym, he has a trainer that he meets with twice per month. Knowing that the man has difficulty staying motivated when the exercises are physically challenging, the trainer can teach the man how to use self-talk to help him get through the difficult parts of the workout. Finally, in the context of injury rehabilitation, athletes typically meet with a therapist on a regular basis and also perform exercises or stretches in the interim. To help an injured athlete recovering from ACL surgery understand the steps in the road to recovery, a therapist might use observational learning techniques to demonstrate to the athlete how the range of motion in the athlete's knee is set to improve over time. She might then encourage the athlete to use imagery while performing the at-home exercises and stretches to imagine the next step in recovery.

Despite the potential for trainers and therapists to deliver psychological interventions on a consistent basis, many trainers do not feel adequately prepared to do so. For example, Moulton, Molstad, and

Turner (1997) surveyed Division I-certified athletic trainers in the United States Collegiate sports system and found that although trainers perceived that their role exceeded the prevention and treatment of athletic injuries and included sports and rehabilitation psychology counseling, most did not feel personally qualified to do so. Moulton et al. (1997) also reported that none of the athletic trainers involved in the study had access to a sport psychologist for support. In another study, Larson, Starkey, and Zaichkowsky (1996) examined responses from 482 members of the National Athletic Trainers' Association. Almost half of these trainers (47%) reported that they thought their injured athletes suffered psychological trauma as a result of their injury, but only 25% of respondents had access to a sport psychologist as a part of their athletic therapy team. These two studies point to the need for athletic therapists to be educated and trained in psychological counseling techniques that could assist their athletes in injury rehabilitation. Indeed, a need for training in psychological intervention techniques is widespread across trainers and therapists in sport, exercise, and injury rehabilitation.

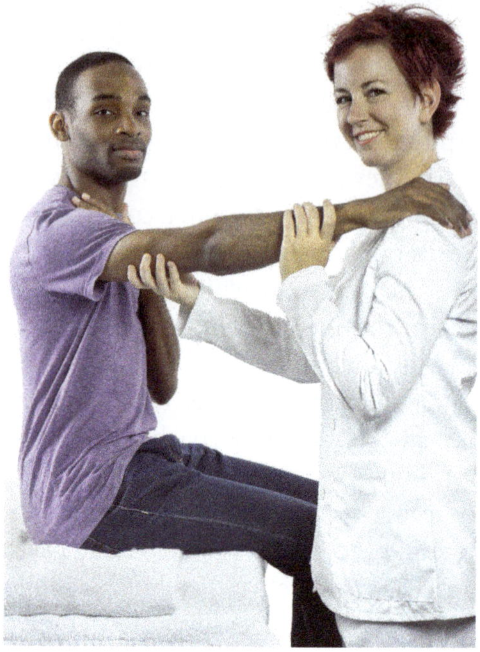

Image © Rommel Canlas, 2014. Used under license from Shutterstock, Inc.

Researchers

Although researchers do not represent a typical member of a sport, exercise, or rehabilitation training team, many of the psychological interventions being developed and implemented are a part of a research program. Athletes and sports teams, exercisers and exercise facilities, and rehabilitation clinics that participate in or have partnerships with researchers often benefit from having access to emerging psychological interventions. The goal of research on psychological interventions in sport, exercise, and injury rehabilitation is to develop and test interventions that can be implemented into actual practice. However, while those interventions are being tested (i.e., before effective intervention strategies are disseminated to the general public), athletes, exercisers, and organizations who participate in the research may receive some immediate benefit from access to a new intervention technique.

In the sport domain, effective interventions are relatively easily disseminated into actual practice. Because coaches, especially those of more elite athletes, endorse psychological skills training as an integral part of athlete development, they often seek out the latest research. There are numerous textbooks, websites, and other resources available for coaches who wish to implement effective psychological interventions into their practices and competitions. This widespread endorsement of psychological interventions, however, does not occur in the domains of exercise and injury rehabilitation. Although psychological interventions are not absent from these domains, many exercise trainers and athletic therapists are either skeptical about the importance of psychological interventions or simply are undereducated on how to implement them. Therefore, exercisers who participate in studies testing psychological interventions often are exposed to interventions that they would not have access to through traditional personal training or exercise instruction approaches. For example, in a research study, Stanley and Cumming (2010) demonstrated among 75 exercisers that individuals who imagined enjoying exercise while riding a stationary bike reported significantly more post-exercise enjoyment compared to individuals who imagined either feeling energized from exercise or who imagined exercising with perfect technique. These findings have potentially-important implications given that the way someone feels post-workout can influence their likelihood of engaging in subsequent exercise sessions.

Although Stanley and Cumming demonstrated a strategy that may be important for increasing perceived enjoyment of exercise, these findings are not in widespread use in the exercise community. Until psychological interventions are more commonly accepted in the domain of exercise, effective psychological strategies for increasing exercise participation may not be disseminated to the general public. In the domain of injury rehabilitation, we have seen that physical therapists do not feel adequately educated to deliver psychological interventions (Moulton et al., 1997). This finding suggests that injured athletes who participate in research studies may have access to psychological interventions that are not a part of traditional therapy.

Where Are Psychological Interventions Delivered?

As you will see in the upcoming chapters, psychological interventions can be delivered in a variety of settings. We will discuss the typical setting for the delivery of psychological interventions in the sport, exercise, and rehabilitation domains separately.

In Sport

In the domain of sport, the two most common settings for the delivery of psychological interventions are practice and competition. Although athletes also use psychological skills outside of sporting arenas, it is most common for interventions to be delivered in the context of practice or competition and for those skills to be practiced both inside and outside actual sporting venues. The optimal setting in which to intervene depends largely on the intervention strategy. For example, because goal setting occurs early in a season and involves a prospective look toward the competitive portion of the season, goal-setting interventions occur primarily during practice. In contrast, mental imagery is often used to help control arousal levels that can often be heightened during competition. Thus, although mental imagery skills may be taught during practice time, it may be more appropriate to use certain mental imagery interventions during competition.

In Exercise

In the context of exercise, psychological interventions are most commonly administered in the exercise setting. Unlike the sport domain, there is typically only one venue in which exercise sessions take place (e.g., a gym or an aerobics studio); thus, this is the natural setting for intervention delivery. For example, exercisers may use self-presentational strategies during a workout at the gym to help them feel more confident. In addition, the exercise setting is typically the location in which exercisers have access to trainers who are likely administrators of the interventions. Conducting interventions inside the actual exercise setting is ideal because exercisers can learn and practice new psychological skills and strategies in the context in which they are intended.

Exercise psychology interventions also can take place in more real-world settings such as at home or in a primary care clinic. As psychological interventions are becoming more common in the exercise domain, researchers and practitioners are becoming increasingly creative with respect to how these interventions can be delivered. As we have seen, physical activity counseling as part of a primary care team are becoming increasingly popular. In addition, interventions delivered over the phone or in small group sessions outside the actual exercise setting are alternatives to conducting in-house interventions. Delivering interventions outside the actual exercise facility can be ideal for helping exercisers develop their motivation as they plan and prepare for upcoming workouts.

In Rehabilitation

Athletes recovering from an injury may use psychological interventions in a wide variety of settings. Perhaps the most obvious place for the delivery of rehabilitation psychology interventions is in the actual rehabilitation environment. For example, athletes may use self-talk to help guide them through their routine of exercises or biofeedback to ensure that they are engaged in the appropriate intensity of rehabilitation exercises. Injured athletes may also use psychological interventions outside the rehabilitation setting at home or in their typical practice environment. For example, athletes recovering from an injury may use imagery to help them mentally rehearse skills they are not able to physically perform in their injured state. They also may attend practice sessions to observe their teammates as they learn and practice new skills and strategies. This opportunity to engage in observational learning in the sport environment may help athletes get back up to speed once they have made a full recovery. Finally, many of the psychological skills discussed in this book can be implemented outside the rehabilitation and training environments to help athletes maintain the motivation to finish their rehabilitation and return to play.

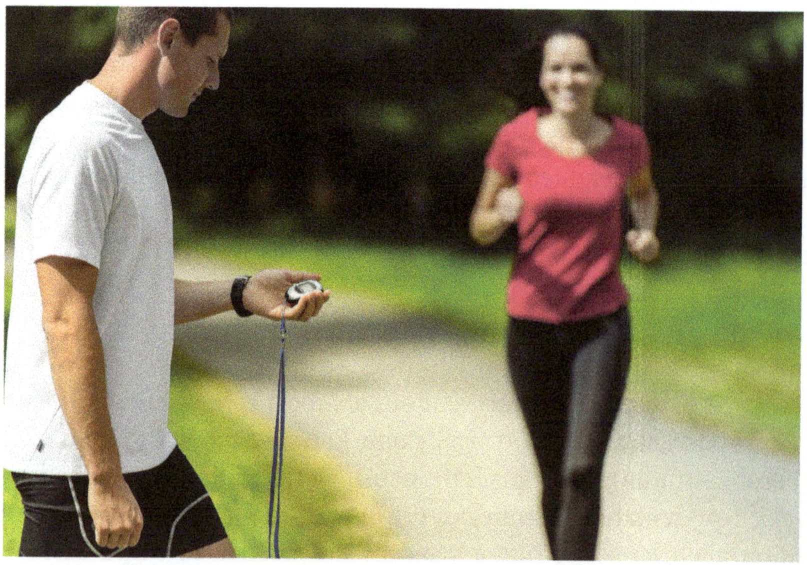

How Are Psychological Interventions Delivered?

Although psychological interventions are delivered in a variety of ways, one common approach entails three phases: education, acquisition, and practice. In the education phase, using sport as an example, athletes learn to recognize the importance of mental skills in sport and how these skills influence performance. There are various approaches to accomplishing this; however, one of the simplest ways is to ask athletes about the importance of mental skills in sport. Although most athletes realize the importance of the mental side of sport, very few actually spend time developing these skills in comparison with the time spent on technical skills. In the acquisition phase, the focus is placed on helping athletes acquire the various psychological skills and learn how to most effectively employ them. In the practice phase, the goals are to have the athletes automate the various psychological skills through over-learning and to implement these skills in practice and competition.

Previously in this chapter other aspects of how to deliver interventions were considered such as delivering interventions one-on-one versus to a whole team, and the delivery of interventions by a SP/SPC versus a coach or therapist. As we review interventions for specific psychological skills (e.g., goal setting, imagery) in the following chapters, we will see the various ways researchers and practitioners have delivered them. One critical determinant of how interventions are delivered is the length of the intervention. Delivering a very short intervention of one or two sessions is very different than delivering an intervention consisting of many sessions spread throughout an entire competitive season.

Which Intervention Technique Should Be Delivered?

As you will see in the upcoming chapters, there are specific benefits to each intervention technique or skill. For example, self-talk can be applied quickly without any extra resources; thus, an exerciser in need of a quick boost in motivation to push through an intense workout may easily apply some self-talk. Biofeedback, however, requires more resources to operate and is more appropriate for facilitating learning over the long term; thus, biofeedback is particularly well-suited for an injury rehabilitation session. Considering what the objective is when undertaking a psychological intervention is critical in determining which skill or combination of skills is optimal. In most cases, a combination of multiple psychological skills is ideal. Consider the sport psychology needs of a collegiate-level volleyball player. Early in the season it will be critical for the player to establish goals. In addition, the early season is a time for skill-learning in which observational learning and biofeedback may be particularly helpful techniques. As a long season of practices and games continues, the player may require some extra motivation to help her stay motivated to train and compete. In this situation, self-talk and imagery may be the best skills to use. If the player is injured over the course of the season, recovering from the injury and returning to play will require still another set of psychological skills. Given the unique benefits that the various psychological techniques can have in improving performance and the experience of the participants, combining psychological skills to deliver a maximally-effective, holistic intervention is often the best approach.

CHAPTER SUMMARY

There are numerous considerations that must be made when planning the delivery of psychological interventions in sport, exercise, and injury rehabilitation. For example, who should deliver the intervention? Where should the intervention be delivered? And, what are the most appropriate psychological skills to include in the intervention? The answers to these questions depend on the specific goals of the psychological intervention, on the specific expertise of the personnel (i.e., coaches, trainers, or therapists) involved, and on the resources available for conducting the intervention. With regard to who should deliver psychological interventions, there are numerous options. It is common for sport psychologists or sport psychology consultants to deliver interventions. Intervention delivery by SPs or SPCs is ideal because of the extensive knowledge, training, and experience accrued by these individuals. When SPs or SPCs are not available, or available resources do not allow for them to be employed, interventions may also be delivered by coaches, trainers, or therapists. Although delivery of psychological interventions by coaches, trainers, and therapists can help to ensure that psychological skills training is incorporated into everyday practice, these individuals often lack the specific training and confidence to deliver psychological interventions effectively.

Determining the optimal setting for intervention delivery depends largely on the desired outcome of the intervention. For example, whereas certain psychological interventions are ideally suited for a practice environment, others have a stronger impact when they are administered in competition. Finally, selecting the appropriate psychological techniques to include in the intervention also depends on the goals of the intervention. When there is a specific issue to be addressed by an intervention, such as an exerciser experiencing social physique anxiety in a gym setting or an injured athlete who is experiencing extreme hesitation returning to regular play after their injury rehabilitation, a single intervention approach may be appropriate. In contrast, when a coach wishes to provide an athlete or a team with optimal training conditions, combining psychological techniques to facilitate learning and help maintain motivation may be best. Regardless of who delivers the intervention, in what setting the intervention is delivered, and which intervention approach that is selected, the best psychological interventions are carefully planned to address the specific needs and challenges of the recipient.

REVIEW QUESTIONS

1. Who is typically responsible for delivering psychological interventions in the context of injury rehabilitation?
2. What are the advantages of an exercise psychology intervention being delivered by a personal trainer? What are some potential disadvantages?
3. List three common preferences that coaches have when working with a sport psychologist or sport psychology consultant.
4. In what circumstances might it be ideal to apply a single sport psychology skill, rather than a combination of multiple skills?

SUGGESTED READINGS

Fortier, M. S., Tulloch, H., & Hogg, W. (2006). A good fit: Integrating physical activity counselors into family practice. *Canadian Family Physician, 52*, 947–951.

Zakrajsek, R. A., Steinfeldt, J. A., Bodey, K. J., Martin, S. B., & Zizzi, S. J. (2013). NCAA Division I coaches' perceptions and preferred use of sport psychology services: A qualitative perspective. *The Sport Psychologist, 27*, 258–268.

REFERENCES

Abramson, S., Stein, J., Schaufele, M., Frates, E., & Rogan, S. (2000). Personal exercise habits and counseling practices of primary care physicians: a national survey. *Clinical Journal of Sport Medicine, 10*, 40–48.

Fortier, M. S., Tulloch, H., & Hogg, W. (2006). A good fit: Integrating physical activity counselors into family practice. *Canadian Family Physician, 52*, 947–951.

Gould, D., Damarjian, N., & Medbery, R. (1999). An examination on mental skills training in junior tennis coaches. *The Sport Psychologist, 13*, 127–143.

Gould, D., & Eklund, R. C. (1991). The application of sport psychology for performance optimizations. *Journal of Sports Sciences, 1*, 10–21.

Gould, D., Medbery, R., Damarjian, N., & Lauer, L. (1999). A survey of mental skills training knowledge, opinions, and practices of junior tennis coaches. *Journal of Applied Sport Psychology, 11*, 28–50.

Gould, D., Murphy, S., Tammen, V., & May, J. (1989). *An assessment of psychological programs and personnel in U.S. amateur sports (1984–1988). A report to the U.* Colorado Springs, Colorado: S. Olympic Committee.

Grobbelaar, H. W. (2007). A survey of South African provincial netball coaches' opinions, abilities and limitations regarding mental skills training. *South African Journal for Research in Sport. Physical Education and Recreation, 2*, 27–39.

Larson, G. A., Starkey, C., Zaichkowsky, L. D. (1996). Psychological aspects of athletic injuries as perceived by athletic trainers. *The Sport Psychologist, 10*, 37–47.

Martens, R. (2004). Planning for teaching. In R. Martens (Ed.), *Successful coaching: America's best-selling coach's guide* (3rd ed., pp. 235–260). Champaign, IL: Human Kinetics.

Moulton, M. A., Molstad, S., & Turner, A. (1997). The role of athletic trainers in counseling collegiate athletes. *Journal of Athletic Training, 32*, 148–150.

Nupponen, R. (1998). What is counseling all about—basics in the counseling of health-related physical activity. *Patient Education Counseling, 33*, S61–67.

Orlick, T., & Partington, J. (1988). Mental links to excellence. *The Sport Psychologist, 2*, 105–130.

Ottley, M. (2000). Knowledge, attitudes, and perceptions of selected Trinidad and Tobago coaches and athletes regarding sport psychology consultation. *Dissertation Abstracts International Section A: Humanities and Social Sciences, 61*(3-A), 932.

Petrella, R., & Wright, D. (2000). An office-based instrument for exercise counseling and prescription in primary care. The step test exercise prescription (STEP). *Archives of Family Medicine, 9*, 339–344.

Reade, I., Rodgers, W., Holt, N., Dunn, J., Hall, N., Stolp, S., Jones, L., Smith, J., & Baker, T. (2008). A report of the status of coaches of carded athletes in Canada: A summary of the findings. *Submitted to the Coaching Association of Canada.*

Ritchie, C., Stetson, B., Bass, P., & Adams, K. (2002). Physical activity counseling: an educational exercise for medical students. *Nutrition in Clinical Care, 5*, 103–114.

Stanley, D. M., & Cumming, J. (2010). Are we having fun yet? Testing the effects of imagery use on the affective and enjoyment responses to acute moderate exercise. *Psychology of Sport and Exercise, 11*, 582–590.

Sullivan, J., & Hodge, K. P. (1991). A survey of coaches and athletes about sport psychology in New Zealand. *The Sport Psychologist, 5*, 140–151.

Tulloch, H., Fortier, M., & Hogg, W. (2006). Physical activity counseling in primary care: Who has and who should be counseling? *Patient Education and Counseling, 64*, 6–20.

Walsh, J., Swangard, D., Davis, T., & McPhee, S. (1999). Exercise counselling by primary care physicians in the era of managed care. *American Journal of Preventive Medicine, 16*, 307–313.

Yarnell, K., Pollak, K., Ostbye, R., Krause, K., & Michener, L. (2003). Primary care: is there enough time for prevention? *American Journal of Public Health, 93*, 635–641.

Zakrajsek, R. A., Steinfeldt, J. A., Bodey, K. J., Martin, S. B., & Zizzi, S. J. (2013). NCAA Division I coaches' perceptions and preferred use of sport psychology services: A qualitative perspective. *The Sport Psychologist, 27*, 258–268.

Chapter 3

Expertise and Psychological Interventions

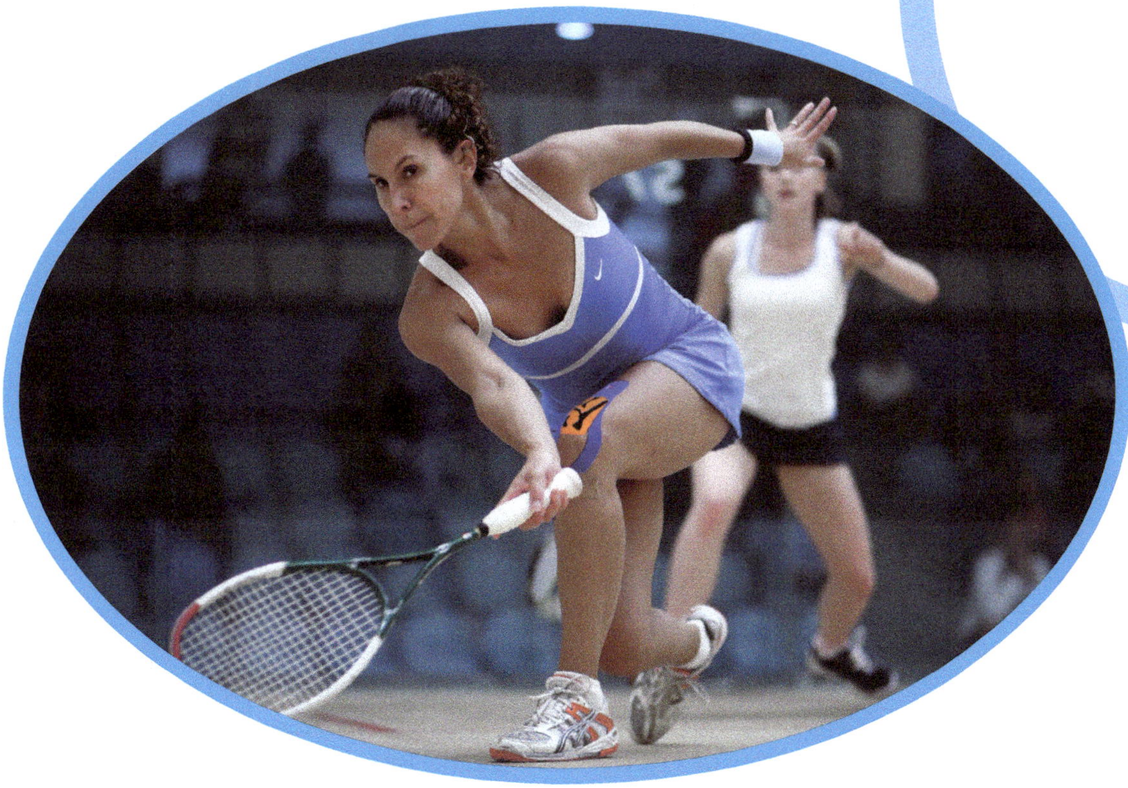

Introduction

It can be argued that in many physical activity contexts three general components come into play: technical, physical, and mental. Taking the sport of squash as an example, to be an elite player one must have the shots and strategies (i.e., technical), the speed, strength and endurance (i.e., physical), and be motivated, mentally tough and highly confident (i.e., mental). If you have a weakness in one of these components your likelihood of being successful is greatly diminished. While expert performers such as world squash champion Ramy Ashour are certainly compelling to watch, researchers have been keenly interested in the development of expertise since there is strong scientific rationale for studying it. An understanding of the features that limit performance at the highest levels of sport can increase our understanding of the factors that influence human achievement across other domains (Williams & Ericsson, 2005). Such knowledge may be used to test general theories of expertise and skill acquisition. In addition, knowledge of the mechanisms underpinning expertise provides a foundation for determining what types of practice are most likely to be beneficial for performance improvement, and why some people improve at different rates compared to others or reach much higher levels of achievement (Ericsson, 2006). This knowledge is relevant when designing appropriate training interventions, including psychological interventions (Williams & Reilly, 2000).

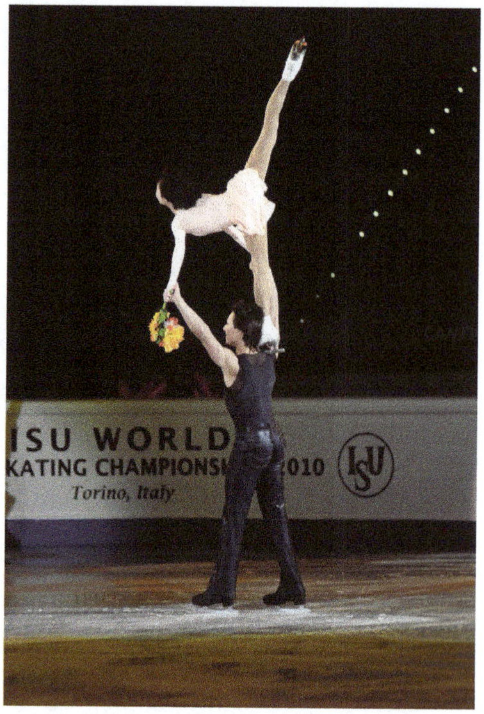

Expertise has been studied in a variety of domains including music, chess, education, physics, mathematics, and business. With respect to physical activity domains, most of the expertise research has considered sport. Some of the sports in which expertise have been investigated include field hockey, figure skating, soccer, and wrestling. Consequently, sport will serve as the focus of this chapter.

Expertise in Sport

Ericsson, Prietula, and Cokely (2007, p. 2) asked the question "How, then, can you tell when you're dealing with a genuine expert?" They argued that real expertise must pass three tests. First, it must produce performance that is consistently superior to that of the expert's peers. Second, real expertise leads to concrete results. Third, true expertise can be replicated and measured. Skill in some domains, such as swimming, is relatively easy to measure as competitions are standardized so that everyone competes in a similar environment. Moreover, all competitors have the same start and finish, so that everyone can agree on who came in first. This standardization permits comparisons among individuals over time.

In line with this concept of what is an expert, researchers for over three decades have sought to better understand the psychological factors that distinguish between expert and non-expert athletes (Abernethy, 1987; Starkes & Ericsson, 2003). Typically, these two groups of athletes are compared on a number of perceptual and cognitive tasks that are specific to a given sport. Overall, research has demonstrated that experts, when compared to non-experts, visually detect and locate objects and patterns in the visual field faster and more accurately, use situational probability information better, have more elaborate task knowledge, make more use of available information, encode and retrieve relevant information more efficiently, and make more rapid and appropriate decisions (Hodges & Starkes, 1996; Mann, Williams, Ward, & Janelle, 2007; Singer & Janelle, 1999; Starkes & Ericsson, 2003).

So how does someone become an expert? Baker and Horton (2004) reviewed the research investigating the acquisition of sport expertise. The three factors having a primary influence on expertise were identified as genetic (hereditary characteristics), psychological, and training (practice) factors. Much of the research examining the genetic factor has used twins and/or family members and these studies show that cardiovascular measures, and perhaps more importantly an athlete's response to exercise training, is influenced by his or her genetic makeup. In addition, some measures of intelligence and personality have also been associated with inherited characteristics [for detailed information see the HERITAGE (Health, Risk Factors, Exercise Training and Genetics) family study and the MISTRA (Minnesota Study of Twins Reared Apart) research].

With respect to the psychological factor, investigators (Gould, Diffenbach, & Moffett, 2002; Williams & Krane, 2001) have identified the mental characteristics of successful athletes. In the Gould et al. study, 10 U.S. Olympic champions (winners of 32 Olympic medals) were interviewed, as was one of their coaches, and a parent, guardian, or significant other. A number of psychological inventories were also administered to the athletes. Not surprisingly, the mental characteristics identified included strong motivation, high self-confidence, good concentration, superior coping skills, and the effective use of imagery and self-talk. More recently, McNamara, Button, and Collins (2010) considered the role of psychological characteristics in facilitating the development of elite performance. Seven elite athletes and a parent of each of these athletes were interviewed regarding their own (their son's/daughter's) development in sport. They established a range of psychological factors that facilitated the translation of potential into talent which they termed Psychological Characteristics of Developing Excellence. These were:

- Competitiveness
- Commitment
- Vision of what it takes to succeed
- Imagery
- Importance of working on weaknesses
- Coping under pressure
- Game awareness
- Self-belief

They concluded that although sporting achievement was conceptualized as being multidimensional, psychological factors were emphasized as the key determinants of athletes who emerged as talented and maintained excellence. Accordingly, they argued that greater emphasis should be placed on the development and application of psychological factors at an early stage to optimize both the improvement and performance of athletes.

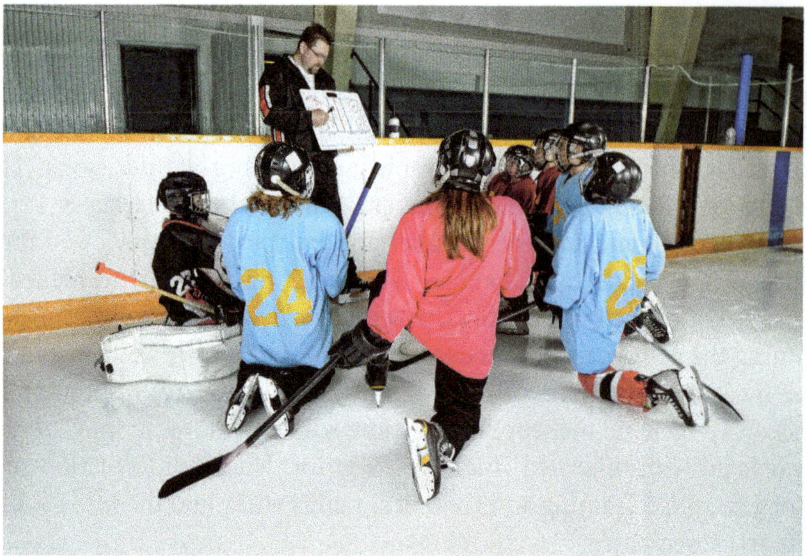

Image © Lorraine Swanson, 2014. Used under license from Shutterstock, Inc.

Training, the third factor categorized by Baker and Horton (2004), seems to have the strongest association with expertise. Some researchers such as Ericsson et al. (2007) propose that experts are always made and never born. Furthermore, it will take at least a decade of deliberate practice to achieve expertise. Deliberate practice involves considerable, specific, and sustained effort to work on things you cannot do well or even at all. It entails working on your weaknesses and not your strengths (Ericsson et al., 2007).

Deliberate Practice

In the theory of deliberate practice, Ericsson and his colleagues (Ericsson, 2006; Ericsson, Krampe, & Tesch-Römer, 1993) argued that an individual's level of attainment is directly proportional to the amount of practice hours accumulated within a domain. This does not imply that extensive experience within a domain (e.g., sport) will inevitably lead to expertise. Continued improvements in performance depend on deliberate efforts to improve important aspects of performance rather than the repetitive execution of routine work. Deliberate practice consists of activities that require effort and attention, but are not inherently enjoyable. Furthermore, the activity must be a well-defined task with an appropriate level of difficulty for the individual, provide informative feedback, and opportunities for repetition and for corrections of errors. Finally, the amount of time that an individual is engaged in deliberate practice activities is predicted as being monotonically related to that individual's acquired level of performance.

To initially test their framework, Ericsson et al. (1993) examined the perceptions of three different skill levels of violinists. More specifically, the participants were requested to rate different types of violin and everyday activities along three dimensions: (1) the relevancy to improving performance; (2) the inherent enjoyment of the activity; and (3) the amount of effort required to perform the activity. Three different activities were defined as deliberate practice based on the violinists' high ratings of relevance and effort, and comparably lower rating for enjoyment: practice alone with the violin, taking violin lessons, and engaging in solo practices. Also, a comparison across skill levels revealed that all the participants had similar perceptions of the importance of practice, but the "best" violinists engaged in significantly more deliberate practice than violinists in the other two lower skill levels. Finally, the basic tenet of Ericsson et al.'s theory was supported with the finding that performance was monotonically related to the amount of deliberate practice done by the violinist, and that the time spent in practice was a critical determinant of the level of performance.

Subsequently, this framework was tested in various sport populations and similar results were found, except activities rated by athletes as being highly relevant to sport performance were also perceived as being enjoyable (Helsen, Starkes, & Hodges, 1998; Hodges & Starkes, 1996). Based on these findings, a sport specific deliberate practice framework was proposed to include activities that are highly relevant to improving performance, require a great deal of effort to perform, and are perceived as being enjoyable (Helsen et al., 1998; Hodges & Starkes, 1996). Moreover, the sport specific deliberate practice framework differentiates between the amount of physical and mental effort required to perform various practice activities. Some activities demand a great deal of physical effort, but very little mental concentration to perform; therefore it is difficult for athletes to interpret a composite term consisting of both physical effort and mental concentration (Starkes, Deakin, Allard, Hodges, & Hayes, 1996). Accordingly, a fourth dimension was added to the framework to consider the amount of concentration required to perform the activity, and it has been shown to be highly correlated with the relevance to enhancing performance, and is clearly separate from the dimension of physical effort (Helsen et al., 1998; Hodges & Starkes, 1996).

In support of the sport specific definition of deliberate practice, research has investigated athletes' perceptions of the relevance, effort, concentration, and enjoyment of different practice, leisure, and everyday activities (Starkes, 2000). Generally, practice activities identified as being: (1) highly relevant to performance, (2) requiring a great deal of mental concentration and/or physical effort, and (3) seemingly enjoyable to perform were those activities that most closely reflected what the athletes are required to do in competition. For example, deliberate practice activities for wrestling were identified as sparring with a partner and working with a coach; for figure skating these were on-ice activities and lessons with a coach; and for middle distance running, these were speed work and time trials activities. For team sports, such as soccer and field hockey, deliberate practice activities consisted of training drills that recreated game conditions and tactics.

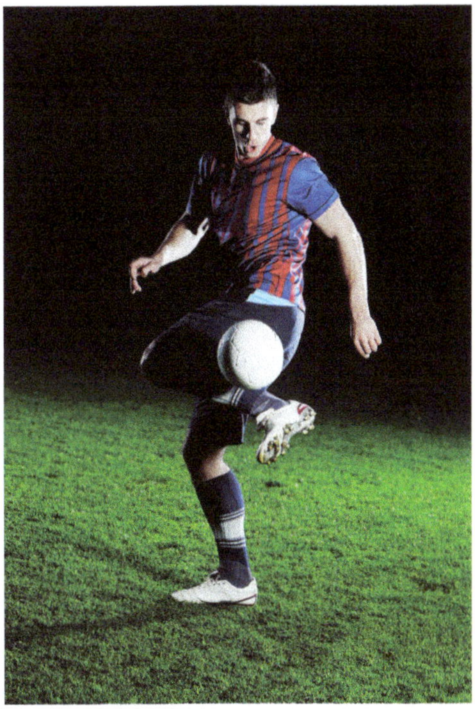

Deliberate Imagery Practice

In an extension to the deliberate practice research, Cumming and Hall (2002) examined mental imagery as another form of deliberate practice. It was their contention that imagery should be considered as deliberate practice because of the functional equivalence that exists between physical and imagery practice (Holmes & Collins, 2001). Mental imagery is often considered to be the visualization of an object, scene, or sensation as though it were occurring in overt, physical reality (Denis, 1985). We discuss mental imagery in detail in chapter 6.

Cumming and Hall (2002) predicted that athletes would perceive imagery as being highly relevant to improving their performance, requiring a great deal of effort, and that it is enjoyable to perform. A total of 150 Canadian athletes, 78 male and 72 female, participated in their study. The athletes were from a broad range of sports and participated at one of three different competitive levels: recreational, provincial, and national.

The athletes were asked to complete the Deliberate Imagery Practice Questionnaire that was based on the methodology employed in previous deliberate practice research (e.g., Hodges & Starkes, 1996). First, the athletes were asked to provide biographical information concerning age, gender, sport, and competitive level. Second, the athletes were asked to rate imagery practice along the different dimensions of deliberate practice on an 11-point Likert scale (0 = *not at all*, 10 = *highly*). More specifically, the athletes were asked to rate to what extent imagery is relevant to improving their performance, relevant to competing effectively, enjoyable to perform regardless of the result, and how much mental effort is required to perform the activity. Third, the athletes were asked to estimate the amount of time (minutes) they spent practicing different types of imagery in a current typical week for their training cycle. The different types of imagery that were listed in the questionnaire were skills, strategies, the obtainment of goals, the stress and excitement of performing, and imagery of being confident, mentally tough, positive, and/or focused. In the fourth and final part of the questionnaire, the athletes were asked to estimate the number of hours per week that they spent on imagery for each year that they participated in their sport, starting with the first year, and continuing until the present time.

Previous research (Helsen et al., 1998; Hodges & Starkes, 1996) had found that no differences exist between international, national, and provincial level athletes' perceptions of practice according to the dimensions of relevance, effort, and enjoyment. Similar to this previous research, Cumming and Hall (2002) found no differences between three competitive levels (i.e., national, provincial, and recreational) in their perceptions of effort and enjoyment. Athletes at the national level, however, perceived imagery as being more relevant to improving their performance and competing effectively than recreational level athletes. The explanation they offered for this difference was that lower level athletes do not understand the value of mental imagery and its relevance to performing to the same extent as higher level athletes. Cumming and Hall also showed that national level athletes accumulated the most hours of imagery practice, followed in order by provincial and recreational level athletes. This was the case even when numbers of years in the sport was accounted for. Based on these findings, Cumming and Hall concluded that mental imagery is another practice activity that can be considered as deliberate practice given that it fits the criteria established in previous research.

CHAPTER SUMMARY

For athletes to achieve the elite level in their sports they must work on the technical, physical, and mental components. Research on the development of expertise has demonstrated that this requires working on weaknesses. Athletes must make deliberate efforts to improve important aspects of performance that they cannot do well. Even athletes at the very top of their sport believe they still have room for improvement. They can do most things in their sport extremely well, but still believe there are some areas in which they can make further improvements. Serena Williams, considered the top female tennis player at the time, in a media interview stated that she felt she could take her game to even a higher level. While she could usually beat all her opponents, most very handily, she still saw weaknesses in her game that could be improved.

The research on deliberate imagery practice shows that mental skills should be treated the same as technical and physical skills. Athletes need to identify their mental weaknesses and then make deliberate efforts to improve them. This entails working on these weaknesses on a regular and structured basis. When Ramy Ashour and Serena Williams practice, which takes place most days of the week (i.e., regular practice), they have a plan for what they need to accomplish. That is, their practice is structured with most of their effort aimed at improving their weaknesses. In the following chapters we talk about psychological interventions for specific mental skills such as goal setting and imagery. These interventions need to take the deliberate practice approach. Weaknesses in mental skills need to be identified and then these weaknesses need to be regularly worked on. Athletes and coaches know the value of regular and structured practice sessions, so taking this same approach when it comes to practicing mental skills is really just a logical extension of what they already do with technical and physical skills.

REVIEW QUESTIONS

1. Why are researchers interested in studying expertise?
2. What were the three factors that Baker and Horton (2004) found primarily influenced the development of sport expertise?
3. The sport specific definition of deliberate practice has four dimensions. List the four dimensions.
4. What did Cumming and Hall (2002) conclude after examining deliberate imagery practice?

SUGGESTED READINGS

Cumming, J., & Hall, C. (2002). Deliberate imagery practice: The development of imagery skills in competitive athletes. *Journal of Sport Sciences, 20*, 137–145.

Starkes, J. L. (2000). The road to expertise: Is practice the only determinant? *International Journal of Sport Psychology, 31*, 431–451.

REFERENCES

Abernethy, B. (1987). The relationship between expertise and visual search strategy in a racquet sport. *Human Movement Science, 6*, 283–319.

Baker, J., & Horton, S. (2004). A review of primary and secondary influences on sport expertise. *Higher Education, 15*, 211–228.

Cumming, J., & Hall, C. (2002). Deliberate imagery practice: The development of imagery skills in competitive athletes. *Journal of Sport Sciences, 20*, 137–145.

Denis, M. (1985). Visual imagery and the use of mental practice in the development of motor skills. *Canadian Journal of Applied Sport Sciences, 10*, 4S–16S.

Ericsson, K. A. (2006). An introduction to the Cambridge handbook of expertise and expert performance: its development, organization, and content. In K. A. Ericsson et al. (Eds.), *The Cambridge handbook of expertise and expert performance* (pp. 3–20). New York: Cambridge University Press.

Ericsson, K., Krampe, R., & Tesch-Römer, C. (1993). The role of deliberate practice in the acquisition of expert performance. *Psychological Review, 100*, 363–406.

Ericsson, K. A., Prietula, M. J., & Cokely, E. T. (2007). The making of an expert. *Harvard Business Review, July–August*, 1–7.

Gould, D., Diffenbach, K., & Moffett, A. (2002). Psychological characteristics and their development in Olympic champions. *Journal of Applied Sport Psychology, 14*, 172–204.

Helsen, F. W., Starkes, J. L., & Hodges, N. J. (1998). Team sports and the theory of deliberate practice. *Journal of Sport and Exercise Psychology, 20*, 12–34.

Hodges, N. J., & Starkes, J. L. (1996). Wrestling with the nature of expertise: A sport specific test of Ericsson, Krampe and Tesch-Römer's (1993) theory of deliberate practice. *International Journal of Sport Psychology, 27*, 400–424.

Holmes, P. S., & Collins, D. J. (2001). The PETTLEP approach to motor imagery: A functional equivalence model for sport psychologists. *Journal of Applied Sport Psychology, 13*, 60–83.

McNamara, A., Button, A., & Collins, D. (2010). The role of psychological characteristics in facilitating the pathway to elite performance. Part 1: Identifying mental skills and behaviors. *The Sport Psychologist, 24*, 52–73.

Mann, D. T. Y., Williams, A. M., Ward, P., & Janelle, C. M. (2007). Perceptual-cognitive expertise in sport: A meta-analysis. *Journal of Sport and Exercise Psychology, 29*, 457–478.

Singer, R. N., & Janelle, C. M. (1999). Determining sport expertise: From genes to supremes. *International Journal of Sport Psychology, 30*, 117–150.

Starkes, J. L. (2000). The road to expertise: Is practice the only determinant? *International Journal of Sport Psychology, 31*, 431–451.

Starkes, J. L., Deakin, J. M., Allard, F., Hodges, N. J., & Hayes, A. (1996). Deliberate practice in sports: What is it anyway? In K. A. Ericsson (Ed.), *The road to excellence: The acquisition of expert performance in arts and sciences, sports, and games* (pp. 81–106). Mahwah, NJ: Lawrence Erlbaum Associates, Inc.

Starkes, J. L., & Ericsson, K. A. (2003). *Expert performance in sports: Advances in research on sport expertise*. Champaign, IL: Human Kinetics.

Williams, A. M., & Ericsson, K. A. (2005). Some considerations when applying the expert performance approach in sport. *Human Movement Science, 24*, 283–307.

Williams, A. M., & Reilly, T. (2000). Talent identification and development in soccer. *Journal of Sports Sciences, 18*, 657–667.

Williams, J. M., & Krane, V. (2001). Psychological characteristics of peak performance. In J. M. Williams (Ed.), *Applied sport psychology: Personal growth to peak performance*. Mountain View, CA: Mayfield.

Chapter 4

Modeling

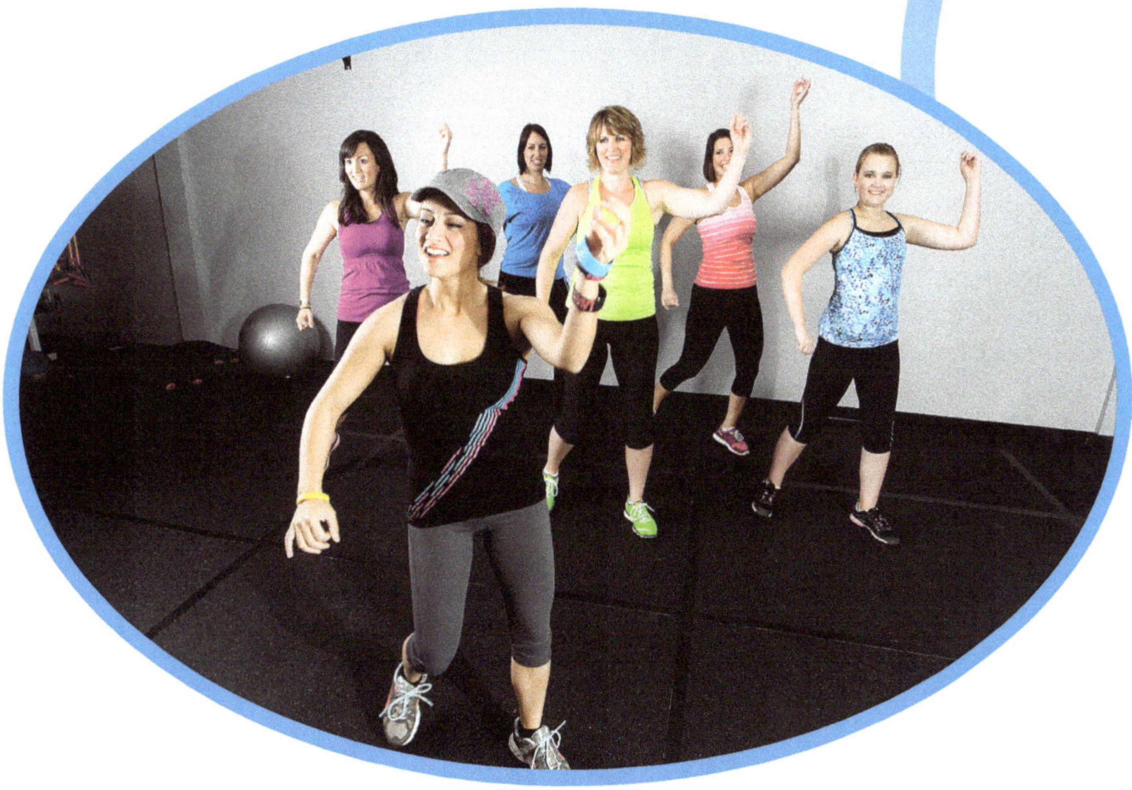

Image © Mat Hayward, 2014. Used under license from Shutterstock, Inc.

Introduction

A long-standing research finding that is not disputed is that we repeat and learn the behaviors of those we have observed. How to label this process is not as clear. A wide variety of terms, such as imitation, emulation, observational learning, and modeling have been used (Williams, Davids, & Williams, 1999). We will term this process modeling and it can be thought of as how observation of others, or the self, can be optimized to assist the learning of motor skills, as well as to enhance motor skill performance (Ste-Marie, Law, Rymal, O, Hall, & McCullagh, 2012).

We are interested in modeling because it is one of the most common methods of teaching. For example, a coach may tell an athlete how to perform a specific skill, but the coach will also likely demonstrate the skill. In addition, there is the opportunity for modeling of motor skills to occur in a variety of situations including sport, exercise, and injury rehabilitation.

Researchers interested in the use of modeling have just recently begun to study the reasons *why* learners engage in observation. Cumming, Clark, Ste-Marie, McCullagh, and Hall (2005) were the first to investigate the functions (i.e., the reasons why athletes, learners, coaches, or other individuals engage in modeling) that modeling may serve in the sport context. They investigated these reasons through their development of the Functions of Observational Learning Questionnaire (FOLQ). They found that athletes use modeling for motor skill acquisition and execution (i.e., the skill function), to develop and execute sport strategies (i.e., the strategy function), and to reach optimal arousal levels and mental states for physical performance (i.e., the performance function). Their research and subsequent studies employing the FOLQ (Hall, Munroe-Chandler, Cumming, Law, Ramsey, & Murphy, 2009; Hancock, Rymal, & Ste-Marie, 2011; Law & Hall, 2009; Wesch, Law, & Hall, 2007) have demonstrated that athletes of all skill levels employ the skill function most frequently, followed by the strategy function, and then the performance function. In addition, individual and independent sport athletes report greater use of the skill and performance functions, and team and interactive sport athletes report greater use of the strategy function.

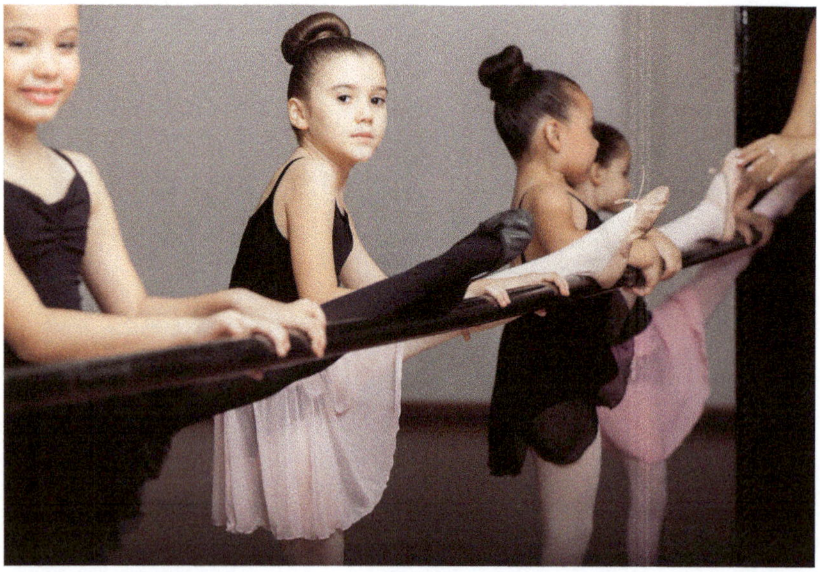

When should a model demonstrate? The most common approach in research studies is to have the model demonstrate both before and during physical practice, and given the positive effects of modeling, this appears to be effective (Ste-Marie et al., 2012). Is it the optimal approach? At this point we really do not know because of the lack of research examining when a model should demonstrate.

Many researchers have been interested in *who* is the most beneficial model to observe. The two basic model types are others or the self (Ste-Marie et al., 2012). With respect to observing others, these can be grouped into peer (i.e., matched gender and age between observer and model) and non-peer models. Within these two model types, there is also the consideration of whether the model is a skilled model (shows proper execution of skill) or an unskilled model (execution of skill contains errors). Another level of variation is in terms of coping and mastery models. A coping model is viewed across a number of trials and progresses from verbalizations concerning difficulty performing the skill and feeling a lack of confidence concerning the ability to do the skill to verbalizations that demonstrate confidence and ease in performing the skill. Coupled with these verbalizations is a change in the physical execution of the skill from an unskilled to a skilled performance. In contrast, mastery models begin with confident statements in their ability to do the skill and expressing the ease with which the skill is performed and always show a skilled execution. In terms of observing the self as a model, one can view the self from a self-observation (basic video replay) or self-modeling technique (edited video replay techniques).

Ste-Marie et al. (2012) recently developed an applied model that can guide practitioners in the use of modeling (see Figure 4–1). At the forefront of the applied model are observer (e.g., age) and task (e.g., complexity) characteristics. These two variables would influence the implementation of a modeling intervention. At the second level of the applied model, it is proposed that the practitioner should consider the environment in which the observer is situated (i.e., where), and the functions they anticipate the use of modeling will serve (i.e., why). After acquiring a good appreciation of these first four components (observer/task/where/why), the practitioner is in a better position to consider

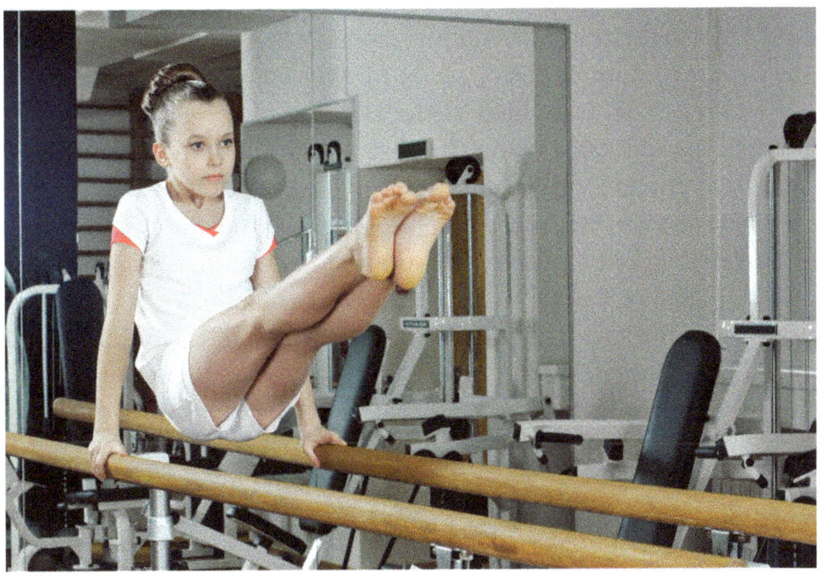

FIGURE 4–1 The Applied Model

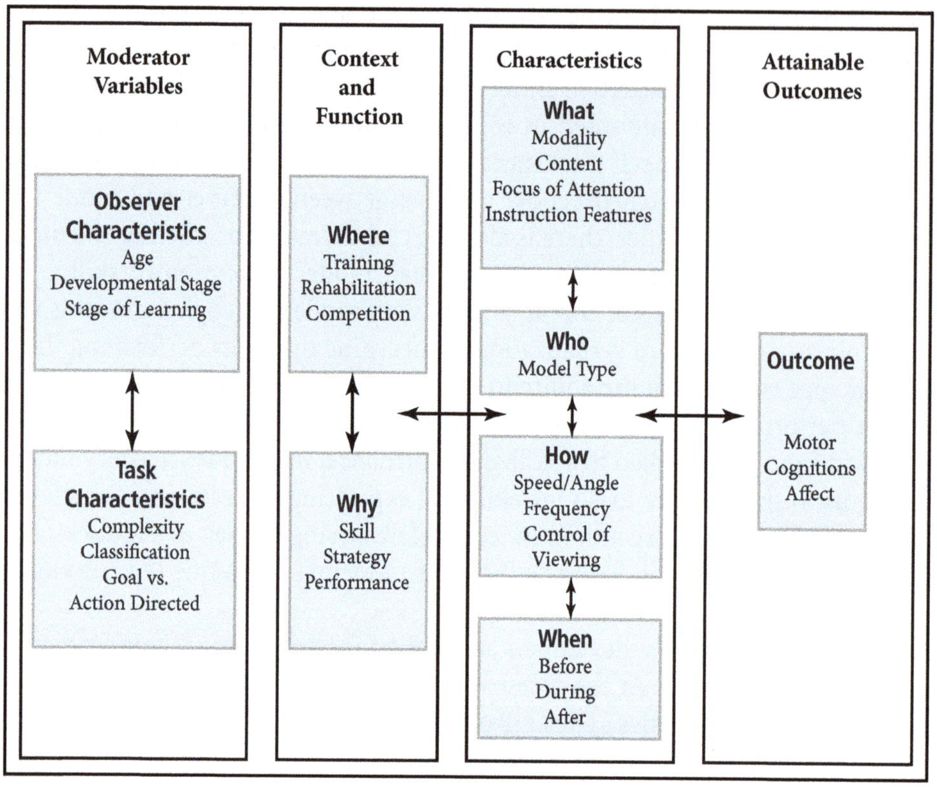

Ste-Marie et al. (2012)

the choices involved in manipulating the characteristics in the next level of the applied model, namely *Who* is the model, *What* information is the model conveying, *When* should the model demonstrate, and *How* should the demonstration be delivered. The final level of the model is the outcome the practitioner wants the observer to achieve, such as the learning of a skill, an increase in the observer's confidence, or an increase in the satisfaction the observer has in doing the task.

Ste-Marie et al. (2012) provide some scenarios of modeling interventions, outlining the observer/task characteristics, where and why the intervention is being used, and how the intervention may unfold given the situation provided. In one example they consider a novice dancer, Jessica, who is six years old and is learning a dance sequence within a dance class. The outcome focus in this situation is on skill learning. They suggest it is likely that Jessica would benefit from a live, skilled model (i.e., a dance instructor) who provides metaphors for the movements during the dance sessions. They also suggest it may be best for the instructor to provide an objective view when modeling the dance and to perform the dance in real time.

In the following sections we will consider modeling interventions in sport, exercise, and injury rehabilitation and as we discuss these interventions keep this applied model in mind.

Modeling in Sport

Modeling in sport can take place both in training and competition. Most of the intervention research has been conducted in the training context. With respect to who is the model, McCullagh and Meyer (1997) compared a group that received only knowledge of results (KR; i.e., no observation provided) to a peer skilled model plus KR, and two peer unskilled model groups, one receiving KR and one not receiving KR, during the learning of a free weight squat. For free weight squat form, all groups did better over time but the groups with observation plus KR did better than the peer unskilled without KR. After reviewing the literature, Ste-Marie et al. (2012) concluded that observers viewing skilled and unskilled models do not seem to differ much on physical performance measures, given those watching the unskilled model receive feedback.

Clark and Ste-Marie (2002) investigated the acquisition of a diving skill, as well as self-efficacy and perceived difficulty. Participants either viewed a peer mastery model, a peer coping model or no model. They found that the peer mastery model group performed the dive better than the peer coping and control groups, though this only approached statistical significance. Perceived task difficulty of those in the peer coping model group decreased, indicating that a mastery model may be better for physical performance changes, but coping models provide more change to psychological factors. Other research has supported this finding suggesting that for peer models, mastery and coping models may affect physical and psychological measures differentially. However, non-peer models show a similar pattern for both of these measures (Ste-Marie et al., 2012).

Of the research that has included comparisons of the self as a model, the majority of research has been related to self-observation techniques, with very few investigating self-modeling. Some studies have shown positive effects for the self-observation video (e.g., Clark & Ste-Marie, 2007; Onate, Guskiewic, Marshall, Giuliani, Yu, & Garrett, 2005; Van Wieringen, Emmen, Bootsma, Hoogesteger, & Whiting, 1989), but one study found it to be less effective (Zetou, Fragouli, & Tzetzis, 1999), and another reported no differences between self-observation and other model types (Emmen, Wesseling, Bootsma, Whiting, & Van Wieringen, 1985). As for the research investigating self-modeling, the results are again mixed. Some research has found that self-modeling is more effective than other model types (Clark & Ste-Marie, 2007; Dowrick & Raeburn, 1995; Starek & McCullagh, 1999), whereas others have shown no learning differences from self versus other models (Barzouka, Bergeles, & Hatziharistos, 2007).

Skill Learning Interventions

We will discuss the various interventions conducted in the sport context using as headings the three functions that modeling may serve for the athlete (Cumming et al., 2005). The majority of the modeling intervention research has examined the skill function; that is, effectiveness of skill-based modeling experiences on motor skill learning. Although many of these studies have employed laboratory tasks (e.g., computer keyboard, knock-down barrier, stabilometer tasks), many also have been conducted on specific sports skills.

An example of an intervention aimed at increasing skilled performance via modeling is one conducted by Wulf, Raupach, and Pfeiffer (2005). They compared the effectiveness of a condition in which the learner has control over the model presentation schedule (i.e., self-control modeling) with that of a control condition. Each participant in the self-control group was yoked to a partner in the control condition; therefore, the frequency and scheduling of the model presentations were, on average, identical for both groups. The only difference between the conditions was that self-control participants had control over the model presentations, whereas yoked participants did not. The skill was a basketball jump shot. Participants were randomly assigned to the self-control and control conditions, with the restriction that each self-control participant was paired with a yoked participant of the same sex. All participants were told that they would (a) have to practice the basketball jump shot, (b) have 25 practice trials, and (c) be retested one week later. The instructions also emphasized the importance of the quality of the movement (form) as well as accuracy. Participants were able to see a video model and asked to try to imitate the movements of the model as closely as possible. Their shots were videotaped for later analysis.

The subsequent instructions differed for participants in the self-control and control conditions. Self-control participants were told they were free to watch the video at any time as often as they wanted during the practice phase. Control participants were informed that the video model would be shown again from time to time during the practice phase. Two experimenters recorded the accuracy score of each shot and the number of model presentations. One week later, all participants performed a retention test consisting of 10 trials, at which time no video model was available.

It was found that giving learners the opportunity to decide when and how often they saw the model can be effective. After the 7-day retention interval, the self-control group clearly outperformed the control group on form, and showed a similar trend for accuracy. The investigators concluded that their findings added to the evidence for the learning advantages of self-controlled motor learning (e.g., Chiviacowsky & Wulf, 2002), and additionally demonstrated that the benefits of self-control learning generalize to modeling.

Ste-Marie and colleagues (2012) recently summarized the intervention research investigating the effectiveness of skill-based modeling experiences on motor skill learning. They concluded that studies have demonstrated significant outcomes related to skill learning in terms of both acquisition (short-term) and retention (long-term) effects. These physical performance tests have demonstrated modeling benefits for movement outcomes, as well as the quality and coordination of movements (i.e., movement dynamics).

Strategy Learning Interventions

There has been limited research on the effectiveness of modeling interventions to perform and learn sport strategies. A study by Granados and Wulf (2007) is one of the few to consider this issue. It has been shown that practice in dyads, as compared to individual practice, can increase learning as well as enhance the efficiency of practice as two participants can be trained at the same time. Granados and Wulf examined the difference between dyads observing and just discussing strategies that can be used in speed cup stacking. The participants used two hands to build a 3 × 6 × 3 cup stack based on the instructions developed by the World Sport Stacking Association.

Participants were randomly assigned to one of four groups. In the observation/dialogue group, participants practiced in alternating dyad format. More specifically, while one partner performed a trial, the other observed. This was followed by a dialogue period of 10 seconds in which both participants were asked to discuss the trial by sharing possible strategies they might have used (to remember the correct sequence, for example). Then the second partner practiced while the first observed. This sequence of physical practice, observational practice, and dialogue (strategy discussion) continued until both partners had completed 20 practice trials. The observation/no dialogue group was similar to the first group in that participants practiced physically and observationally in an alternating format. In this group, however, no strategy discussion was allowed during the break between trials. In the no observation/dialogue group, participants also practiced in dyads but they were not allowed to observe each other perform. When one partner practiced, the other was instructed to turn around, and vice versa. During the breaks, participants were instructed to engage in a strategy discussion similar to the observation/dialogue group. Finally, there was a control group (no observation/no dialogue) in which participants practiced individually. The dependent measure was the movement time for each trial. All participants performed 20 practice trials on day 1. One day later, they performed a retention test that consisted of five trials performed individually in the same manner the practice trials were performed.

Granados and Wulf demonstrated that participants practicing with a partner benefited most from observing their partners, rather than engaging in a strategy discussion (dialogue) with them. The two groups that included observing a partner, with or without strategy discussion (observation/dialogue, observation/no dialogue), performed more effectively than those who did not observe another person (no observation/dialogue, no observation/no dialogue). In contrast, strategy discussion with a partner provided no additional benefit, compared to no strategy discussion, and this was the case for both the practice phase and retention test. Therefore, the advantages of observing a partner during practice transferred to a situation in which the partner was no longer present (i.e., in retention) and thus represented learning effects. Although these results and others (e.g., Meaney, Griffin, & Hart, 2005) are promising, future research is warranted before definite conclusions can be drawn about the utility of modeling interventions for sport strategy learning.

Performance Interventions

There have been no studies specifically designed to investigate the impact of a modeling intervention on psychological variables (i.e., the performance function) alone. Rather, researchers often measure the

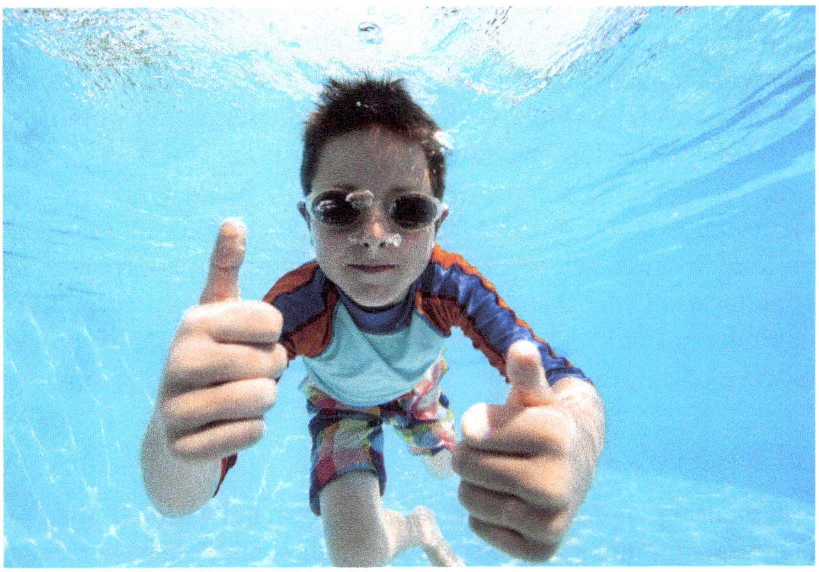

influence of their skill-based modeling interventions by assessing psychological variables (e.g., self-efficacy) as well as physical performance. Research that has assessed changes in psychological variables generally supports positive modeling effects on self-efficacy, motivation, and other self-regulatory variables in sport (Clark & Ste-Marie, 2007; Kitsantas, Zimmerman, & Cleary, 2000).

We will consider the Clark and Ste-Marie study in more detail. They investigated the effect of two modeling interventions on three self-regulatory processes (self-efficacy, intrinsic motivation, and self-satisfaction), as well as physical performance. The two interventions were self-modeling (i.e., viewing oneself perform an edited behavior; the video is edited in an attempt to remove all errors in the performance) and self-observation (i.e., viewing oneself perform at current skill level). There was also a control condition. Thirty-three children were randomly assigned to one of the three conditions. The experimental protocol took place over 8 days and consisted of three phases: pre-test, intervention, and retention phases. During the pre-test phase a swimming stroke to learn was selected for each swimmer, each participant was videoed performing this stroke, and each swimmer completed self-efficacy, motivation, and self-satisfaction measures.

The intervention was conducted across six consecutive days, with each swimmer participating in six swimming lessons, each lasting approximately 30 minutes. Before the beginning of each lesson, swimmers were first shown their self-modeling video, self-observation video, or control group video. The self-modeling and self-observation videos consisted of four 15-second clips of the swimming stroke chosen for the study. The children were instructed to pay close attention while watching their video. Next, the swimmers engaged in a swimming lesson that was specific to the experimental swimming stroke identified and was led by a certified swimming instructor. The swimming instructor provided verbal feedback to each participant on skill execution following a set feedback schedule. This ensured that all participants received similar feedback. In addition, the instructor was responsible for ensuring that each swimmer had the same amount of practice time. At the end of the swim lesson, each swimmer was asked to perform the swimming stroke to the best of his or her ability for a 10-meter distance and their performance was videoed. This performance was used to update the self-modeling and self-observation videos throughout the experiment, as well as for evaluation of physical performance. In addition, the swimmers completed the measures of self-efficacy, motivation, and self-satisfaction according to a set schedule over the course of the intervention phase. Twenty-four hours after the intervention phase, the retention test was administered. This entailed completion of the self-efficacy and motivation measures, performance of the selected swimming skill (videotaped), and completion of the self-satisfaction measure. No video or instructor intervention was used during this session.

Analyses of the retention scores revealed significant differences for all four dependent measures, self-efficacy, intrinsic motivation, self-satisfaction, and swimming performance. The self-modeling group consistently performed better than the self-observation and control groups, with the two latter groups performing similarly. Clark and Ste-Marie concluded that their results provide support for the implementation of self-modeling interventions with children when teaching motor skills.

Measurement of Modeling in Sport

Based on the applied model by Ste-Marie et al. (2012), as shown in Figure 4-1, there are three basic outcomes that can be measured in modeling intervention studies: motor behavior, cognitions, and affect.

Moreover, the measured outcomes within an experiment arise as a result of the specific function(s) that the researchers target in their intervention. Basically, the functions (i.e., the reasons why athletes are engaging in modeling) can be considered the intended focus or desired outcome of the modeling experience, whereas the outcome can be considered as the actual effects of the observation experience on key performance variables (i.e., the physical and/or psychological effects of the modeling experience on the learner's behavior, cognitions, and affect).

Motor behavior can be measured in various ways with two of the common outcome measures being the speed and accuracy of performance. Another approach is to assess the movement dynamics, or the quality and coordination of movements. Literature reviews have demonstrated that in terms of skill-related outcomes, the use of observation appears to produce greater changes in movement dynamics than movement outcomes (Ashford, Bennett, & Davids, 2006). Cognitions and affect are typically measured using questionnaires. For example, in the Clark and Ste-Marie (2007) study described above, the measure used to rate the swimmer's self-efficacy consisted of five circles ranging in size from small, representative of low feelings of self-efficacy, to progressively larger circles, representing greater feelings of self-efficacy. The swimmers selected the circle that best represented their current level of self-efficacy. To measure self-satisfaction a single question was employed. Swimmers rated from 1 to 10 "how satisfied are you with your performance of the (selected swimming skill) today?" with a higher score representing greater satisfaction.

Some General Recommendations

The applied model of Ste-Marie et al. (2012) can be used to guide the development of modeling interventions. It is clear that modeling interventions can improve skill performance and learning, and the cognitions and affect associated with training and competition. To be most effective, however, interventions should account for as many of the factors in the applied model as possible.

Some other general recommendations for sport modeling interventions are:

- Demonstration frequency should be determined by the observer (athlete).
- Athletes benefit from watching both skilled and unskilled models, but unskilled models need to be accompanied with feedback.
- Younger children seem to need some sort of verbal information beyond mere visual demonstrations for enhanced performance (Ste-Marie et al., 2012).
- Skill learning can be improved when modeling is combined with other mental skills such as imagery (Hall & Erffmeyer, 1983).

Modeling in Exercise

In the exercise domain, observation of individuals or groups has the capacity to influence physical activity participation. In the sport domain, modeling is used most frequently for skill and strategy acquisition (Hall et al., 2009; Hancock et al., 2011; Law & Hall, 2009; Wesch et al., 2007) whereas in the exercise domain, research has focused on the performance, or motivational functions of modeling. Because research on modeling in exercise is concentrated in the area of performance/motivation, we structure

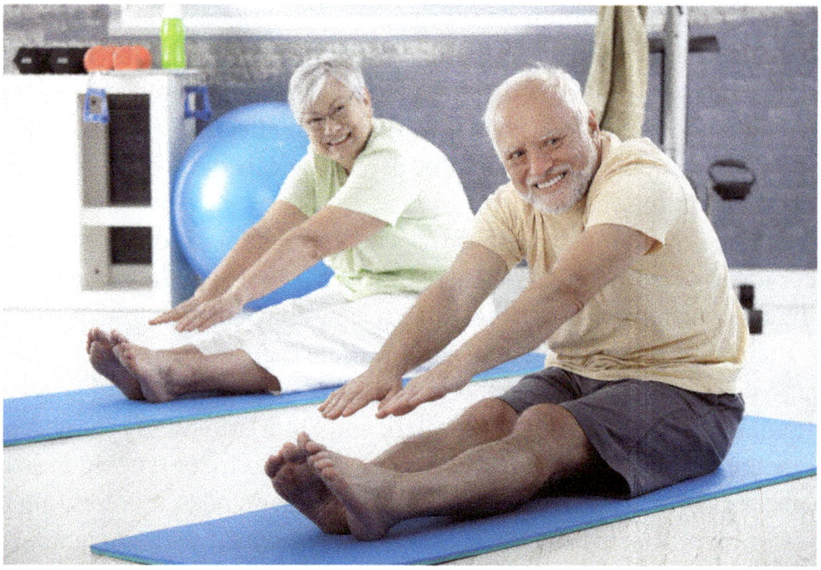

this section of the chapter to explain the why, who, and when of modeling interventions in exercise settings, rather than discussing modeling interventions for separate functions of modeling.

Why Use Modeling in Exercise Settings?

Our understanding of modeling in exercise is largely grounded in self-efficacy theory (Bandura, 1986). Modeling is a form of vicarious experience which Bandura identified as a strong source of self-efficacy. Exercise models, such as aerobics instructors, personal trainers, and other exercisers, have the ability to positively influence exercise participation (Franklin, 1988). Thus, in an exercise context, individuals may use exercise models as role models or to assist them in acquiring self-efficacy for exercise. We provide examples of each, below.

Role modeling. Fitness leaders serve as role models for health and fitness behaviors (Worsley, 1989). For example, in a study conducted by Crozier (2012) college-aged men ($N = 99$) with minimal experience engaging in weight training were assigned randomly to complete a 1-RM chest and leg press with a male trainer who was either (a) visibly muscular and described as an expert or (b) physically lean and described as a novice trainer. The results revealed that the group assigned to the muscular, expert trainer attained higher 1-RM scores than the group assigned to the lean, novice trainer for both the chest and leg press exercises. Although the design of this study does not allow us to distinguish between the influences of the models' physicality and knowledge on the performance of the participants, we can reasonably conclude that characteristics of a model can influence the actual behavior of individuals in an exercise setting.

Instilling self-efficacy. Consistent with Bandura's (1986) suggestion that modeling can influence the development of self-efficacy, Bray, Gyurcsik, Culos-Reed, Dawson, and Martin (2001) demonstrated that fitness leaders may play an important role in instilling confidence in female exercise participants. In this study, Bray et al. (2001) recruited 127 women who were enrolled in a 10-week structured group fitness program to complete self-report measures of self-efficacy and proxy efficacy (i.e., participants' confidence in their fitness instructors' communication, teaching, and motivating capabilities). The measures were completed in the third week and attendance was recorded through the remainder of the program. The results revealed a significant correlation between self- and proxy-efficacy and a significant influence of both types of efficacy on subsequent class attendance. The findings from this study demonstrate that the perceived capabilities of the instructor are related to self-efficacy of the exercise participants and that may also be an important predictor of exercise behavior.

In addition to expert models (i.e., fitness leaders), peer models may also be influential for increasing self-efficacy for exercise. Maddison, Prapavessis, Armstrong, and Hill (2008) conducted an intervention aimed at increasing self-efficacy and optimal performance (i.e., effort) during a peak oxygen uptake (VO2) test among 20 patients with chronic heart failure. The peak VO2 test assesses exercise tolerance and requires the participant to exercise at maximum effort. All participants in the study underwent two peak VO2 tests, conducted one week apart. Between the two tests, patients were assigned randomly to either an intervention or control group. Participants in the intervention group watched a 10-minute coping-model DVD which included (a) clips of patients performing a peak VO2 test, (b) patient demonstrations and verbalizations about acquiring confidence to perform the test, (c) patients offering strategies to cope with the required effort and overcome discomfort that occurs during the test, and (d) clips of a cardiologist who outlined the purpose of a peak VO2 test, the importance of the diagnostic information, the importance of pushing for maximal effort, and information about the safety of the test. Patients in the control group did not view the DVD. The results of this study revealed that compared to participants in the control group, those patients in the intervention group achieved higher levels of self-efficacy for engaging in the exercise test as well as higher peak V02 scores. These findings demonstrate that peer models can be used to increase self-efficacy and behavior among individuals in an exercise setting.

When Are Exercise Models Used?

Modeling of physical activity and exercise behavior occurs both inside and outside formal exercise environments. As discussed above, Crozier (2012) demonstrated that exercise trainers who model a muscular physique and expert knowledge can influence actual exercise behavior among men during weight training sessions. Additionally, Maddison et al. (2008) demonstrated that peer exercise models can be used to influence the self-efficacy and behavior of patients undergoing an exercise test.

The effects of modeling in an exercise context may not all be positive, however. Models who exemplify physical ideals may undermine the self-perceptions of exercisers who do not have ideal physiques. For example, Fleming and Martin Ginis (2004) recruited 101 women to watch an exercise video that featured either exercisers with physiques that match the female cultural ideal (i.e., ultra-thin and ultra-toned), or exercisers who were considered more "normal-looking." The participants completed a measure of self-presentational efficacy (SPE) one week before watching the video as well as measures of SPE and intentions immediately after watching the video. After controlling for pre-video self-presentational efficacy, the findings showed that women who saw the perfect-looking models had lower post-video self-presentational efficacy than women who saw the more "normal-looking" exercise models. Additionally, participants who did not exercise regularly reported lower self-presentational efficacy after seeing either type of model. The results also showed that self-presentational efficacy was also a significant predictor of intentions to exercise. The findings from this study suggest that exposure to exercise models in commercial exercise videos may undermine SPE and subsequently, intentions to exercise. These findings also point to the importance of considering both model and observer characteristics when designing and implementing modeling interventions in exercise. We will discuss this point further in the section on the *who* of exercise modeling.

Exercise models may exert an influence on the thoughts, feelings, and behaviors of observers outside formal exercise settings. For example, parents who are physically active regularly model a physically active lifestyle to their children. Although some studies demonstrate that parent modeling of physical activity significantly influences activity levels of their children, other studies do not support this finding; thus, findings in this area remain inconclusive (Gustafson & Rhodes, 2006). There is also some evidence of peer-modeling of physical activity and exercise behavior. For example, in a cross-sectional study, Voorhees et al. (2005) found that adolescent girls who have more physically active friends report engaging in more physical activity themselves. Due to constraints of the research design, Voorhees et al. could not determine if this association was due to the effects of peer modeling, to peers simply engaging in shared physical activities, or both. Researchers have yet to determine if a friendship-based physical activity modeling intervention can increase physical activity participation.

As is the case inside formal exercise settings, exercise modeling may have negative impacts on exercise-related cognitions and behavior outside of formal exercise settings. Berry, McLeod, Pankratow, and Walker (2013) sought to determine the impact of exercise-related segments from *The Biggest Loser*, a popular reality TV show that often depicts exercise as difficult and painful, on attitudes toward exercise. Berry et al. (2013) presented 138 university students with a clip from either *The Biggest Loser* or *American Idol* (control) reality TV shows and then had them complete assessments of implicit and explicit attitudes toward exercise. Berry et al. reported that compared to participants who viewed a clip of *American Idol*, participants who saw a clip from *The Biggest Loser* reported significantly lower explicit (but not implicit) attitudes toward exercise. This finding highlights the potential influence of exercise models in the "real world." The impact of negative exercise modeling in popular media on the behavior of individuals who consume these media is not known.

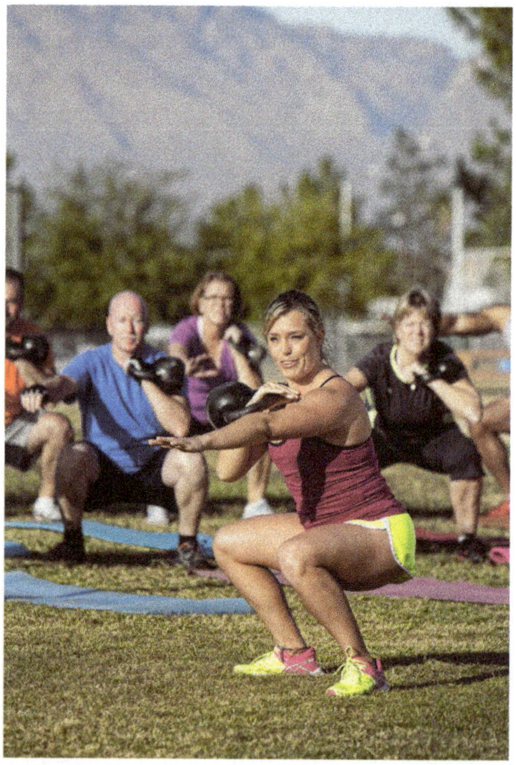

Image © CREATISTA, 2014. Used under license from Shutterstock, Inc.

Who Can Be an Exercise Model?

In the exercise domain, many of the other people around us can serve as models. So far we have discussed the role of fitness leaders such as personal trainers or aerobics instructors as models during in-person or video exercise instruction. In fact, fitness leaders have been cited as the single most important determinant of continued participation in exercise (Franklin, 1988). We have also suggested the possibility of peers and family members as models and demonstrated the impact of a peer modeling intervention on self-perceptions and behavior during an exercise test (Maddison et al., 2008).

It is also possible to use one's self as an exercise model via video feedback or by using mirrors in the exercise environment. Videotaping exercise sessions is not a common practice; however, many gyms and exercise facilities have large mirrors on the walls which provide an opportunity for exercisers to view and correct their own technique. Mirrored walls also allow exercisers to make evaluative decisions about themselves as exercisers; which can have both positive and negative influences on their self-perceptions. For example, Katula and McAuley (2001) recruited 43 female undergraduates to perform 20 minutes of aerobic exercise either in front of, or in the absence of, a full-length mirror. Self-efficacy was assessed before entry into the experimental setting, immediately before the exercise session, immediately following the exercise session, and 20 minutes after the exercise session. In the no-mirror condition, participants did not report changes in self-efficacy from pre-exercise to either of the post-exercise time points; however, in the mirror condition, participants reported moderate increases in self-efficacy immediately following the exercise session and large increases 20 minutes later. These results suggest using the self as a model during aerobic exercise may increase one's perceptions of capabilities. In contrast to these findings, Martin Ginis, Jung, and Gauvin (2003) demonstrated that exercising in front of a mirror had no impact on the body image or self-efficacy of undergraduate research participants; however, it did have a negative impact on their feelings. Because of the mixed research findings in this area, we recommend that practitioners take caution and consider the unique needs of individual exercisers (or groups of exercisers) when determining whether self-modeling via mirrors is appropriate.

Recently, some researchers have begun to examine the potential utility of virtual exercise models. Using avatars, Fox and Bailenson (2009) examined the differential impacts on exercise behavior of viewing (a) a virtual representation of the physical self running on a treadmill, (b) a virtual representation of the physical self loitering, or (c) a virtual representation of another person on a treadmill. The researchers recruited 73 university students to view one of the three representations for 5 minutes and 20 seconds. Twenty-four hours after the participants viewed the video they were asked to self-report all of the physical activity they had done since the experiment ended. The results revealed that the participants who viewed the virtual representation of the physical self running on a treadmill had significantly higher levels of exercise than participants who viewed the other two videos. These findings suggest that an exercise model doesn't have to be a real person to impact the behavior of an observer.

Measurement of Modeling in Exercise

In the exercise literature, the impact of modeling is typically assessed by measuring the desired outcome of the modeling intervention. Perhaps the most important outcome of any intervention in the exercise domain is an actual increase in exercise behavior; thus, the success of many exercise modeling interventions is determined by assessing the impacts of the intervention on behavior. Whereas modeling interventions in the sports domain are frequently focused on improving skills and strategies among athletes, modeling in exercise is more frequently focused on motivational outcomes. Thus, self-perceptions such as self-efficacy and self-presentational efficacy are among the most common outcomes in the exercise modeling literature.

Some General Recommendations

Based on the available literature, it appears that modeling is most often used in the exercise domain for increasing self-efficacy among exercisers. We propose some recommendations for effectively increasing exercise self-efficacy via modeling.

- Models are most effective when they are similar to the observer (i.e., they are similar in age, ability, experience, or they have similar physical limitations) or when they are perceived by the observer as knowledgeable and credible (e.g., Crozier, 2012).
- Characteristics of the model should be tailored to the needs of the observer. For example, exercise videos that portray exercisers with "perfect looking" physiques may undermine the self-efficacy of women who are "normal looking" or who have anxiety surrounding their physical appearance. In contrast, exercisers who perceive themselves as relatively fit may experience a motivational boost if they observe themselves in a mirror during an exercise session.
- Modeling should be positive in nature. Researchers have demonstrated that when people view negative models (i.e., video clips of models struggling during an exercise session) they subsequently report more negative attitudes toward exercise (Berry et al., 2013).

Modeling in Sport Injury Rehabilitation

In the same way that modeling can be used to acquire motor skills and modulate psychological responses in sport and exercise, it can also be beneficial during injury rehabilitation (Heil, 1993; Flint, 1999). It is logical that, especially for athletes who are recovering from their first major injury, observational learning is a crucial component of performing novel exercises and regaining movement patterns. Yet, less than 5% of the research literature examining the effectiveness of modeling in sport has been

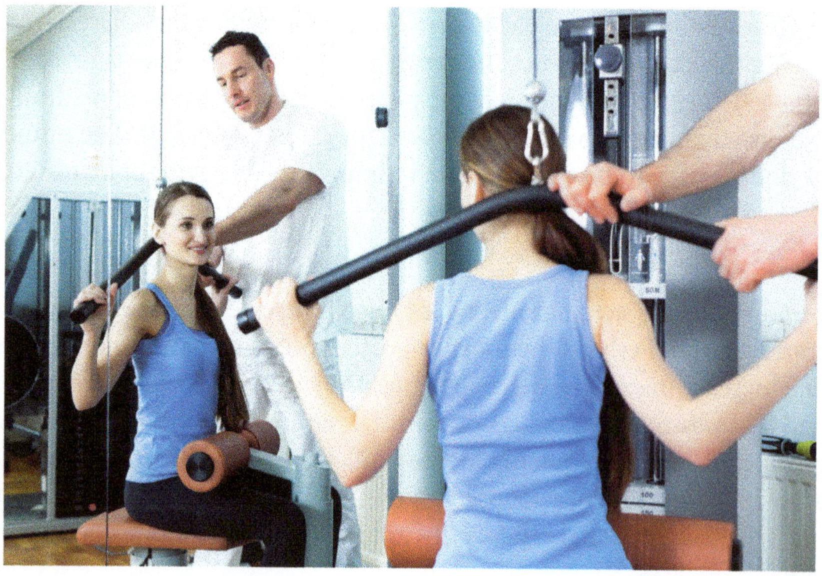

conducted in rehabilitation settings (Ste-Marie et al., 2012). Despite this limitation, however, the scant evidence we do have suggests that modeling can be an effective strategy for improving injury outcomes.

Types of Modeling in Rehabilitation

Mastery models. Generally, mastery models are effective in situations where an individual is working toward a given level of physical performance. This can be particularly salient when an injured athlete is attempting a new rehabilitation exercise and is focusing on acquiring the correct technique. Therapists often demonstrate these exercises themselves, or they may use pictures to illustrate, but athletes may also seek cues from injured peers. Watching another athlete successfully execute the movement can be an important method of gaining information about correct body positioning, speed, and coordination patterns (Williams, Davids, & Williams, 1999).

Although the effect of mastery peer modeling has not been well examined in rehabilitation, two studies have used mastery self-modeling to improve the physical performance of children with physical disabilities (Dowrick & Dove, 1980; Dowrick & Raeburn, 1995). These authors used edited video of study participants demonstrating only adaptive behaviors related to the acquisition of physical skills such as walking, swimming, and other activities of daily living. They found that those who received the mastery self-modeling video intervention performed significantly better compared to those who were not exposed to the intervention (Dowrick & Dove, 1980; Dowrick & Raeburn, 1995). It was also noted that using a self-model paradigm may be more effective than using other children as models because those with disabilities are faced with unique challenges, and therefore do not easily identify with their able-bodied peers (Dowrick & Raeburn, 1995).

The value of mastery modeling in rehabilitation is somewhat intuitive, although using self-modeling is not likely to be feasible. In rare cases, athletes who sustain re-injuries may benefit from video recording of their previous rehabilitation sessions, but this will not apply to the majority of cases. Additionally, there is some suggestion that mastery models may have limited effect in treatment settings. For example, Ng and colleagues found that mastery modeling had no effect on self-efficacy for patients with chronic obstructive pulmonary disease (COPD) (Ng, Tam, Yew, & Lam, 1999). Athletes who view a mastery model may become discouraged at their inability to perform at the desired level, particularly early in rehabilitation. Such frustration may lead to a reduction in motivation and adherence, alongside a decrease in self-confidence. Coping models may therefore provide greater benefit following injury.

Coping models. Whereas mastery models are good for assisting in physical skill development, coping models have the advantage in promoting psychological changes and emotional regulation. When attempting to guide athletes through the struggles of pain and distress management after a significant injury, it can be helpful to refer to peers who have encountered similar difficulties en route to successful recoveries.

Maddison and colleagues (2006) examined the effect of peer modeling on perceptions of preoperative anxiety and pain, as well as postoperative self-efficacy and functional outcomes, in a sample of 58 patients undergoing anterior cruciate ligament (ACL) reconstruction. The investigators developed two coping model videos for this study. Video 1 addressed the preoperative period through two weeks post-surgery and video 2 dealt with the period between two and six weeks post-surgery. Both videos depicted time-matched rehabilitation exercises and edited interviews, and models were matched by gender and age to the study participants. Compared to those in the control condition, patients who watched

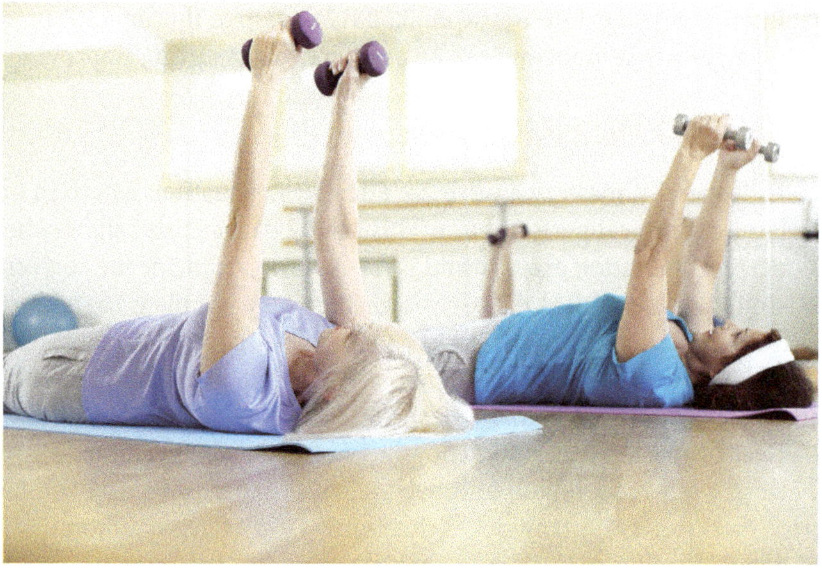

the modeling videos reported significantly lower perceptions of expected pain before surgery and significantly greater self-efficacy for walking and using crutches after surgery; however, the intervention had no effect on anxiety. Intervention patients also demonstrated significantly better objective functional outcome scores compared to controls (Maddison, Prapavessis, & Clatworthy, 2006).

Similarly, Flint (1999) conducted interviews with athletes recovering from ACL injuries. After viewing several coping model videos, these individuals supported the idea that peer modeling can bolster self-confidence in coping ability during the recovery process. Using these models may be particularly effective when they are time-matched to specific recovery periods or milestones. There is also qualitative evidence that athletes use observational learning to understand the norms of sport groups to which they are affiliated (Law, 2008). By extension, it is possible that injured athletes might use peer coping models to establish the range of typical responses to various rehabilitation obstacles, although this has yet to be empirically demonstrated.

Formal versus informal models. In the rehabilitation setting, both formal and informal models may be useful. Informal modeling occurs frequently within the context of the clinic, as therapists may point out other individuals with the same injury who are successfully progressing through treatment. This type of modeling may also occur during return to sport, where coaches or team trainers may identify a previously injured athlete to act as an example for others (Flint, 1999). In most cases, informal models fall under the coping domain, and can serve a motivational function.

When the modeling process is formalized, it allows for the standardization and control of the content that is being delivered. Models can thus provide specific behavioral demonstrations and verbal cues that are designed to effect particular changes (Flint, 1999). For research purposes, and when offering modeling as part of a larger rehabilitation program, structured interventions are critical.

Who Should Model?

Because recovery is impacted by numerous personal factors, including physiological, psychological, and situational characteristics, self-modeling can be a powerful tool during rehabilitation. Previously injured athletes tend to exhibit greater perceived self-efficacy during treatment (Shaffer, 1991), largely because they can draw on their prior experiences. This is especially useful for re-injury situations, when athletes can view themselves as both mastery models (i.e., while performing exercises) and coping models (i.e., when overcoming setbacks), as needed. In such cases, modeling may be conducted through various media, including videos, diaries, mental imagery, and guided interviews.

As one of the only available frames of reference for first-time injured athletes, peer modeling provides meaningful information about rehabilitation skills, as well as possible approaches to dealing with stressors that arise through the phases of recovery. As with any peer modeling scenario, it is important that injured athletes are matched as closely as possible with models who are similar in gender, age, sport played, competitive level, injury type, and injury severity. It may also be helpful to match based on the type of therapeutic intervention required, so that the model can address salient issues that accompany specific treatments. Importantly, the benefits of peer modeling are not restricted to those who have never been injured before. Although previously injured athletes will have developed some of the necessary skills for successful recovery, they may be asked to perform novel exercises or encounter setbacks that are unfamiliar. A peer model may therefore be useful for aiding the athlete through these challenges.

Sometimes a peer model can be identified from the athlete's own team. By using a previously injured teammate as the comparator, it is possible to also account for factors that are unique to the athlete's playing environment, such as competitive schedules, team dynamics, and coaching. Athletes may identify better with models whom they know personally, as there is an inherent level of trust that will lend credibility to the model's assessment of given rehabilitation situations. When feasible, this can be a particularly good approach to modeling for children and young adolescents. There is considerable evidence that younger individuals tend to rely on parents and classmates for information regarding physical competence (Weiss, 2003; Horn, 2004; Smith, 2003), so familiar models are likely more meaningful to these athletes. Conversely, older adolescents and adults are more likely to use self-referenced sources of competence information (i.e., self-improvement) (Weiss, 2003; Horn, 2004; Smith, 2003), suggesting that self-modeling may be more appropriate in these age groups.

There is also a belief that the use of multiple, diverse models can improve the learning of new behaviors (Flint, 1999). In this modeling strategy, several individuals who differ in terms of physical characteristics and physical attributes demonstrate the target behavior. It is hoped that the injured athlete will bond with one or more of the models, eliciting a motivational effect whereby the athlete will want to "be like" one of the models (Flint, 1999).

When Should They Model?

Although no research has directly investigated *when* modeling should occur, it is reasonable to suggest that it can play a role at all stages of recovery, from initial diagnosis through return to play. As we have seen in sport and exercise settings, modeling appears to be effective when employed before the athlete attempts a new behavior, as well as during the attempt. This pattern is likely to hold in rehabilitation as well.

While considering the timing of modeling interventions, we must also ask how frequently modeling should be used. There have been a limited number of studies in this area, but the effectiveness of self-selected viewing frequencies is promising (Wrisberg & Pein, 2002; Wulf et al., 2005). Presenting models through video therefore holds an advantage over live modeling, as it allows athletes to review the session as needed.

Modeling and Adherence

There is a paucity of information concerning the relationship between modeling and adherence to rehabilitation. It has been suggested that peer modeling can improve adherence, but this has not yet been empirically investigated (Fisher, 1990; Weiss & Troxel, 1986). Based on the motivational effects of modeling, it is reasonable to hypothesize that coping models would be capable of influencing treatment adherence, but future studies will be required to address this issue.

Modeling and Return to Play

There is also limited information about the effects of modeling during the return to play period. The transition back into sport can be difficult for many athletes, as they may not be confident in their health or their abilities, and re-injury fear can emerge. A model who has successfully returned to play can be a valuable source of motivation for these athletes, and can help to provide strategies for coping with competitive anxiety and negative emotional responses during this time.

How Is It Measured?

Just as in sport and exercise, the three basic outcomes that can be measured in rehabilitation modeling interventions are motor behavior, cognitions, and affect. In this context, motor behavior can be assessed by measuring movement dynamics, (e.g., the quality and coordination of movements). Cognitions and affect can be measured using questionnaires that specifically target aspects of treatment, such as patient satisfaction, pain, or health-related quality of life. Indexes of anxiety and self-efficacy have also been used (Maddison et al., 2006).

Special Considerations in Injury Rehabilitation

The biggest concern for athletes following injury is whether or not they will successfully recover. Although models can provide information about the correct performance of motor skills and what to expect from different kinds of treatment, their most important role is to show the injured athlete that it is possible to get through treatment and return to a state of health. We do not yet know the ideal combination of mastery and coping modeling to attain this outcome, and it may vary from athlete to athlete, but it should always be the primary goal of any modeling intervention in this setting.

It is essential that the model strike a balance between the amount of detailed information provided to the athlete, and the amount of emotional support given. To illustrate, overwhelming an athlete with details before going in for surgery can actually create a fear response, and the athlete may consequently feel an insurmountable loss of control over the situation (Flint, 1999). This may have the undesired effect of undermining the athlete's self-confidence, which will negatively impact rehabilitation outcomes. Models are a key component of enhancing self-efficacy, which may be best achieved through providing enough details to ensure accurate expectations alongside vicarious learning from a similar other who has already been through the process (Bandura, 1986; Flint, 1999; Weiss & Troxel, 1986).

Some General Recommendations

When using modeling during rehabilitation, it is important to account for the experience and age of the injured athlete. For example, those who have a history of injury may require different modeling content than those who have no previous rehabilitation experience. When dealing with youth athletes, we must also consider that younger children may require more instruction along with observational learning than adults do. Additionally, children often have difficulty processing concurrent verbal and visual cueing, so instruction should be given prior to or after a behavioral demonstration (Ste. Marie, Clark, & Latimer, 2002).

Some additional factors to consider are:

- Verbal cues generally influence the qualitative aspects of performance, but not the quantitative aspects, so they are unlikely to affect adherence (McCullagh, Stiehl, & Weiss, 1990; Weiss, Ebbeck, & Rose, 1992).
- Visual modeling supported by imagery rehearsal can enhance learning, and may help to facilitate recovery (Gray, 1990; Onestak, 1997).

CHAPTER SUMMARY

Modeling is a useful intervention in a number of settings, including sport, exercise, and injury rehabilitation. It serves functions of skill and strategy acquisition, motivation, and performance enhancement, and can be used by practitioners to improve motor, cognitive, and affective outcomes. Although there is little research to guide when a model should demonstrate, or who that model should be, substantial evidence suggests that both peer modeling and self-modeling strategies can be effective when used to augment learning objectives.

This chapter has highlighted the disparity in modeling research between the domains of sport, exercise, and injury rehabilitation. Using the Applied model proposed by Ste-Marie et al. (2012) as a foundation, we see that both coping and mastery models have been used to improve motor skill development and self-regulatory variables in sport, whereas models in exercise are primarily used only for the performance function. In injury rehabilitation, there has been little research into the effects of modeling, despite its intuitive benefit for patients. Considering the successful use of observational learning in many educational settings, the value of modeling as a psychological intervention cannot be ignored; however, much research is needed to determine the optimal type, timing, and methods of delivery in sport and recreation contexts.

REVIEW QUESTIONS

1. Give the reasons *why* learners engage in modeling that were identified by Cumming et al. (2005).
2. What is the difference between a coping model and a mastery model?
3. When Ste-Marie and colleagues (2012) summarized the intervention research investigating the effectiveness of skill-based modeling experiences on motor skill learning, what did they conclude?
4. What are the main findings from research that has assessed the effects of modeling interventions on changes in psychological variables in sport?
5. Outline how the effects of modeling interventions are measured in sport.
6. Why might peer modeling work to encourage exercise behavior?
7. Discuss a situation where exercise modeling may have negative or undesirable consequences for the observer.
8. What is the difference between informal and formal modeling?
9. How can coping models help an athlete during the beginning, middle, and end stages of rehabilitation?

SUGGESTED READINGS

Clark, S. E., & Ste-Marie, D. M. (2007). The impact of self-as-a-model interventions on children's self-regulation of learning and swimming performance. *Journal of Sports Sciences, 25*, 577–586.

Flint, F. A. (1999). Seeing helps believing: Modeling in injury rehabilitation. In D. Pargman (Ed.), *Psychological bases of sport injuries* (3rd ed., pp. 221–234). Morgantown, WV: Fitness Information Technology.

Maddison, R., Prapavessis, H., Armstrong, G. P., & Hill, C. (2008). A modeling intervention in heart failure. *Annals of Behavioral Medicine, 36*, 64–69.

Maddison, R., Prapavessis, H., & Clatworthy, M. (2006). Modeling and rehabilitation following anterior cruciate ligament reconstruction. *Annals of Behavioral Medicine, 31*(1), 89–98.

Ste-Marie, D. M., Law, B., Rymal, A. M., O, J., Hall, C., & McCullagh, P. (2012). Observational interventions for motor skill learning and performance: An applied model for the use of observation. *International Review of Sport and Exercise Psychology, 5*, 145–176. doi:10.1080/1750984x.2012.665076

REFERENCES

Ashford, D., Bennett, S. J., & Davids, K. (2006). Observational modeling effects for movement dynamics and movement outcome measures across differing task constraints: A meta-analysis. *Journal of Motor Behavior, 38*, 185–205.

Bandura, A. (1986). *Social foundations of thought and action: A social cognitive theory.* Englewood Cliffs, NJ: Prentice-Hall.

Barzouka, K., Bergeles, N., & Hatziharistos, D. (2007). Effect of simultaneous model observation and self-modeling of volleyball skill acquisition. *Perceptual & Motor Skills, 104*, 32–42.

Berry, T. R., McLeod, N. C., Pankratow, M., & Walker, J. (2013). Effects of *Biggest Loser* exercise depictions on exercise-related attitudes. *American Journal of Health Behavior, 37*, 96–103.

Bray, S. R., Gyurcsik, N. C., Culos-Reed, S. N., Dawson, K. A., & Martin, K. A. (2001). An exploratory investigation of the relationship between proxy efficacy, self-efficacy and exercise attendance. *Journal of Health Psychology, 6*, 425–434.

Chiviacowsky, S., & Wulf, G. (2002). Self-controlled feedback: Does it enhance learning because performers get feedback when they need it? *Research Quarterly for Exercise and Sport, 73*, 408–415.

Clark, S. E., & Ste-Marie, D. M. (2002). Peer mastery versus peer coping models: Model type has differential effects on psychological and physical performance measures. *Journal of Human Movement Studies, 43*, 179–196.

Clark, S. E., & Ste-Marie, D. M. (2007). The impact of self-as-a-model interventions on children's self-regulation of learning and swimming performance. *Journal of Sports Sciences, 25*, 577–586.

Crozier, S. A. (2012). The effect of trainer muscularity and expertise on self-presentational concerns, body image, and performance in college men during one-repetition maximum testing (Master's thesis). Brock University, St. Catharines, Canada.

Cumming, J., Clark, S. E., Ste-Marie, D. M., McCullagh, P., & Hall, C. (2005). The functions of observational learning questionnaire (FOLQ). *Psychology of sport and exercise, 6*, 517–537.

Dowrick, P. W., & Dove, C. (1980). The use of self-modeling to improve the swimming performance of spina bifida children. *Journal of Applied Behavior Analysis,* 13, 51–56.

Dowrick, P. W., & Raeburn, J. M. (1995). Self-modeling: Rapid skill training for children with physical disabilities. *Journal of Developmental and Physical Disabilities, 7*, 25–37.

Emmen, H. H., Wesseling, L. G., Bootsma, R. J., Whiting, H. T. A., & Van Wieringen, P. C. W. (1985). The effect of video-modelling and video-feedback on the learning of the tennis service by novices. *Journal of Sports Sciences, 3*, 127–138.

Fisher, A. C. (1990). Adherence to sports injury rehabilitation programmes. *Sports Medicine, 9*, 151–158.

Fleming, J. C., & Martin Ginis, K. A. (2004). The effects of commercial exercise video models on women's self-presentational efficacy and exercise task self-efficacy. *Journal of Applied Sport Psychology, 16*, 92–102.

Flint, F. A. (1999). Seeing helps believing: Modeling in injury rehabilitation. In D. Pargman (Ed.), *Psychological bases of sport injuries* (3rd ed., pp. 221–234). Morgantown, WV: Fitness Information Technology.

Fox, J., & Bailenson, J. N. (2009). Virtual self-modeling: The effects of vicarious reinforcement and identification on exercise behaviors. *Media Psychology, 12*, 1–25.

Franklin, B. A. (1988). Program factors that influence adherence. In R. K. Dishman (Ed.), *Exercise adherence: Its impact on public health* (pp. 237–258). Champaign, IL: Human Kinetics.

Granados, C., & Wulf, G. (2007). Enhancing motor learning through dyad practice: Contributions of observation and dialogue. *Research Quarterly for Exercise & Sport, 78*, 197–203.

Gray, S. W. (1990). Effect of visuo-motor rehearsal with videotaped modeling on racquetball performance of beginning players. *Perceptual & Motor Skills, 70*, 379–385.

Gustafson, S. L., & Rhodes, R. E. (2006). Parental correlates of physical activity in children and early adolescents. *Sports Medicine, 36*, 79–97.

Hall, C. R., Munroe-Chandler, K. J., Cumming, J., Law, B., Ramsey, R., & Murphy, L. (2009). Imagery and observational learning use and their relationship to sport confidence. *Journal of Sports Sciences, 27*(4), 327–337.

Hall, E. G., & Erffmeyer, E. S. (1983). The effect of visuo-motor behavior rehearsal with videotape modeling on free throw accuracy of intercollegiate female basketball players. *Journal of Sport Psychology, 5*, 343–346.

Hancock, D. J., Rymal, A. M., & Ste-Marie, D. M. (2011). A triadic comparison of the use of observational learning amongst team sport athletes, coaches, and officials. *Psychology of Sport and Exercise, 12*, 236–241.

Heil, J. (1993). Psychology of sport injury. Champaign, IL: Human Kinetics Publishers.

Horn, T. S. (2004) Developmental perspectives on self-perceptions in children and adolescents. In: M. R. Weiss (Ed.), *Developmental sport and exercise psychology: A lifespan perspective.* Morgantown, WV: Fitness Information Technology.

Katula, J. A., & McAuley, E. (2001). The mirror does not lie: Acute exercise and self-efficacy. *International Journal of Behavioral Medicine, 8*, 319–326.

Kitsantas, A., Zimmerman, B., & Cleary, T. (2000). The role of observation and emulation in the development of athletic self-regulation. *Journal of Educational Psychology, 92*, 811–817.

Law, B. (2008). A description of athletes' observational learning use in sport (Unpublished doctoral dissertation). The University of Western Ontario, London, ON.

Law, B., & Hall, C. (2009). Observational learning use and self-efficacy beliefs in adult sport novices. *Psychology of Sport and Exercise, 10*(2), 263–270.

Maddison, R., Prapavessis, H., Armstrong, G. P., & Hill, C. (2008). A modeling intervention in heart failure. *Annals of Behavioral Medicine, 36*, 64–69.

Maddison, R., Prapavessis, H., & Clatworthy, M. (2006). Modeling and rehabilitation following anterior cruciate ligament reconstruction. *Annals of Behavioral Medicine, 31*(1), 89–98.

Martin Ginis, K. A., Jung, M. E., & Gauvin, L. (2003). To see or not to see: Effects of exercising in mirrored environments on sedentary women's feeling states and self-efficacy. *Health Psychology, 22*, 354–361.

McCullagh, P., & Meyer, K. (1997). Learning versus correct models: Influence of model type on the learning of a free-weight squat lift. *Research Quarterly for Exercise & Sport, 68*, 56–61.

McCullagh, P., Stiehl, J., & Weiss, M. (1990). Developmental modeling effects on the quantitative and qualitative aspects of motor performance. *Research Quarterly for Exercise & Sport, 61*, 344–350.

Meaney, K., Griffin, L. K., & Hart, M. (2005). The effect of model similarity on girls' motor performance. *Journal of Teaching in Physical Education, 24*, 165–178.

Ng, J. Y. Y., Tam, S. F., Yew, W. W., & Lam, W. K. (1999). Effects of video modeling on self-efficacy and exercise performance of COPD patients. *Social Behavior and Personality, 27,* 475–486.

Onate, J. A., Guskiewic, K. M., Marshall, S. W., Giuliani, C., Yu, B., & Garrett, W. E. (2005). Instruction of jump-landing technique using videotape feedback altering lower extremity motion patterns. *American Journal of Sports Medicine, 33*, 831–842.

Onestak, D. M. (1997). The effect of visuo-motor behaviour rehearsal (VMBR) and videotaped modeling (VM) on the free-throw performance of intercollegiate athletes. *Journal of Sport Behaviour, 20,* 185–198.

Shaffer S. M. (1991). Attributions and self-efficacy as predictors of rehabilitative success (Masters thesis). University of Illinois: Champaign-Urbana.

Smith, A. L. (2003). Peer relationships in physical activity contexts: a road less traveled in youth sport and exercise psychology research. *Psychology of Sport and Exercise, 4,* 25–39.

Spink, K. S., & Carron, A. V. (1992). Group cohesion and adherence in exercise classes. *Journal of Sport & Exercise Psychology, 14,* 78–86.

Spink, K. S., & Carron, A. V. (1994). Group cohesion effects in exercise classes. *Small Group Research, 25,* 26–42.

Starek, J., & McCullagh, P. (1999). The effect of self-modeling on the performance of beginner swimmers. *The Sport Psychologist, 13*, 269–287.

Ste-Marie, D. M., Clark, S. E., & Latimer, A. E. (2002). Contributions of attention and retention processes in the observational learning of a motor skill by children. *Journal of Human Movement Studies, 42,* 317–333.

Ste-Marie, D. M., Law, B., Rymal, A. M., O, J., Hall, C., & McCullagh, P. (2012). Observational interventions for motor skill learning and performance: An applied model for the use of observation. *International Review of Sport and Exercise Psychology, 5,* 145–176. doi:10.1080/1750984x.2012.665076

Van Wieringen, P. C. W., Emmen, H. H., Bootsma, R. J., Hoogesteger, M., & Whiting, H. T. A. (1989). The effect of video-feedback on the learning of the tennis service by intermediate players. *Journal of Sports Sciences, 7*, 153–162.

Voorhees, C. C., Murray, D., Welk, G., Birnbaum, A., Ribisl, K. M., Johnson, C. C., Allor Pfeiffer, K., Saksvig, B., & Jobe, J. B. (2005). The role of peer social network factors and physical activity in adolescent girls. *American Journal of Health Behavior, 29,* 183–190.

Weiss, M. R. (2003). Psychological aspects of sport-injury rehabilitation: a developmental perspective. *Journal of Athletic Training, 38*(2), 172–175.

Weiss, M. R., Ebbeck, V., & Rose, D. (1992). 'Show and tell' in the gymnasium revisited: Developmental differences in modeling and verbal rehearsal effects on motor skill learning and performance. *Research Quarterly for Exercise & Sport, 63,* 292–301.

Weiss, M. R, & Troxel R. K. (1986). Psychology of the injured athlete. *Athletic Training, 21,* 105–109.

Wesch, N. N., Law, B., & Hall, C. R. (2007). The use of observational learning by athletes. *Journal of Sport Behavior, 30*, 219–231.

Williams, A. M., Davids, K., & Williams, J. G. (1999). *Visual action and perception in sport.* New York, NY: Routledge.

Worsley, A. (1989). Perceived reliability of sources of health information. *Health Education Research, 4,* 367–376.

Wrisberg, C. A., & Pein, R. L. (2002). Note on learners' control of frequency of model presentation during skill acquisition. *Perceptual & Motor Skills, 94,* 792–794.

Wulf, G., Raupach, M., & Pfeiffer, F. (2005). Self-controlled observational practice enhances learning. *Research Quarterly for Exercise & Sport, 76*, 107–111.

Zetou, E., Fragouli, M., & Tzetzis, G. (1999). The influence of star and self modeling on volleyball skill acquisition. *Journal of Human Movement Studies, 37*, 127–143.

Chapter 5

Goal Setting

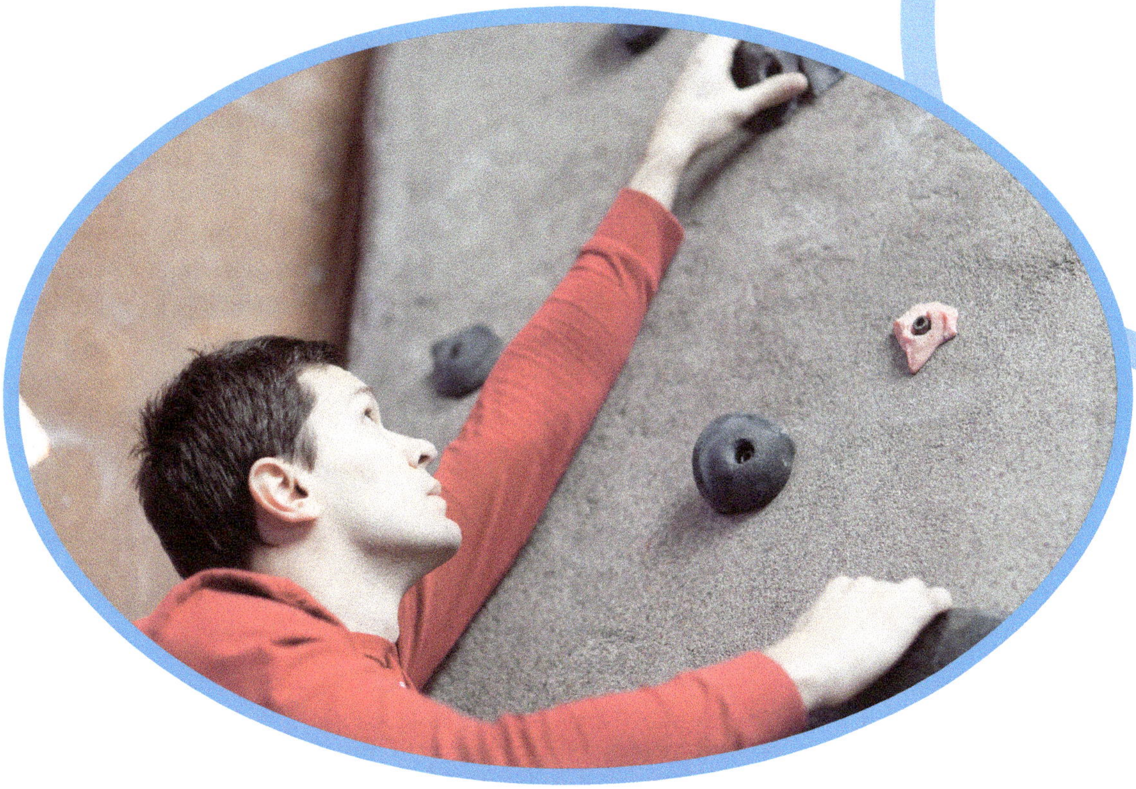

Introduction

A goal can be defined as "that which one wants to accomplish; it concerns a valued, future end state" (Lee, Locke, & Latham, 1989, p. 299). Thus, because a goal represents a valued objective to individuals, goal setting should act as an incentive toward behavior change. Goal setting has been a topic of interest in psychology for decades and has been examined in many domains including business, education, and sport. Locke, Shaw, Saari, and Latham (1981), after reviewing the literature concluded that "the beneficial effect of goal setting on task performance is one of the most replicable findings in the psychology literature" (p. 145).

There are three types of goals that individuals can set. ***Outcome goals*** focus on social comparison and standards of success, such as receiving a bonus for being the most productive stock trader. Thus, outcome goals are often dependent on the ability and performance of others. ***Performance goals*** focus on improving and attaining personal performance standards with an example being increasing your own sales from last year. Finally, ***process goals*** focus on specific procedures an individual wants to improve (e.g., spend more time studying). Research suggests that all three types of goals should be included when developing a goal-setting program (Filby, Maynard, & Graydon, 1999).

Goals must be specific, challenging, and proximal in order to provide effective motivation for individuals to change their behavior (Bandura, 1997). The acronym SMART has been recommended to help individuals remember five important guidelines for effective goal setting (Weinberg & Gould, 2003). Goals should be specific, measurable, adjustable, realistic, and timely. These five guidelines are described in Table 5–1. With respect to setting challenging goals, they encourage you to stretch a little farther, and accomplish more. Keep in mind, however, that goals need to be realistic—the only thing worse than a goal that is not challenging enough is one that proves to be too challenging. The element of proximity is especially important and refers to increasing the temporal nearness of a goal to increase motivation (Latham & Seijts, 1999). One approach is reducing large, distant goals into smaller sub-goals that are more easily achieved and through which the larger goal can be attained. Reducing large goals into proximal sub-goals is frequently encouraged and has been suggested as a means of assisting individuals in achieving their ultimate objectives (Steel & Konig, 2006).

TABLE 5–1 Setting SMART Goals

Specific	Set a goal that is specific (e.g., increase free throw shooting in basketball percentage by 5%) rather than vague (e.g., to improve).
Measurable	Be sure you can measure your goal in order to assess progress.
Adjustable	Adjust your goal if necessary (i.e., if progressing faster or slower than expected).
Realistic	Set a goal that is moderately difficult. If a goal is too easy, it is of little value. If a goal is too difficult, it may lead to a decrease in confidence or even abandoning the goal.
Timely	Identify a point in time at which the goal is to be achieved, thereby increasing motivation.

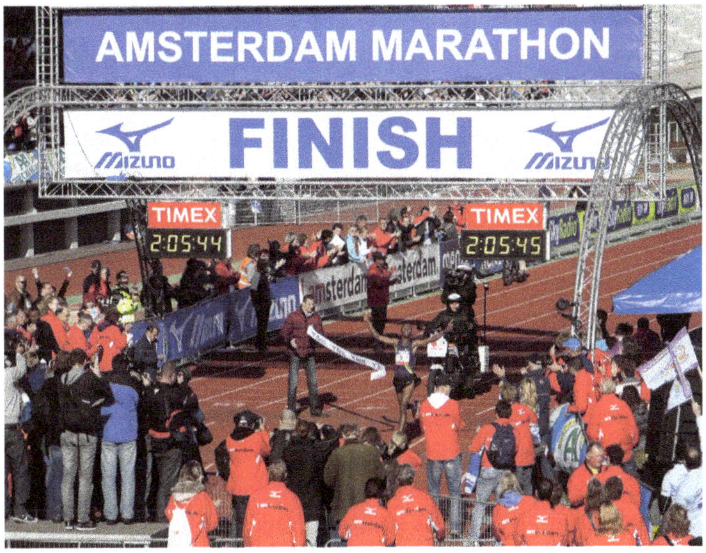

Image © Gertan, 2014. Used under license from Shutterstock, Inc.

Why is goal setting effective? Researchers argue there are four main reasons why goal setting works:

1. It directs action by focusing attention
2. It increases effort and intensity
3. It encourages persistence in the face of adversity or failure
4. It promotes the development of new task or problem solving strategies

Goal Setting in Sport

In 1989, Gould, Tammen, Murphy, and May suggested that goal setting was the most commonly used performance enhancement strategy in sport psychology and this is probably still true today. Interestingly, most athletes rate their goals as being only moderately effective in enhancing sport performance (Burton, Naylor, & Holliday, 2001). This may be due to athletes being uncertain about how to effectively set goals, and as a result they do not think that goal setting works that well. Various reviews (e.g., Kyllo & Landers, 1995) have concluded that goal setting in sport is indeed effective and that moderately difficult goals are best. Burton et al. (2001) noted that 78% of sport and exercise studies have shown moderate-to-strong effects on behavior.

Burton et al. (2001) proposed that goals likely serve different functions in training versus competition, thus suggesting the types of goals set in these situations must be different. They proposed that enhanced learning is usually the primary focus in practice situations, whereas performing optimally or outperforming one's opponent is the main focus in competitive situations. Because practice situations generally foster minimal evaluation and social comparison as compared to competition, the function of practice goals may be on skill development/improvement, as opposed to arousal goals and mental toughness goals, which may be more prominent in competition. Given this rationale, Munroe-Chandler, Hall, and Weinberg (2004) proposed that athletes would set primarily learning oriented goals in practice and execution oriented goals in competition. Athletes (N = 249, representing 18 different sports) were asked about the goals they set in both training and competition. Some support for this hypothesis was found as athletes reported setting more improvement-oriented goals for both skills and strategies in training than in competition. However, the frequency with which they set execution-oriented goals for skills was actually higher in training than in competition. Therefore, their results only provided partial support for the proposal by Burton et al. (2001) that in practice, athletes set goals that tend to focus on learning, whereas in competition they set goals that tend to focus on execution.

Individual Goal-Setting Interventions

Goal-setting interventions targeting individual athletes have been conducted in a variety of sports. A good example is the research by Mellalieu, Hanton, and O'Brien (2006) in which goal setting effects on selected performance behaviors of five male collegiate rugby players were measured over an entire competitive season. The players were between 21 and 24 years of age, were all starting players on a team competing in the National Collegiate Rugby Union Championships, and all had a minimum of 10 years playing experience. Five performance behaviors were assessed. *Number of ball carries* was employed to determine the frequency with which a player attempted to gain yardage with the ball carried in hand. *Number of tackles* (either *made* or *missed*) was used to measure the player's success or failure in preventing an opponent from carrying the ball. A *successful kick* was defined as a kick out of hand from a player with the aim of successfully putting the ball out of the field of play. Finally, *number of turnovers won* was used to measure the frequency with which a player managed to steal possession of the ball from the opposing team.

The intervention consisted of three stages: goal determination, goal setting, and goal reviewing. In the goal-determination stage, each participant selected one of the five behaviors for improvement (e.g., tackles made). The frequency of each participant-selected performance behavior was then recorded for the first half of the competitive season. At the midseason break, the goal-setting took place. Based on the mean values for each participant's performance from the first half of the season, a series of numerical values (goals) for the targeted performance was generated for the second half of the season. In the goal-reviewing stage, the researcher met individually with the players 48 hours before each match in the second half of the season and reviewed their numerical scores for the target behaviors.

The intervention proved to be effective. For all participants, post intervention performance showed a desired change in behavior. More specifically, player 1 demonstrated a 77% increase in ball carries per game. Participant 2 exhibited an increase of 32% for the number of tackles made, while player 3 demonstrated a desirable decrease of 55% in tackles missed. Player 4 showed a 26% increase for successful kicks, and finally participant 5 demonstrated a 118% increase in turnovers won. The researchers concluded that their results support previous research and show that goal-setting interventions can be effective for the enhancement of specific performance behaviors in rugby players.

Team Goal-Setting Interventions

Goal-setting interventions focused on the team have not been researched to the same extent as interventions for individual athletes. Team goal setting extends individual goal setting in that it also attempts to foster respect and cohesiveness among the team members, while helping the team with its focus and direction. It has been argued that team goals without accompanying individual goals may reduce performance by prompting social loafing (Burton & Weiss, 2008). Social loafing is a phenomenon in which people working together on a task tend to exert less individual effort than when they perform the same task alone.

A study by Senécal, Loughead, and Bloom (2008) is an example of a team goal-setting intervention. The purpose of this research was to determine if a season-long team goal-setting intervention influenced team cohesion. The participants were 86 female high school senior basketball players from 8 teams. Four teams were randomly assigned to a goal-setting condition and the remaining four teams to a control condition. For the teams in the goal-setting condition, a three stage protocol for implementing a team goal-setting program originally proposed by Eys, Patterson, Loughead, and Carron (2006) was employed and is outlined in Table 5–2. The goal-setting sessions took place before a practice in the team's facility and took 20–30 minutes to complete. Similar to the players in the intervention, the players in the control condition were asked to complete a measure of cohesion before the start of the season and after the season ended. However, they received no additional information.

TABLE 5–2 An Overview of the Team Goal Setting Program

Principle	Implementation Strategy
Selecting the team goals	1. Players are provided with a list of performance indices (e.g., turnovers, steals, blocked shots, free throw shooting percentage). 2. From the list, each player independently identifies the four most important indices to establish for team goals. 3. Subunits of five players agree on the four most important performance indices that should be set for team goals. 4. The team as a whole then agrees on the four performance indices for which the team goals will be set.
Establishing the target	1. Each player independently identifies the target levels for each of the four team goals. 2. Subunits of five players agree on the target levels. 3. The team as a whole agrees on the target levels.
Coaches remind players of the team's goals	The goals are posted in the team's locker room.
Evaluation, feedback, and reevaluation are essential	The sport psychology consultant meets with the team to review and discuss the team's goals after each block of three games. Modifications to the team's goals or target levels are made if deemed necessary.

It was found that although players in both conditions reported similar levels of team cohesion prior to the intervention, following the season-long intervention the goal-setting players were significantly higher in cohesion than the control participants. This finding was a result of the control players experiencing a decrease in cohesion while the players in the goal-setting condition maintained their levels of cohesion over the course of the season. It was concluded that team goal-setting interventions are effective for influencing cohesiveness in sports teams.

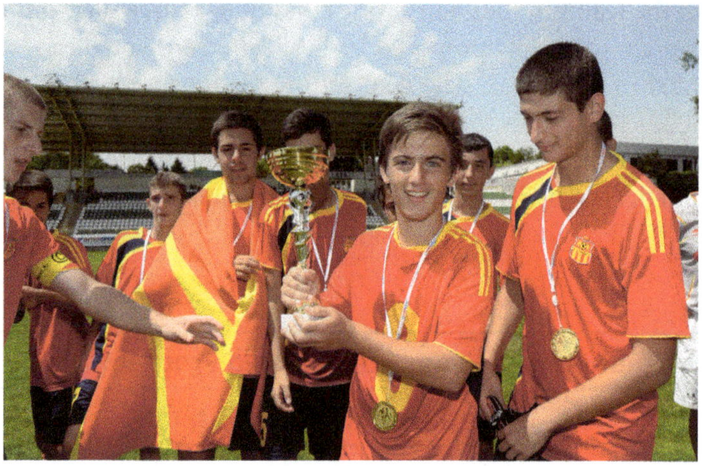

Measurement of Goal Setting in Sport

If athletes are to set measurable, quantifiable goals, they need to determine what these goals should be and what are their current performance standards (i.e., how they presently perform with respect to each target goal). One possible approach to obtain this information is to use performance profiling (Butler & Hardy, 1992). The traditional performance profiling procedure follows three simple steps. In the first step, a completed performance profile, either in the form of a circular target or column chart, is presented to the athlete to reinforce the basic procedure and to emphasize what will be gained from the process. An example of a completed performance profile is presented in Figure 5–1. Step two involves the generation of qualities that underpin athletic performance in the sport in question. This is accomplished by having the athlete answer the following question: 'What in your opinion are the qualities or characteristics of an elite athlete in your sport?' (Butler & Hardy, 1992, p. 256). The athlete generates a list of qualities across technical, physical, psychological, and tactical attributes.

The third step entails the athlete's self-assessment of their ability in each of the chosen performance attributes. Athletes typically rate their current perception of their ability in each quality via a scale of 1 ('lowest possible ability') to 10 ('ideal level of performance'). Other rating scales can be employed, but the key issues are that the scale is meaningful to the athlete, the athlete has a good understanding for what constitutes a 1 and a 10 rating, and that the rating scales are clear and specific. The resultant completed profile provides a useful visual display as to the athlete's perceived strengths and weaknesses, from which goals can be set around the athlete's weaknesses.

FIGURE 5–1 Psychological Performance Profile Including Self and Coach Assessments

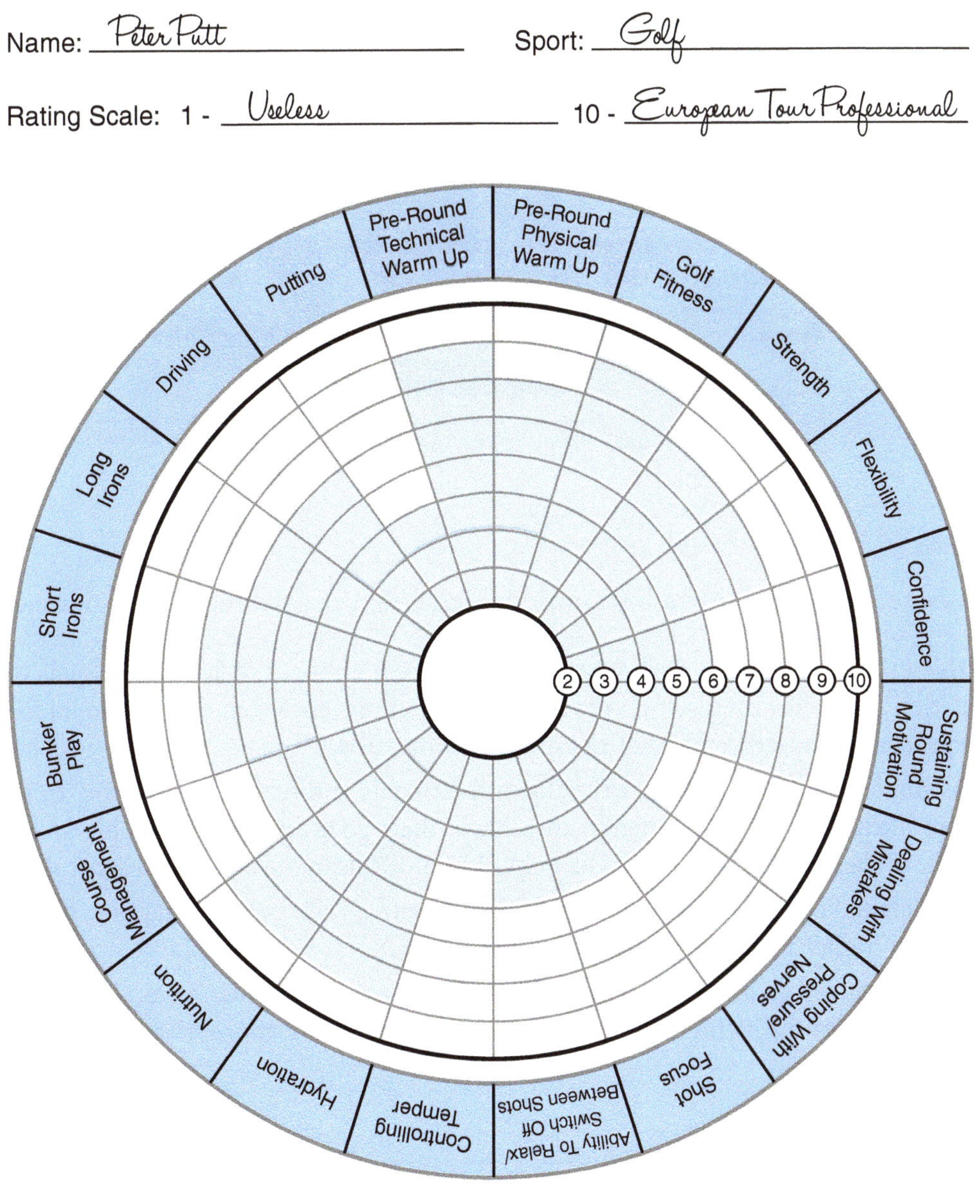

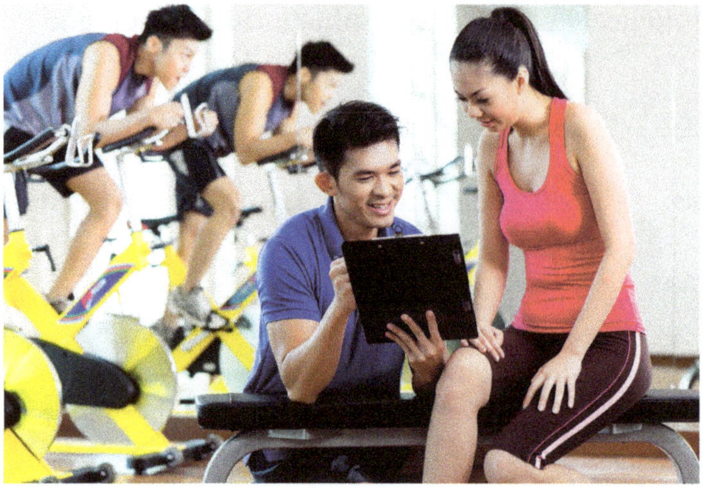

Some General Recommendations

Some general recommendations for both individual and team goal-setting interventions are:

- Athletes should set goals for both practice and competition. Often athletes focus only on competition goals; however, setting practice goals is important when one considers the time spent in practice compared with the time spent in competition.
- It is important for athletes to write down their goals and make them public. In doing so, it is more likely that they will attempt to achieve their goals, given that people around them are aware of their objectives and can be helpful in motivating the athletes to accomplish them.
- Goals should be stated positively, rather than negatively: "I want to run the best 100-metre time possible" rather than "I don't want to come in last in the 100-metre."
- Progress toward goal achievement should be reviewed on a regular basis. Conducting this regular review allows athletes to identify whether their goals are appropriate.

Goal Setting in Exercise

For many decades goal setting has been a frequently-used tool in health education programs (Strecher et al., 1995). More recently, research regarding the effectiveness of goal setting in exercise promotion has begun to expand rapidly. Overall, researchers have found goal-setting interventions to be effective for increasing exercise behavior in the general population as well as in many clinical populations (e.g., Kyllo & Landers, 1995; Pearson, 2012; Shilts, Horowitz, & Townsend, 2004; Strecher et al., 1995; Weinberg, 1994). It is not surprising that goal-setting interventions are effective for promotion of exercise given that goal setting works by directing attention, effort, and motivation toward the task and that lack of effort and motivation are significant barriers to regular exercise. Indeed, exercise participants often report having some type of goal regarding the level of exercise participation to which they aspire (Poag-

DuCharme & Brawley, 1994). Additionally, frequent exercisers value their exercise-related goals and spend more time pursuing them compared to less frequent exercisers (Jung & Brawley, 2010).

Properties of Goals in Exercise

As we identified in the introduction, goals should be specific, challenging, and proximal (Bandura, 1997). With respect to specificity, a review of goal-setting interventions to encourage physical activity and healthy eating in community-based samples of individuals with overweight or obesity identified that most interventions involve specific goals exclusively, or a combination of general and specific goals. Although early lab-based studies failed to provide evidence for the goal difficulty-performance relationship in physical activity settings (e.g., Weinberg, Bruya, Garland, & Jackson, 1990; Weinberg, Bruya, Jackson, & Garland, 1987), more recent studies of goal setting for health behavior change (including exercise and healthy eating) have shown that people do perform better when their goals are more challenging (e.g., Shilts et al., 2004; Strecher et al., 1995). For example, Jeffery, Wing, Sherwood, and Tate (2003) randomly assigned 202 overweight men and women to a standard behavior therapy treatment for obesity with either a standard exercise goal or a high exercise goal. At 6-, 12-, and 18-month assessments, the group assigned to the high exercise goals reported engaging in more physical activity than the group assigned to the standard exercise goals. It should be noted, however, that setting goals that are too complex can undermine self-efficacy for a given behavior and impair subsequent task performance (Strecher et al., 1995). Therefore, the best exercise goals are challenging yet attainable (Shilts et al., 2004).

Goals can focus on either short-term or long-term processes or outcomes. In general, short-term goals are encouraged because they provide people with immediate cues to action whereas long-term goals allow people to procrastinate in their efforts toward goal achievement. Indeed, researchers have shown that people who set a short-term goal are more likely to succeed in a task compared to people who set a long-term goal (Bodenheimer & Handley, 2009). In the exercise domain, however, empirical tests of short- versus long-term goals have been inconclusive (Dubbert & Wilson, 1984; Martin, Dubbert, Katell, et al., 1984). Although short-term goals allow people to immediately organize and enable their aspirations and skills, long-term goals may be helpful in helping people focus on the bigger picture and stay motivated to continue pursuing short-term goals after each successive accomplishment. Thus, researchers have suggested that setting a series of short-term goals that will lead to the accomplishment of a longer-term goal can be effective for encouraging exercise behavior (Kyllo & Landers, 1995).

Content of Goals in Exercise

It has been said that "all goals are not created equal" (Ryan, Sheldon, Kasser, & Deci, 1996, p. 7). That is, the content of goals can vary, and the foci of different goals may result in substantially different affective, cognitive, or behavioral outcomes (Vanseenkiste, Lens, & Deci, 2006). A considerable amount of the literature regarding goal content is grounded in self-determination theory (SDT: Deci & Ryan, 2000). According to this theory, goal content may be intrinsic or extrinsic in nature. Intrinsic goals are focused on internal indicators such as developing personal interests and values and are inherently satisfying to pursue. Extrinsic goals are focused on the pursuit of external worth such as wealth, fame, and material possessions. In the exercise domain, intrinsic goals are related to health management, skill development, and social affiliation whereas extrinsic goals are related to image improvement and social recognition (Sebire, Standage, & Vansteenkiste, 2008).

With respect to the pursuit of general life goals, intrinsic goals tend to be positively associated with well-being (e.g., satisfaction, vitality) and negatively associated with ill-being (e.g., depression), whereas extrinsic goals tend to have the opposite associations (Kasser, 2002; Vansteenkiste, Neyrinck, Niemiec, Soenens, De Witte, & Van den Broeck, 2007; Vansteenkiste, Soenens, & Duriez, 2008). A similar pattern of findings emerges with respect to intrinsic and extrinsic exercise goals. Specifically, intrinsic exercise goals are positively associated with exercise class attendance and workout enjoyment (Ryan et al., 1996), behavioral persistence (Vansteenkiste, Simons, Soenens, & Lens, 2004), and self-determined motivation (Gillison, Standage, & Skevington, 2006), and are negatively associated with social physique anxiety (Crawford & Eklund, 1994). In contrast, extrinsic goals are positively related to indices of ill-being (Maltby & Day, 2001), social physique anxiety (Crawford & Eklund, 1994) and negatively related to self-esteem (Maltby & Day, 2001), attendance at exercise sessions, exercise adherence, enjoyment (Ryan et al., 1996), and self-determined motivation (Gillison et al., 2006).

How Goal Setting Works in Exercise

As you learned in the introduction to this chapter, goal setting works by (a) focusing attention on a given task, (b) providing impetus to increase effort and intensity, (c) encouraging persistence, and (d) promoting the development of strategies for problem solving related to the target behavior. Self-efficacy, a person's confidence that he or she can execute the necessary steps to obtain a desired outcome, plays an important role in translating personal goals into effort expenditure, perseverance, and behavior (Bandura, 1989; 1997). In the exercise domain, researchers have demonstrated that goal efficacy (i.e., the degree to which a person is confident in his or her ability to meet a goal) is positively related to perceptions of goal achievement. Poag and McAuley (1992) demonstrated that people who were more confident in their ability to meet their exercise goals at the outset of an 8–10 week exercise program perceived themselves as more successful in obtaining those goals at the end of the program. Self-efficacy has also been identified as a mediator of the influence of personal goal setting on behavior. Dawson and Brawley (2000) demonstrated that when people rate their exercise goals as influential, those goals impact their self-efficacy to engage in exercise and, in turn, that self-efficacy leads to more frequent exercise participation.

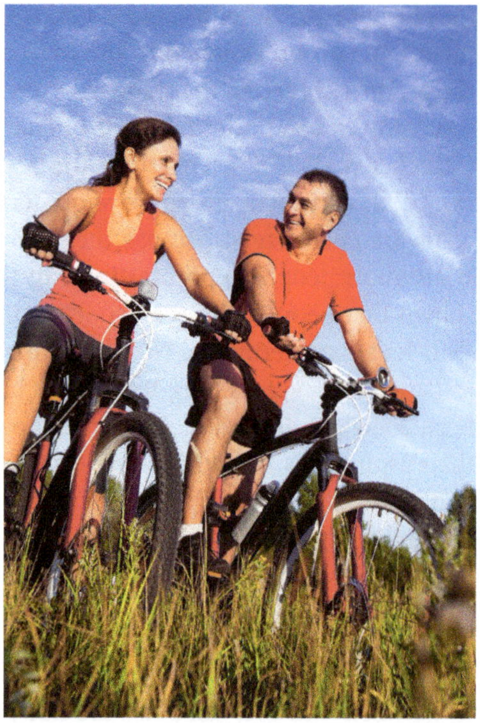

Image © YanLev, 2014. Used under license from Shutterstock, Inc.

Components of Goals in Exercise

Feedback. Among the strongest findings in the goal-setting literature is the importance of providing feedback (Strecher et al., 1995). Receiving feedback allows goal setters to determine their progress, adjust their effort, and stay motivated to achieve their goals. Goal setting and feedback have a reciprocal relationship in which setting a goal provides a context in which to acquire and understand feedback and, in turn, that feedback can be used to revive motivation toward the goal or to adjust the goal to make it more or less challenging, as necessary.

In the exercise domain there are numerous sources of feedback. Personal sources of feedback can be achieved through self-monitoring of physiological, affective, and emotional states as well as behavior. Personal feedback can be achieved simply through self-reflection or more deliberately by using tools such as exercise logs, pedometers, and weight scales. Interpersonal feedback can be achieved through praise, support, encouragement, reinforcing messages, discussions and problem solving, and the provision of information. As technology evolves, opportunities to derive both personal and interpersonal feedback through technological means are becoming increasingly prevalent. For example, there are numerous mobile telephone applications that allow people to use GPS technology to map their walks or jogs, or to use social-networking websites to post details of their workouts, allowing friends to comment.

Feedback can be provided in reference to one's self (i.e., whether one is doing better, worse, or the same as a previous performance or whether one is making good progress toward a personal goal) or in reference to others (i.e., whether one is doing better, worse, or the same as others). With respect to feedback in reference to others, Bandura and Jourden (1991) demonstrated that when people are told they are making better progress than others they report higher levels of self-efficacy, more satisfaction with their performance, and better actual performance, and they subsequently set more challenging goals. In contrast, when people are told they are doing worse than others, they report lower levels of self-efficacy, less satisfaction with their performance, and poorer actual performance, and they subsequently set less challenging goals.

Rewards. Synonymous with achieving a goal is the acquisition of some type of reward. Rewards can be either internal (e.g., feelings of pride or satisfaction) or external (e.g., recognition, money, etc.). Rewards can serve as a motivating factor in the pursuit of goals. Research examining the impact of adding reward schemes to goal-setting interventions for physical activity and health behavior change has been equivocal (Locke & Latham, 2002; Shilts et al., 2004; Strecher et al., 1995). A review of goal-setting interventions to increase physical activity and healthy eating among overweight and obese community-based samples demonstrated that very few interventions included rewards as an intervention component. Indeed, attaching external rewards to goals can be detrimental because it may lead to a decrease in self-efficacy and subsequent performance if the goal is not reached and the reward is not obtained. Additionally, in "the real world" external rewards for exercise and health behavior change may not be in place; thus, providing external rewards in such interventions may set people up for failure (i.e., relapse) if they have come to expect external rewards for their behavior and they are no longer available when the intervention is complete.

Acquisition of Goals in Exercise

One factor that may impact how successfully a goal can be obtained is who sets the goal. Goals that are designed and chosen by the participant are called self-set goals. People may be more likely to be committed and motivated to achieving a self-set goal because the parameters of the goal can be tailored to meet the specific needs and desires of the individual. Self-set goals can be problematic, however, in cases where the individual is relatively unfamiliar with the behavioral domain in which they are setting a goal and thus "off base" in terms of what kind of goal would be realistic. Goals can also be assigned or prescribed, which means that they are designed and chosen for the individual by someone else, usually a practitioner with expertise in the behavioral domain. In contrast to self-set goals, assigned goals are likely to be realistic but may not have as much buy-in from the individual. Collaborative goals are those that are designed and chosen by the individual and a practitioner, collectively. Finally, group-set goals are designed and chosen by a group of individuals. With group-set goals, the attainment of the goal depends on the collective outcomes of all of the group members. Research on goal acquisition in the organizational psychology domain has found that task performance remains relatively constant regardless of whether goals are self-set or assigned. This finding does not seem to hold in the health behavior literature. With respect to goals for exercise and other health behaviors, there is increasing evidence that self- and collaboratively set goals are better than assigned goals (Estabrooks, Nelson, Xu, King, Bayliss, Gaglio, et al., 2005).

Concurrent Management of Exercise and Other Goals

Although exercise is important for many people, family, work, friends, and other recreational or creative pursuits are also important priorities for most people. Most studies of goal-directed behavior focus on different types of goals independently; however, in the real world we pursue many goals simultaneously (Jung & Brawley, 2010). Understanding how exercise goals can be either conflicting or congruent with our other life goals may help to determine how we design and select goals in each of these areas.

It has been suggested that exercise goals may be inhibited by the pursuit of non-exercise goals (Jung & Brawley, 2010). For example, in a cross-sectional study, Gebhardt and Maes (1998) asked 980 people of varying exercise levels to indicate the degree to which their exercise goal conflicted with 16 other personal goals. Sedentary participants anticipated that exercise goals would interfere with their other goals significantly more than frequent exercisers (i.e., participants who exercised more than three times per week). In another study, undergraduate students were asked to identify both an exercise goal and the life goal that most interfered with that exercise goal. The findings revealed that regular exercisers maintained an equivalent focus on both goals whereas irregular exercisers valued, monitored, planned, socially compared, and self-rewarded their progress toward their interfering goal more than their exercise goal (Karoly, Ruehlman, Okun, Lutz, Newton, & Fairholme, 2005).

More recently, researchers have deviated from the notion that "other" goals must be in conflict with exercise goals and instead have begun to test the idea that exercise and other goals might be mutually facilitative. For example, in a 5-month study of exercise behavior, Riediger and Freund (2004) showed that the degree to which participants indicated that their concurrent (one exercise and three non-exercise) goals facilitated one another at month 1 predicted the amount of exercise they did at months 4 and 5. Additionally, Jung and Brawley (2010) reported that frequent exercisers have higher levels of self-regulatory efficacy to manage concurrent, highly-valued goals, have greater persistence to achieve exercise and non-exercise goals, and perceived the pursuit of concurrent goals more positively than less frequent exercisers.

Tools for Goal Setting in Exercise

Although laboratory research on goal setting examines goal-setting interventions in isolation, in the real world, goal-setting interventions are rarely, if ever, conducted in the absence of some other intervention component. A recent review of goal-setting interventions for weight-loss behaviors (including physical activity and healthy eating) identified a number of other tools that are frequently offered in combination with goal setting. Self-monitoring in forms such as diaries, scales, contracts, action plans, and exercise logs, is a common addition to goal-setting interventions. Educational resources outlining benefits, recommendations, tips, and problem-solving strategies are also common additions to goal-setting interventions. Again, recent technological advancements such as apps for mobile telephones are allowing these additional goal-setting tools to be easily accessible to exercisers on a day-to-day basis.

Some General Recommendations

Based on the goal-setting research in exercise, some general recommendations can be put forth.

- Ensure that exercise goals are challenging enough to increase effort, motivation, and persistence but not so complex that failure to achieve them is likely.
- Set specific exercise goals, rather than general, "do your best" goals, to ensure that actionable steps and indicators of progress are established within the goal.
- Avoid extrinsic goals and goals that provide external reward, when possible.
- Goal setting for exercise is more effective when it is combined with other behavioral or motivational tools such as educational resources or self-monitoring.

Goal Setting in Injury Rehabilitation

Rehabilitation presents a number of challenges to injured athletes, often leaving them with a sense of low personal control over their recovery (Kobasa, Maddi, & Kahn, 1982). To alleviate this feeling, research has shown that coping strategies aimed at both problem solving and affective regulation are more helpful than emotion-focused coping alone (Wiese & Weiss, 1987). Goal setting can facilitate both problem solving and affective regulation and is therefore one of the most common approaches to maintaining positive affect through the rehabilitation process (Cupal, 1998).

Although it seems obvious that return to sport is the ultimate objective of many rehabilitation programs, a single long-term goal is often insufficient to keep an athlete motivated during a protracted recovery period. A structured program of both short- and long-term goals is therefore necessary for facilitating a successful return to sport.

Setting Short-Term and Long-Term Goals

Just as short- and long-term goals can be effective for improving sport performance, they can also be extremely beneficial during rehabilitation. Particularly for severely injured athletes who have weeks or months of therapy ahead of them, return to play can seem like a distant and overwhelming prospect. It is helpful to complement this long-term goal with short-term functional goals that the athlete can work toward on a daily basis (Worrell, 1992). The achievement of short-term goals provides positive reinforcement that recovery is progressing, which gives the athlete a sense of control and a more positive outlook on his or her situation (Worrell, 1992). The importance of setting realistic, achievable, short-term goals has therefore been advocated by athletic trainers and therapists (Wiese, Weiss, & Yukelson, 1991), as well as athletes (Ievleva & Orlick, 1991).

Regularly reaching small goals can enhance motivation to keep pushing through difficult stretches of treatment, and can maintain the athlete's drive to ultimately return to competition. As Evans and Hardy (2002b) reported, athletes may feel as though they have little to focus on while they are not able to compete. For example, one athlete in their study stated:

> "I haven't had anything to train for so I haven't trained as much as perhaps I should have..."
>
> **(injured athlete; Evans & Hardy, 2002b)**

Goals can provide meaningful objectives for athletes to focus on, and there is evidence that setting short-term (even daily) goals facilitates recovery.

It is important that short-term goals include a variety of process and performance objectives (Evans, Hardy, & Fleming, 2000). Early in rehabilitation, process goals may be more salient as athletes work on executing specific movements, such as range of motion or basic mobility exercises. Later in the program, performance goals may be set to reflect milestones like achieving a given strength level or running for a length of time on a treadmill. Regardless of the goal type, however, it is essential that the goal-setting program itself be flexible (Evans et al., 2000). Athletes may experience setbacks during rehabilitation, and not all athletes will recover at the same rate. Some individuals will therefore require a greater emphasis on process goals early on, whereas others may begin meeting performance goals much sooner. It may also be necessary to set additional intermediate process goals if an athlete is struggling to reach

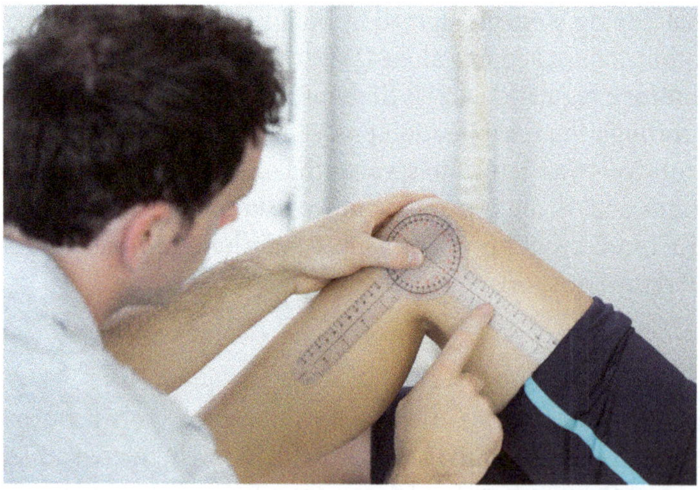

a set performance goal. The athlete and his or her therapist must work together to evaluate treatment progress, and may have to negotiate changes in the types of goals set, and the timing of those goals, in order for the athlete to be successful (Sanderson, 1996).

How Goal Setting Works in Injury Rehabilitation

Goal setting is most effective when it is conducted using a systematic approach (Wayda, Armenth-Brothers, & Boyce, 1998). By setting a series of short-term goals that all contribute to a larger, long-term goal, the process is broken into manageable steps. It is essential that athletes take a leading role in selecting the goals to be set, in order to ensure that they are meaningful (Danish, Petitpas, & Hale, 1992); however, this approach may result in more goals being set, but not necessarily being achieved (Dalton, Farrell, De Souza, Wujanto, McKenna-Slade, Thompson, et al., 2011). Under ideal conditions, goals also have the effect of holding athletes accountable for their effort, which is crucial during rehabilitation.

Researchers have proposed a number of potential mechanisms through which goal setting might improve rehabilitation outcomes, including reducing anxiety, increasing focus, promoting greater perceptions of control, and fostering more positive outcome attributions (i.e., athletes attribute progress to their own effort, rather than external factors; Danish et al., 1992; Evans & Hardy, 2002b; Gilbourne & Taylor, 1998; Wayda et al., 1998). There is also some evidence that achieving one goal leads to the setting of more difficult goals, which in turn leads to measurable progress in rehabilitation (Evans & Hardy, 2002b). Additionally, Gilbourne and Taylor (1998) have suggested that goal setting can encourage stronger task orientation, or give athletes a "mastery" experience. It is believed that the resulting boost to self-confidence has a positive impact on motivation and, consequently, rehabilitation progress.

Goal setting may also improve performance during rehabilitation. Theodorakis and colleagues investigated the relationship between goal setting and knee extension strength in a sample of 92 university-aged female athletes (Theodorakis, Malliou, Papaioannou, Beneca, & Filactakidou, 1996). Participants were divided into three groups, including one experimental group of 32 knee injured women (Group 1), one experimental group of 29 healthy women (Group 2), and one control group of 30 healthy women (Group 3). All three groups performed four trials of a knee extension task on an isokinetic dynamometer. The two experimental groups (Groups 1 and 2) set personal performance goals between trials 2 and 3. Based on feedback they received after trial 3, they set another performance goal before completing trial 4. The study showed that both goal-setting groups performed better on trials 3 and 4 compared to the control group, and there was a significant correlation between performance, self-efficacy, and self-satisfaction. It is believed that greater self-efficacy likely prompts individuals to set higher personal goals, which are associated with improved performance. Goal setting combined with strategies that encourage self-efficacy may therefore help athletes decrease recovery time (Theodorakis et al., 1996).

There is some evidence that goal setting can help to speed up recovery following sport injury (Ievleva & Orlick, 1991), although it may be most useful when combined with other interventions. Johnson (2000) conducted a trial comparing injured athletes who received a combination psychological intervention (consisting of stress management, relaxation/guided imagery, and goal-setting) to injured athletes in a control group. The study demonstrated that those in the intervention group had a significant improvement in overall mood at the midpoint and end of rehabilitation, and also felt more prepared to return to competition than the control athletes. There was, however, no effect of the goal-setting component on its own, suggesting that optimal benefit may be achieved using a multimodal approach.

Social support can have a major influence on injury rehabilitation, and much of that support comes from the athlete's therapist or trainer. Receiving feedback from these individuals regarding progress toward set goals, or even the process of setting goals together, can help to mitigate the negative effects of setbacks during treatment (Evans & Hardy, 2002b). Social support networks, including coaches, teammates, family, and friends can also be instrumental in helping the athlete meet his or her goals through the provision of feedback and encouragement. The key to a successful goal-setting program is to ensure that the individuals around the athlete are committed to facilitating his or her goal achievement (Wade, 1998).

Goal Setting and Adherence

Although there is limited evidence to suggest that goal setting increases rehabilitation adherence in the broader acquired disability literature (Levack, Taylor, Siegert, & Dean, 2006), researchers have found that goal setting is quite effective at improving adherence to sport injury therapy (Duda, Smart, & Tappe, 1989; Evans & Hardy, 2002b). Evans and Hardy (2002a) investigated the effect of a goal-setting intervention on rehabilitation adherence among 77 injured athletes and found that goal setting significantly improved adherence and increased self-efficacy for rehabilitation. The authors suggested that enhanced self-efficacy may prompt athletes to invest greater effort and perseverance in the face of rehabilitation obstacles, therefore leading to greater adherence. This explanation is consistent with Self-Efficacy Theory (Bandura, 1977), and is a possible mechanism through which goal setting acts on adherence, although another similar study found no significant difference in self-efficacy between a goal-setting intervention group and a control group (Theodorakis et al., 1996).

There is a prevailing belief in the rehabilitation community that goal setting is a successful strategy for improving adherence. Fisher and colleagues examined the beliefs of 187 Certified Athletic Trainers regarding factors that influence adherence to sport injury rehabilitation programs (Fisher, Mullins, & Frye, 1993). Approximately 32% of their respondents indicated that goal setting was a valuable tool for boosting adherence, particularly because it can help athletes to see the immediate results of their efforts. Athletes have reported that short-term goal setting in particular can maintain their motivation to stick with their treatment plan (Evans & Hardy, 2002b), lending support to the regular use of goal setting in the rehabilitation setting:

> "...you need to feel you are achieving something. If my goal initially had been to get back on a tennis court and play match tennis, I think I would have been knocked back so many times, because it's such a long-term goal."
>
> **(injured athlete; Evans & Hardy, 2002b).**

Goal Setting and Return to Play

When athletes are preparing to return to sport following an injury, goal setting is a fundamental and intuitive strategy for helping them transition from recovery to performance (Podlog & Dionigi, 2010). Return to sport goals should not be made only at the end of treatment; Johnson (1997) found that athletes who ultimately did not return to sport following injury had fewer "comeback" goals throughout the rehabilitation process than did successfully-returning athletes. It is therefore important to set a long-term return to sport goal early during rehabilitation, complemented by shorter-term performance goals at the end of treatment.

Coaches often use goal setting as a "road map" to guide training and to motivate their athletes to prepare for competition. They can apply similar techniques to facilitate an injured player's return to sport. Using in-depth interviews with eight Australian high-performance coaches, Podlog and Dionigi (2010) found that coaches recognize goal setting as the most important strategy that they can use to help injured players transition back into competition. Coaches in the study reported that, for them, goal setting was an ongoing and adjustable process, with an emphasis on process goals as athletes get back to their training schedules at the end of rehabilitation. Although not all coaches view post-injury goal setting as one of their ordinary responsibilities, their participation in the process can be a major influence on successful return to sport. Coaches and athletes should set process and performance goals together, and continue to evaluate progress until the athlete has fully recovered and has reached desired performance levels.

Perceptions About Goal Setting in Injury Rehabilitation

Of all the psychological interventions that can be incorporated into an injury rehabilitation program, goal setting is the most widely accepted and most frequently used. There is a prevailing opinion amongst therapists and athletic trainers that goal setting is an important part of their skill set, and should be taught as part of their certification curriculum (Gordon, Potter, & Ford, 1998; Wiese et al., 1991). Even though not all therapists have formal psychological skills training, many of them set goals with their patients as part of their everyday clinical practice because it is an effective way to monitor progress and keep athletes motivated through treatment.

Goal setting has been accepted in injury rehabilitation settings to the extent that it is now included in clinical guidelines. For example, a recent consensus statement regarding the treatment of neurological conditions indicated that goal setting is a core component of rehabilitation, and should be part of standard patient care (Playford, Siegert, Levack, & Freeman, 2009). Although the authors acknowledge that medical professionals should not simply prescribe goals, they suggest that patients and therapists can negotiate goals that are both medically achievable and a good fit for the patient's personal priorities.

There is also widespread acceptance of goal setting amongst athletes of all abilities. Brewer et al. (1994) administered a questionnaire to 161 healthy college students who participated in a variety of sports, ranging from recreational to varsity levels (Brewer, Jeffers, Petitpas, & van Raalte, 1994). Participants were asked to indicate their preference for goal setting, guided imagery, or traditional counseling as an adjunct to physiotherapy, supposing they were ever injured. Overall, participants preferred goal setting, although the preference was stronger for females compared to males. The second stage of the study included 20 injured athletes who were given introductory sessions in goal setting, guided imagery, and traditional counseling as part of their rehabilitation program. After trying each of the interventions, the athletes again indicated a preference for goal setting. Because of this level of acceptance, goal setting is an easy way for therapists to actively involve athletes in making decisions about the direction their therapy program will take.

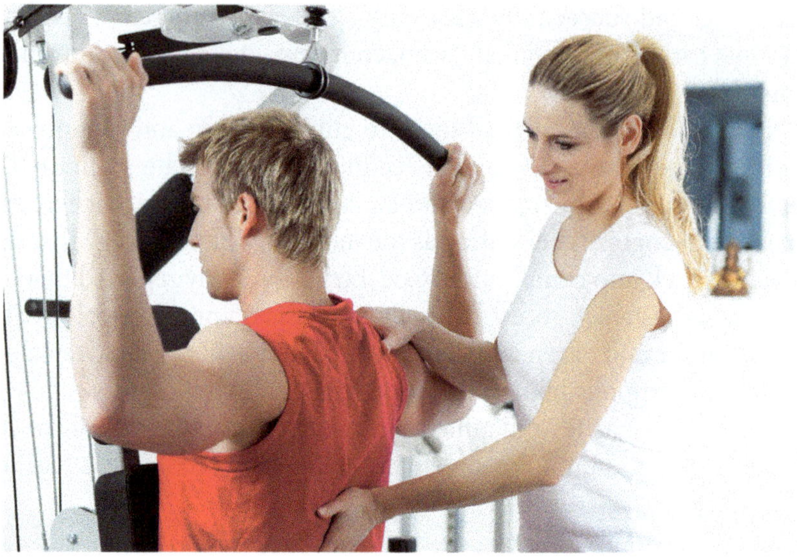

Image © Kzenon, 2014. Used under license from Shutterstock, Inc.

Special Considerations for Goal Setting in Injury Rehabilitation

Using the goal-setting paradigm proposed by Wayda and colleagues (1998), athletes and therapists should follow a three-step process (see Figure 5–2; Wayda et al., 1998). The first step is the *planning phase*, which occurs immediately after the athlete is injured. During this phase, it is important to identify what the expectations are in terms of recovery timelines, rehabilitation milestones, and the ultimate outcome desired by the athlete (i.e., return to sport or simply a return to a healthy state). It is important for the medical team to draw on their clinical expertise to make sure that the athlete has realistic expectations, but also for the athlete to communicate his or her priorities to the therapist. During the planning process, athletes and therapists should also decide together how they will set goals, what their achievement strategy will be, and how they will measure progress. It is crucial that goals are meaningful to both the athlete and the therapist to ensure maximum success.

FIGURE 5–2 Implementation of a Goal-Setting Program

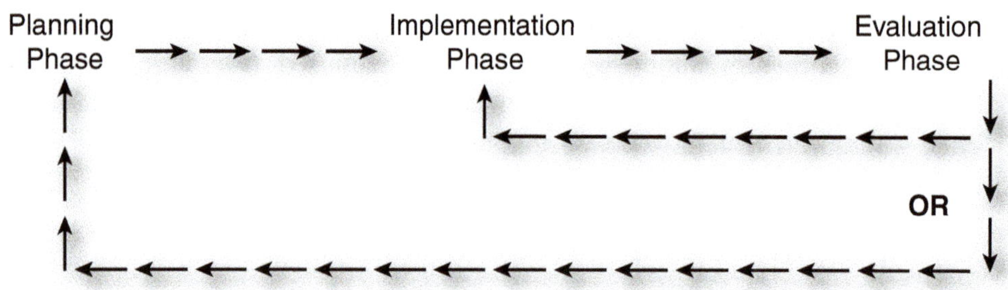

Adapted from Boyce & King, 1993

The second step is the *implementation phase*, during which goals are monitored as the athlete undergoes treatment. Both the athlete and therapist are responsible for supporting the achievement of set goals during this phase. Therapists should make a commitment to facilitating the athlete's success through the design of the rehabilitation program, and athletes must ensure that they invest the effort and time required to achieve the desired outcome.

Finally, the *evaluation phase* consists of measuring progress toward set goals, and the provision of feedback regarding successes and setbacks. If goals have been reached, it is important to set new, perhaps more challenging goals to ensure continued motivation through the rehabilitation process. Goals that are not successfully met should be re-evaluated, and either the timeline for those goals should be altered, or new goals should be set in their place.

It is not only goal achievement that should be evaluated, but also the process of working toward the goals. Feedback about unsuccessful aspects of the rehabilitation program or the goal-setting process itself can be equally beneficial, particularly when recovery is occurring slower than expected or when setting new, more challenging goals.

How Goal Setting Is Measured in Injury Rehabilitation

In rehabilitation settings, there is increasing use of goal attainment scaling as a means of measuring goal achievement (Malec, 1999). This process directs the setting, monitoring, and measurement of goals, and yields scores on a 5-point scale. The "expected" level of achievement is typically designated as a numerical value of 0, and outcomes are defined as: "much less than expected" (–2), "less than expected" (–1), "better than expected" (+1) and "much better than expected" (+2). For example, the measurement of a rehabilitation goal may be evaluated as follows:

Goal: I am able to exercise on a stationary cycle ergometer.

+2	I am able to cycle for 60 minutes at 80% maximum heart rate.
+1	I am able to cycle for 45 minutes at 60–80% maximum heart rate.
0	I am able to cycle for 30 minutes at 60–80% maximum heart rate.
–1	I am able to cycle for 20 minutes at 60–80% maximum heart rate.
–2	I am able to cycle for 15 minutes at 60% maximum heart rate.

Some General Recommendations

Goal setting is one of the first things that should happen in the rehabilitation process. Before therapy begins, the athlete should discuss his or her expectations with the therapist to ensure that they are realistic and achievable. Both parties should then set a combination of short- and long-term goals that are congruent with anticipated rehabilitation milestones. These goals should be put in writing, along with a plan for when and how to evaluate progress. Some other recommendations for goal-setting interventions are:

- Goals should be framed positively to ensure the greatest chance of success (Danish et al., 1992).
- Goals should be matched with specific range of motion, strength, endurance, or cardiovascular fitness processes and outcomes that the athlete is expected to achieve during rehabilitation (Sanderson, 1996).
- Goal setting can impact the relationship between athlete and therapist, which can ultimately affect treatment outcomes. It is therefore important that both parties approach goal setting as a collaborative process (Playford et al., 2009).
- Keeping coaches informed of the athlete's goals and their progress toward those goals can help foster reasonable expectations about the timing of return to play. Coaches can then provide the necessary support for athletes during recovery and can help set performance goals as the player returns to competition (Podlog & Dionigi, 2010).

CHAPTER SUMMARY

Goal setting is a common and effective strategy for improving performance and changing behavior in sport, exercise, and rehabilitation settings. Goal setting impacts behavior because it (a) focuses the goal setter's attention on the desired task, (b) increases the goal setter's effort toward achieving the desired outcome, (c) encourages the goal setter to persist when faced with barriers to achieving the desired outcome, and (d) stimulates the goal setter to strategize and problem-solve in the face of challenges to achieving the desired outcome. Commitment to achieving the goal is an important factor in the effectiveness of goal setting.

Overall, research in all three of these settings supports the suggestion that goal setters should set long-term goals to facilitate motivation over the long term but that short-term goals are essential for ensuring progress toward those long-term goals. In the context of sport, where athletes must perform in both practice and competitive environments, distinct goals can be set for each environment. Across the domains of sport, exercise, and rehabilitation researchers have also demonstrated that for optimal performance/behavioral outcomes, goals should be challenging enough that they inspire motivation but not so challenging that the goal setter comes to believe that attainment of the goal is impossible.

There are special considerations that should be made when setting goals in the domains of sport, exercise, and rehabilitation. In the context of sports teams, setting both team and individual goals can assist in improving overall performance. In exercise settings, care should be taken to set intrinsic, rather than extrinsic goals. In the context of rehabilitation, goal setting should align with the phase of the rehabilitation program.

REVIEW QUESTIONS

1. Why is goal setting effective?
2. How does team goal setting extend individual goal setting?
3. Discuss how performance profiles help athletes set goals.

4. Discuss the relationships between goal setting and self-efficacy in the exercise domain.
5. What are the advantages and disadvantages of attaching external rewards to the accomplishment of exercise goals?
6. Provide an example of when exercise goals should be:
   a. Self-set
   b. Assigned
   c. Collaboratively-set
   d. Group-set
7. What are the benefits of short- and long-term goals during injury rehabilitation?
8. Describe the three-step goal-setting process proposed by Wayda et al. (1998).

SUGGESTED READINGS

Evans, L., & Hardy, L. (2002). Injury rehabilitation: A goal-setting intervention study. *Research Quarterly for Exercise and Sport, 73*, 310–319.

Gilbourne, D., & Taylor, A. H. (1998). From theory to practice: The integration of goal perspective theory and life development approaches within an injury-specific goal-setting program. *Journal of Applied Sport Psychology*, 10, 124–139.

Mellalieu, S. D., Hanton, S., & O'Brien, M. (2006). The effects of goal setting on rugby performance. *Journal of Applied Behavior Analysis, 39*, 257–261.

Strecher, V. J., Seijts, G. H., Kok, G. J., Latham, G. P., Glasgow, R., DeVellis, B., Meertens, R. M., & Bulger, D. W. (1995). Goal setting as a strategy for health behavior change. *Health Education Quarterly, 22*, 190–200.

REFERENCES

Bandura, A. (1977). Self-efficacy: Toward a unifying theory of behavioral change. *Psychological Review, 84*, 191–215.

Bandura, A. (1989). Human agency in social cognitive theory. *American Psychologist, 44*, 1175–1184.

Bandura, A. (1997). *Self-efficacy: The exercise of control.* New York, NY: W. H. Freeman.

Bandura, A. & Jourden, F. (1991). Self-regulatory mechanisms governing the impact of social comparison on complex decision making. *Journal of Personality and Social Psychology, 60*, 941–951.

Bodenheimer, T., & Handley, M. A. (2009). Goal setting for behavior change in primary care: An exploration and status report. *Patient Education Counseling, 76*, 174–180.

Boyce, B. A., & King, V. (1993). Goal-setting strategies for coaches. *Journal of Physical Education, Recreation and Dance, 63*, 65–68.

Brewer, B. W., Jeffers, K. E., Petitpas, A. J., & van Raalte, J. L. (1994). Perceptions of psychological interventions in the context of sport injury rehabilitation. *The Sport Psychologist, 8*, 176–188.

Burton, D., Naylor, S., & Holliday, B. (2001). Goal setting in sport: Investigating the goal effectiveness paradigm. In R. N. Singer, H. A. Hausenblas, & C. M. Janelle (Eds.), *Handbook of sport psychology*, (2nd ed., pp. 497–528). New York: Wiley.

Burton, D., & Weiss, C. (2008). The fundamental goal concept: The path to process and performance success. In T. S. Horn (Ed.), *Advances in sport psychology, 3rd edition* (pp. 339–376). Champaign, IL: Human Kinetics.

Butler, R. J., & Hardy, L. (1992). The performance profile: Theory and application. *The Sport Psychologist, 6*, 253–264.

Crawford, S., & Eklund, R. C. (1994). Social physique anxiety, reasons for exercise, and attitudes toward exercise settings. *Journal of Sport & Exercise Psychology, 16*, 70–82.

Cupal, D. D. (1998). Psychological interventions in sport injury prevention and rehabilitation. *Journal of Applied Sport Psychology, 10*, 103–123.

Dalton, C., Farrell, R., De Souza, A., Wujanto, E., McKenna-Slade, A., Thompson, S., et al. (2011). Patient inclusion in goal setting during early inpatient rehabilitation after acquired brain injury. *Clinical Rehabilitation, 26*, 165–173.

Danish, S. J., Petitpas, A. J., & Hale, B. D. (1992). A developmental-educational intervention model of sport psychology. *The Sport Psychologist, 6*, 403–415.

Dawson, K. A., & Brawley, L. R. (2000). Examining the relationship between exercise goals, self-efficacy, and overt behavior with beginning exercisers. *Journal of Applied Social Psychology, 30*, 315–329.

Deci, E. L., & Ryan, R. M. (2000). The "what" and "why" of goal pursuits: Human needs and the self-determination of behavior. *Psychological Inquiry, 11*, 227–268.

Dubbert, P. M., & Wilson, G. (1984). Goal-setting and spouse involvement in the treatment of obesity. *Behavioral Research and Therapy, 22*, 227–242.

Duda, J. L., Smart, A. E., & Tappe, M. K. (1989). Predictors of adherence in the rehabilitation of athletic injuries: An application of personal investment theory. *Journal of Sport & Exercise Psychology, 11*, 367–381.

Estabrooks, P. A, Nelson, C. C., Xu, S., King, D., Bayliss, E. A., Gaglio, B., et al. (2005). The frequency and behavioral outcomes of goal choices in the self-management of diabetes. *Diabetes Education, 31*, 391–400.

Evans, L., & Hardy, L. (2002a). Injury rehabilitation: A goal-setting intervention study. *Research Quarterly for Exercise and Sport, 73*, 310–319.

Evans, L., & Hardy, L. (2002b). Injury rehabilitation: A qualitative follow-up study. *Research Quarterly for Exercise and Sport, 73*, 320–329.

Evans, L., Hardy, L., & Fleming, S. (2000). Interventions strategies with injured athletes: An action research study. *The Sport Psychologist, 14*, 188–206.

Eys, M. A., Patterson, M. M., Loughead, T. M., & Carron, A. V. (2006). Team building in sport. In J. Duda, D. Hackfort, & J. Ridor (Eds.), *Handbook of research in applied sport psychology: International perspectives* (pp. 219–231). Morgantown, WV: Fitness Information Technology.

Filby, W., Maynard, I., & Graydon, J. (1999). The effect of multiple-goal strategies on performance outcomes in training and competition. *Journal of Applied Sport Psychology, 11*, 230–246.

Fisher, A. C., Mullins, S. A., & Frye, P. A. (1993). Athletic trainers' attitudes and judgments of injured athlete's rehabilitation adherence. *Journal of Athletic Training, 28*, 43–47.

Gebhardt, W. A., & Maes, S. (1998). Competing personal goals and exercise behavior. *Perceptual and Motor Skills, 86*, 755–759.

Gilbourne, D., & Taylor, A. H. (1998). From theory to practice: The integration of goal perspective theory and life development approaches within an injury-specific goal-setting program. *Journal of Applied Sport Psychology, 10*, 124–139.

Gillison, F. F., Standage, M., & Skevington, S. M. (2006). Relationships among adolescents' weight perceptions, exercise goals, exercise motivation, quality of life and leisure-time exercise behaviour: A self-determination theory approach. *Health Education Research, 21*, 836–847.

Gordon, S., Potter, M., & Ford, I. W. (1998). Toward a psychoeducational curriculum for training sport-injury rehabilitation personnel. *Journal of Applied Sport Psychology, 10*, 140–156.

Gould, D., Tammen, V., Murphy, S., & May, J. (1989). An examination of US Olympic sport psychology consultants and the services they provide. *The Sport Psychologist, 3*, 300–312.

Ievleva, L., & Orlick, T. (1991). Mental links to enhanced healing: An exploratory study. *The Sport Psychologist, 5*, 25–40.

Jeffery, R. W., Wing, R. R., Sherwood, N. E., & Tate, D. F. (2003). Physical activity and weight loss: Does prescribing higher physical activity goals improve outcome? *American Journal of Clinical Nutrition, 78*, 669–670.

Johnson, U. (1997). A three-year follow-up of long-term injured competitive athletes: Influence of psychological risk factors on rehabilitation. *Journal of Sport Rehabilitation, 6*, 256–271.

Johnson, U. (2000). Short-term psychological intervention: A study of long-term injured competitive athletes. *Journal of Sport Rehabilitation, 9*, 207–218.

Jung, M. E., & Brawley, L. R. (2010). Concurrent management of exercise with other valued life goals: Comparison of frequent and less frequent exercisers. *Psychology of Sport and Exercise, 11*, 372–377.

Karoly, P., Ruehlman, L. S., Okun, M. A., Lutz, R. S., Newton, C., & Fairholme, C. (2005). Perceived self-regulation of exercise goals and interfering goals among regular and irregular exercisers: A life space analysis. *Psychology of Sport and Exercise, 6*, 427–442.

Kasser, T. (2002). *The high price of materialism.* Cambridge, MA: MIT Press.

Klein, H., Wesson, M., Hollenbeck, J., & Alge, B. (1999). Goal commitment and the goal-setting process: Conceptual clarification and empirical synthesis. *Journal of Applied Psychology, 84*, 885–896.

Kobasa, S. C., Maddi, S. R., & Kahn, S. (1982). Hardiness and health: A prospective study. *Journal of Personality and Social Psychology, 42*, 168–177.

Kyllo, L. B., & Landers, D. M. (1995). Goal setting in sport and exercise: A research synthesis to resolve the controversy. *Journal of Sport and Exercise Psychology, 17*, 117–137.

Latham, G. P. & Seijts, G. H. (1999). The effects of proximal and distal goals on performance on a moderately complex task. *Journal of Organizational Behavior, 20*, 421–429.

Lee, T. W., Locke, E. A., & Latham, G. P. (1989). Goal setting theory and job performance. In L. Pervin (Ed.), *Goal concepts in personality and social psychology* (pp. 291–326). Hillsdale, NJ: Lawrence Erlbaum.

Levack, W. M. M., Taylor, K., Siegert, R. J., & Dean, S. G. (2006). Is goal planning in rehabilitation effective? A systematic review. *Clinical Rehabilitation, 20,* 739–755.

Locke, E. A. & Latham, G. P. (2002). Building a practically useful theory of goal setting and task motivation. *American Psychologist, 57,* 705–717.

Locke, E. A., Shaw, K. N., Saari, L. M., & Latham, G. P. (1981). Goal setting and task performance: 1969–1980. *Psychological Bulletin, 90,* 125–152.

Malec, J. F. (1999). Goal attainment scaling in rehabilitation. *Neuropsychological Rehabilitation: An International Journal, 9,* 253–275.

Maltby, J., & Day, L. (2001). The relationship between exercise motives and psychological well-being. *The Journal of Psychology, 135,* 651–660.

Martin, J. E., Dubbert, P. M., Katell, A. D., et al. (1984). Behavioral control of exercise in sedentary adults: studies 1 through 6 (study 4). *Journal of Consulting and Clinical Psychology, 52,* 795–811.

Mellalieu, S. D., Hanton, S., & O'Brien, M. (2006). The effects of goal setting on rugby performance. *Journal of Applied Behavior Analysis, 39,* 257–261.

Munroe-Chandler, K. J., Hall, C. R., & Weinberg, R. S. (2004). A qualitative analysis of the types of goals athletes set in training and competition. *Journal of Sport Behavior, 27,* 58–74.

Pearson, E. (2012). Goal setting as a health behavior change strategy in overweight and obese adults: A systematic literature review examining intervention components. *Patient Education and Counseling, 87,* 32–42.

Playford, E. D., Siegert, R., Levack, W., & Freeman, J. (2009). Areas of consensus and controversy about goal setting in rehabilitation: a conference report. *Clinical Rehabilitation, 23,* 334–344.

Poag, K., & McAuley, E. (1992). Goal setting, self-efficacy, and exercise behavior. *Journal of Sport & Exercise Psychology, 14,* 352–360.

Poag-DuCharme, K. A., & Brawley, L. R. (1994). Perceptions of the behavioral influence of goals: A mediational relationship to exercise. *Journal of Applied Sport Psychology, 6,* 32–50.

Podlog, L., & Dionigi, R. (2010). Coach strategies for addressing psychosocial challenges during the return to sport from injury. *Journal of Sports Sciences, 28,* 1197–1208.

Riediger, M., & Freund, A. M. (2004). Interference and facilitation among personal goals: Differential associations with subjective well-being and persistent goal pursuit. *Personality and Social Psychology Bulletin, 30,* 1511–1523.

Ryan, R. M., Sheldon, K. M., Kasser, T., & Deci, E. L. (1996). All goals are not created equal: An organismic perspective on the nature of goals and their regulation. In P. M. Gollwitzer & J. A. Bargh (Eds.), *The psychology of action: Linking cognition and motivation to behavior* (pp. 7–26). New York: Guilford Press.

Sanderson, F. (1996). Psychology and injury. In T. Reilly (Ed.), *Science and soccer* (pp. 165–180). Liverpool, UK: Spon Press.

Sebire, S. J., Standage, M., & Vansteenkiste, M. (2008). Development and validation of the Goal Content for Exercise Questionnaire. *Journal of Sport & Exercise Psychology, 28,* 335–354.

Senécal, J., Loughead, T. M., & Bloom, G. A. (2008). A season long team building intervention: Examining the effect of team goal setting on cohesion. *Journal of Sport & Exercise Psychology, 30,* 186–199.

Shilts, M. K., Horowitz, M., Townsend, M. S. (2004). Goal setting as a strategy for dietary and physical activity behavior change: A review of the literature. *American Journal of Health Promotion, 19,* 81–93.

Steel, P. & Konig, C. J. (2006). Integrating theories of motivation. *Academy of Management Review, 31,* 889–913.

Strecher, V. J., Seijts, G. H., Kok, G. J., Latham, G. P., Glasgow, R., DeVellis, B., Meertens, R. M., & Bulger, D. W. (1995). Goal setting as a strategy for health behavior change. *Health Education Quarterly, 22,* 190–200.

Theodorakis, Y., Malliou, P., Papaioannou, A., Beneca, A., & Filactakidou, A. (1996). The effect of personal goals, self-efficacy and self-satisfaction on injury rehabilitation. *Journal of Sport Rehabilitation, 5,* 173–183.

Vansteenkiste, M., Lens, W., & Deci, E. L. (2006). Intrinsic versus extrinsic goal contents in self-determination theory: Another look at the quality of academic motivation. *Educational Psychologist, 41,* 19–31.

Vansteenkiste, M., Neyrinck, B., Niemiec, C. P., Soenens, B., De Witte, H., & Van den Broeck, A. (2007). On the relations among work value orientations, psychological need satisfaction, and job outcomes: A self-determination theory approach. *Journal of Occupational and Organizational Psychology, 80,* 251–277.

Vansteenkiste, M., Simons, J., Soenens, B., & Lens, W. (2004). How to become a persevering exerciser? Providing a clear, future intrinsic goal in an autonomy-supportive way. *Journal of Sport and Exercise Psychology, 26,* 232–249.

Vansteenkiste, M., Soenens, B., & Duriez, B. (2008). Presenting a positive alternative to strivings for material success and the thin-ideal: Understanding the effects of extrinsic relative to intrinsic goal pursuits. In S. J. Lopez (Ed.), *Positive psychology: Exploring the best in people* (Vol. 4, pp. 57–86). Westport, CT: Greenwood Publishing Company.

Wade, D. T. (1998). Evidence relating to goal planning in rehabilitation. *Clinical Rehabilitation, 12,* 273–275.

Wayda V. K., Armenth-Brothers, F., & Boyce, B. A. (1998). Goal setting: A key to injury rehabilitation. *Athletic Therapy Today, 3,* 21–25.

Weinberg, R. S. (1994). Goal setting and performance in sport and exercise settings: A synthesis and critique. *Medicine and Science in Sports and Exercise, 26,* 469–477.

Weinberg, R. S., Bruya, L., Garland, H., & Jackson, A. (1990). Effect of goal difficulty and positive reinforcement on endurance performance. *Journal of Sport Psychology, 12,* 144–156.

Weinberg, R. S., Bruya, L., Jackson, A., & Garland, H. (1987). Goal difficulty and endurance performance: A challenge to the goal attainability assumption. *Journal of Sport Behavior, 10,* 82–92.

Weinberg, R. S., & Gould, D. (2003). *Foundations of sport and exercise psychology* (3rd ed.). Champaign, IL: Human Kinetics.

Wiese, D. M., & Weiss, M. R. (1987). Psychological rehabilitation and physical injury: Implications for the sport medicine team. *The Sport Psychologist, 1,* 318–330.

Wiese, D. M., Weiss, M. R., & Yukelson, D. P. (1991). Sport psychology in the training room: A survey of athletic trainers. *The Sport Psychologist, 5,* 15–24.

Worrell, T. W. (1992). The use of behavioral and cognitive techniques to facilitate achievement of rehabilitation goals. *Journal of Sport Rehabilitation, 1,* 69–75.

Chapter 6

Imagery

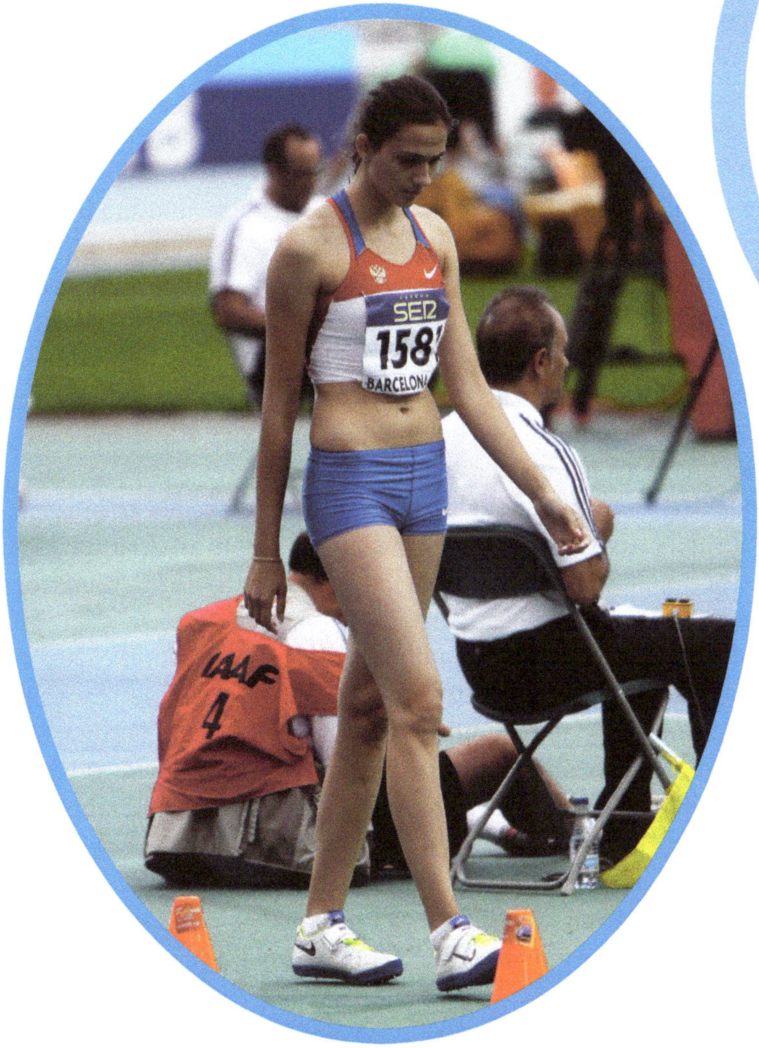

Introduction

Mental imagery, hereafter simply referred to as imagery, is often considered to be the visualization of an object, scene, or sensation as though it were occurring in overt, physical reality (Denis, 1985). However, imagery includes more than just visualization (i.e., seeing something in your mind); it involves the use of one or more of the five senses to generate the object, scene, or sensation. White and Hardy (1998) have defined **imagery** as follows:

> ...an experience that mimics real experience. We can be aware of "seeing" an image, feeling movements as an image, or experiencing an image of smell, tastes, or sounds without actually experiencing the real thing. Sometimes people find that it helps to close their eyes. It differs from dreams in that we are awake and conscious when we form an image (p. 389).

Imagery goes by a variety of names including visualization, mental rehearsal, and mental practice. Imagery has been shown to be an effective technique in a variety of tasks and situations (Hall, 2001; Paivio, 1986; Taylor & Schneider, 1989), and to have powerful effects on behavior, as well as self-confidence and other cognitions (Hall, 2001; Johnson & Lutgendorf, 2002; Paivio, 1986; Taylor, Pham, Rivkin, & Armor, 1998). Imagery can encourage problem-solving and emotional regulation which can then set the stage for turning imagined experience into action (Pham & Taylor, 1999). In this way, it is believed that imagery facilitates goal-directed action by strengthening the links between thought and goal-directed behavior.

Everyone has the ability to create and use imagery; however, some choose not to use it even when it may prove to be beneficial (Hall, 2001). This is partially due to individual differences; some people are better imagers than others. If you are high in imagery ability, you are more likely to use imagery in a given situation. For example, Gregg, Hall, and Nederhof (2005) examined imagery ability and imagery use in a sample of track and field athletes. They found that higher visual and kinesthetic imagery abilities were related to an increased use of imagery.

Betts (1909) conducted one of the first studies that explored the use of imagery. He investigated the spontaneous use of imagery in a variety of tasks including simple association, logical thinking, mental multiplication, and discrimination judgments. He found that people often use imagery in doing these tasks, but that it is more beneficial in doing some tasks than others.

At first glance imagery may seem like a simple mental process. Upon closer inspection, it is multidimensional and entails a number of cognitive processes. We can experience imagery in each of the modalities with visual, kinesthetic, and auditory imagery being most common in physical activity settings. Of course, in many instances these forms of imagery are combined. When we use imagery there are a number of cognitive processes involved. We can create an image from memory (e.g., remembering a winning shot in a hockey game) or create an image of something we have never experienced (e.g., scene from a science fiction novel). We can transform our images in a variety of ways. For example, we can add to an image, subtract from an image, and even rotate an image. See Morris, Spittle, and Watt (2005) for a more elaborate discussion about the nature of imagery.

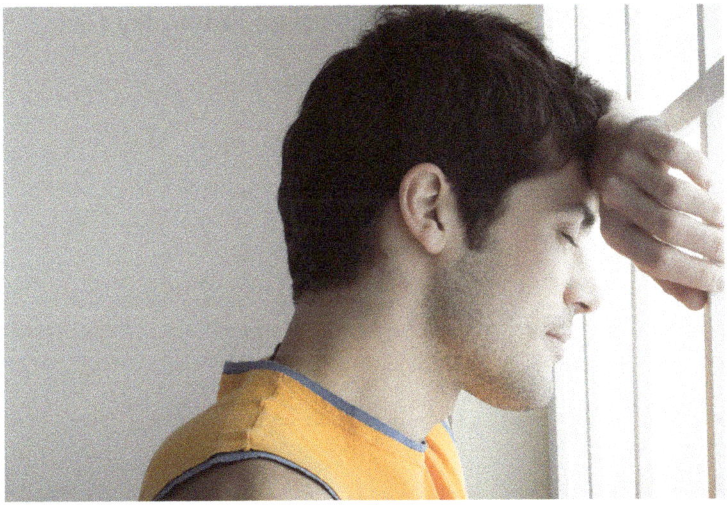

Image © stefanolunardi, 2014. Used under license from Shutterstock, Inc.

Some researchers propose that imagery is a basic way of processing information. According to Paivio (1986), there are two ways a person could expand on learned material: verbal associations and imagery. Dual-coding theory postulates that information can be represented both verbally and by imagery. These two types of information are processed differently and along distinct channels in the human mind, creating separate representations for information processed in each channel. The mental codes corresponding to these representations are used to organize incoming information that can be acted upon, stored, and retrieved for subsequent use. Both verbal and imagery codes can be used when recalling information. Annett (1995) has argued that motor actions are processed and represented primarily in the imagery system.

Imagery in Sport

Researchers have argued that imagery is a "central pillar of applied sport psychology" (Perry & Morris, 1995, p. 339). While imagery and its use in sport has been widely studied by researchers since the 1960s (e.g., Clark, 1960; Start & Richardson, 1964), much of the research conducted over the past two decades has been based on Paivio's (1985) analytical framework, which was the first to conceptualize how imagery operates in different areas of sport performance. According to Paivio, athletes use imagery for both cognitive and motivational functions, operating at either a general or specific level. Hall, Mack, Paivio, and Hausenblas (1998) later expanded this framework into five different imagery functions: cognitive specific (CS; imaging specific skills), cognitive general (CG; imaging strategies of play), motivational specific (MS; imaging specific goals), motivational general-arousal (MG-A; using imagery for the regulation of arousal and anxiety), and motivational general-mastery (MG-M; using imagery to stay in control and be focused, and to increase mental toughness and self-confidence). This expansion into five different imagery functions led to the development of the Sport Imagery Questionnaire (SIQ; Hall et al., 1998), which has become the most prevalent tool for measuring the frequency of imagery use in athlete populations. Paivio's framework and the SIQ have revolutionized imagery research (Short, Ross-Stewart, & Monsma, 2006), and have served as the driving force for imagery interventions.

FIGURE 6–1 Applied Model of Imagery Use

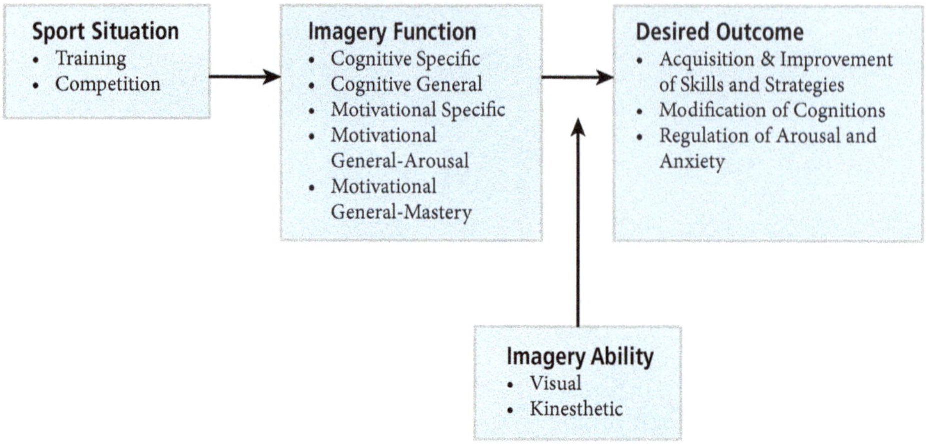

Adapted from Martin, K., Moritz, S., & Hall, C. (1999). Imagery use in sport: A literature review and applied model. *The Sport Psychologist, 13,* 245–268. Human Kinetics, Champaign, IL.

Martin and colleagues (1999) using this framework put forth the Applied Model of Imagery Use in Sport (see Figure 6–1). They identified four key constructs that must be considered when examining imagery use in sport. The model consists of three stages (sport situation, imagery function, and desired outcome) with a moderating variable (imagery ability). The model suggests that for imagery to be most beneficial, the function employed should match the desired outcome (improve skills and strategies, modify cognitions, regulate arousal and anxiety). For example, if athletes want to improve a specific skill, CS imagery should be used; if they need to improve their confidence, MG-M imagery should be employed. The model was summarized nicely by Short and colleagues (2006) in that the model's predictions are essentially "what you see is what you get" (e.g., the imagery of skills would likely improve skill execution). As well, Martin et al. recognized in their model that imagery is used differently in each of the two sport situations (i.e., training and competition). In training the cognitive functions of imagery tend to play a larger role and in competition the motivational functions are emphasized. Imagery ability was included as a moderator given that research has shown that greater ability may lead to greater performance gains (e.g., Goss, Hall, Buckolz, & Fishburne, 1986).

Cognitive Imagery Interventions

The majority of imagery interventions conducted by researchers have targeted the CS function. The standard paradigm employed has consisted of three conditions: (a) a physical practice condition, (b) an imagery condition, and (c) a control condition. Participants are randomly assigned to one of these conditions after being tested on the performance of some skill (e.g., basketball free-throws). Their performance on this skill represents their baseline score. Then the physical practice participants actually practice the skill for a set number of trials or a given amount of time. Those participants in the imagery condition imagine doing the skill (i.e., use CS imagery) for the same number of trials or for the same amount of time that the physical practice participants actually practice. The control participants do not engage in any physical or imagery practice, but rest or practice an unrelated skill. All participants are then retested on the skill and their performance represents their post-intervention score. While a few studies have found imagery practice to be just as effective as physical practice (e.g., Rawlings, Rawlings, Chen, & Yilk, 1972), most investigators have reported the order of performance from best to worst to be physical practice, imagery practice, and control. Taking the results of these studies collectively, it is generally recognized that CS imagery facilitates the learning and performance of motor skills, but not to the same extent as physical practice (Morris, Spittle, & Watt, 2005).

An extension of the above paradigm involves examining the effects of combining physical and imagery practice (e.g., 50% physical and 50% imagery) compared to 100% physical or 100% imagery practice. That is, a certain amount of imagery practice is substituted for physical practice. Durand, Hall, and Haslam (1997) reviewed the research combining physical and imagery practice and concluded that a combination of the two is about as equally effective as 100% physical practice. This conclusion has important implications for athletes. While athletes would not normally substitute imagery practice for physical practice, sometimes circumstances may make this necessary (e.g., injury, fatigue, travel, loss of practice facilities). In these situations, by employing imagery athletes may be able to maintain their usual levels of practice and obtain the positive benefits associated with such practice.

Of course, the usual approach of athletes is to incorporate CS imagery practice into their overall training program. That is, imagery practice is added to regular physical practice. How effective is the addition of CS imagery practice to the regular physical practice undertaken by athletes? To answer this question, Blair, Hall, and Leyshon (1993) measured the performance of elite and non-elite soccer players. Initially, the players were tested on a soccer task designed to include some of the basic skills of the sport (e.g., passing, dribbling, shooting). The players were next randomly assigned to either an imagery practice group or a control group with the only restriction being that equal numbers of elite and non-elite players were in each group. The imagery group received six weeks of imagery practice on the soccer task while the control group spent this time developing a competition strategy for soccer, which should

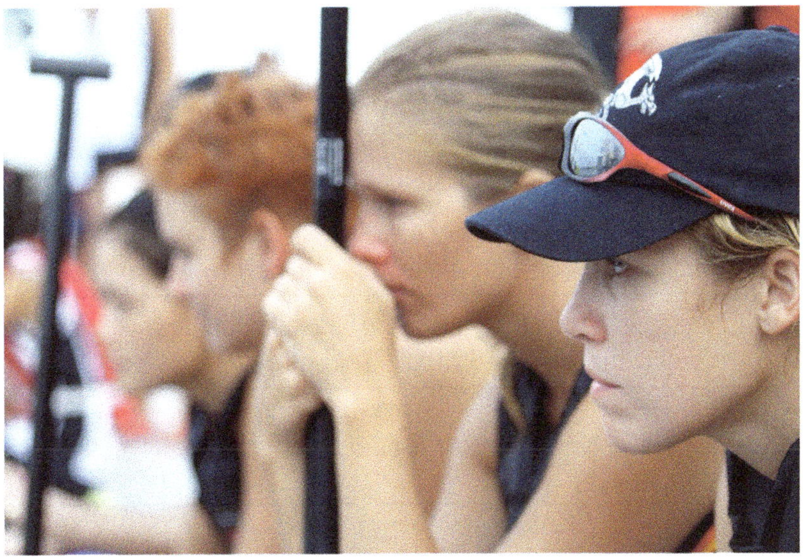

have had no influence on their performance of the soccer task. During this period all players engaged in their regular soccer activities (e.g., team practices). After the six weeks the players were again tested on the soccer task. The imagery group significantly increased their performance on the task while the control group showed no change. The amount of improvement was about the same for both the elite and non-elite players in the imagery group. These findings suggest that athletes should supplement their regular physical practice with CS imagery practice.

There has been considerably less research conducted on CG imagery inventions, likely because of the difficulties associated with measuring strategy performance (Westlund, Pope, & Tobin, 2012). Imagery interventions conducted using CG imagery have found mixed results. Guillot, Nadrowska, and Collet (2009) found their CG intervention for learning tactical movements in basketball to be effective, but Munroe-Chandler, Hall, Fishburne, and Shannon (2005) failed to find a significant effect on performance following their CG imagery intervention for improving soccer strategies. Holmes and Collins (2001) have provided some guidelines in their PETTLEP model that are useful when conducting cognitive imagery interventions (see Table 6-1).

TABLE 6-1 The PETTLEP Model of Imagery

P = Physical	The physical nature of the imagery is dependent upon the task. You must determine whether relaxation or increased arousal is beneficial prior to imaging.
E = Environment	The image should be as real or as close to the actual environment as possible. If you are unfamiliar with a competition venue, video or pictures may enhance your image.
T = Task	Depending on the task, your imagery perspective may vary. Skills that rely on form have been found to benefit most from an external imagery perspective.
T = Timing	The temporal characteristics or timing of the image should be equal to that of your physical performance (e.g., if a gymnastics routine takes 45 seconds to physically execute, so too should the imagery).
L = Learning	The content of the image should change based on the learning of the skill. For example, the content of your image when you are first learning a dive should be different from when you have mastered it.
E = Emotion	Images will be more effective if you attach meaning or emotion to them. If imaging winning a medal, feel the excitement and the joy that is part of it.
P = Perspective	Consider both perspectives, internal (visualizing through your own eyes) and external (visualizing like watching a video), when imaging.

Note: Adapted from Holmes, P. S., & Collins, D. J. (2001). The PETTLEP approach to motor imagery: A functional equivalence model for sport psychologists. *Journal of Applied Sport Psychology, 13,* 60–83. Taylor & Francis, Philadelphia.

Motivational Imagery Interventions

With respect to motivational imagery interventions, most of these have focused on MG-M imagery. An intervention conducted by Callow, Hardy, and Hall (2001) using four elite junior badminton players found some support for the effect of MG-M imagery on self-confidence. Self-confidence data was collected once a week for 21 weeks prior to competitive matches. The imagery intervention consisted of six imagery sessions, two per week for three weeks. The imagery sessions were created around mastery situations in which being in control and confidence were emphasized. The results showed that a 20-week imagery intervention improved the sport confidence for two of the players and stabilized the sport confidence of the third player.

Cumming, Olphin, and Law (2007) examined self-reported psychological states and physiological responses (heart rate) experienced during different MG-M and MG-A imagery scenarios. Forty competitive athletes wore a standard heart rate monitor and imaged five scripts: mastery, coping, anxiety, psyching up, and relaxation. Following each script, the athletes reported their state anxiety and self-confidence. A significant increase in heart rate from baseline to imagery was found for the anxiety, psyching-up, and coping imagery scripts. In addition, the intensity of cognitive and somatic anxiety was greater and perceived as being more debilitative following the anxiety imagery script.

Research suggests that MG-M imagery interventions can increase self-confidence, and MG-A imagery interventions can influence levels of arousal and anxiety. When examining the influence of MG-A imagery in regulating arousal, investigators have often combined imagery with relaxation training (e.g., Cogan & Petrie, 1995). This makes it difficult to determine the exact role imagery plays in producing any treatment effects.

Measurement of Sport Imagery

Hall and colleagues (1998) used Paivio's framework as the basis for developing the Sport Questionnaire (SIQ), which assesses the use of the five functions of imagery by athletes. The validity and reliability of the SIQ have been supported (Hall et al., 1998; Hall, Stevens, & Paivio, 2005). It is composed of 30 questions; six questions per imagery function (CS, CG, MS, MG-A, MG-M). Each item is rated on a 7-point Likert-type scale with anchors of 1 = *rarely* and 7 = *often* use that function of imagery. Hall, Munroe-Chandler, Fishburne, and Hall (2009) modified the SIQ for use with children aged 7–14 years. The SIQ-C is a 21-item questionnaire again assessing the use of the five functions of imagery. Children respond on a 5-point scale with 1 = *not at all* and 5 = *very often.* An example of a CS imagery item is "I can usually control how a skill looks in my head" and "I make up new game plans or routines in my head" is a CG imagery item. The statement "I see myself being mentally strong" is an example of a MG-M imagery item and "In my head, I imagine how calm I feel before I compete" addresses the MG-A imagery function. Finally, "I see myself doing my very best" is an example of a MS imagery item.

Some General Recommendations

For imagery use to be effective, it must be incorporated into a daily routine. Bull, Albinson, and Shambrook (1996) suggest brief sessions (five minutes) once or twice a day for athletes who are just starting to use imagery. As athletes become more comfortable with, and better at, using imagery, they should systematically increase the amount of imagery employed. Cumming and Hall (2002) argue that imagery requires deliberate practice and just as for physical practice, more is better. Given that imagery is a skill and improves with practice, athletes will become better imagers over the course of an imagery intervention. The better imagers they become, the more effective their imagery will likely be.

Some other general recommendations for both cognitive and motivational imagery interventions are:

- Images should be positive; athletes should avoid using negative images (Hall, 2001).
- Athletes should be in a good mood when employing imagery (Gregg, Hall, & Hanton, 2007).
- Athletes need to be encouraged to use imagery during those times when imagery use is typically less frequent, such as in the off-season and early competitive season (Munroe, Hall, Simms, & Weinberg, 1998).
- Athletes of all skill levels and ages can benefit from imagery interventions (Hall, 2001; Munroe-Chandler, Hall, Fishburne, & Strachan, 2007).

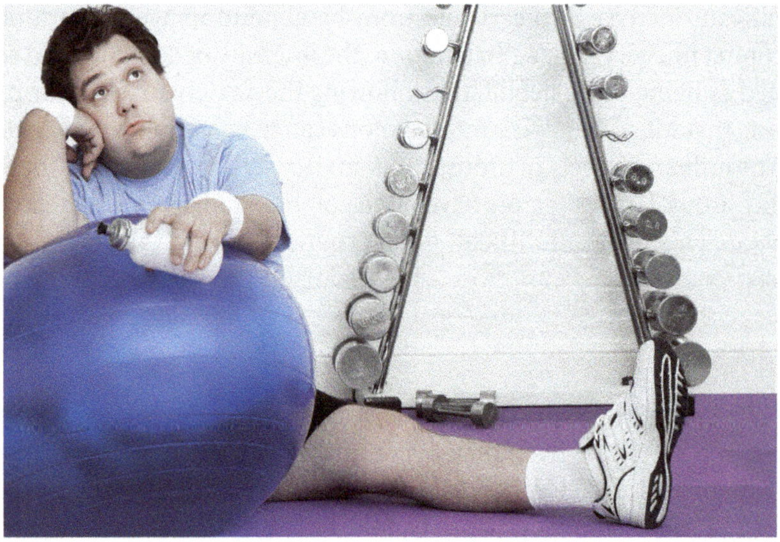

Imagery in Exercise

After findings from decades of research in the sports domain supported the usefulness and importance of imagery among athletes, Hall (1995) proposed that imagery may also be an important determinant of exercise behavior. Initial descriptive investigations of mental imagery in the exercise domain demonstrated that, indeed, more than 75% of regular exercisers report using exercise-related imagery (Hausenblas, Hall, Rodgers, & Munroe, 1999). Subsequent research has also demonstrated that exercise-related imagery is used by individuals who exercise less frequently (Gammage, Hall, & Rodgers, 2000), individuals who do not exercise regularly, and even individuals who do not have any intention of becoming a regular exerciser (Hall, Rodgers, Wilson, & Norman, 2010). Given the prevalence of exercise-related imagery among exercisers and non-exercisers alike, investigations into the content of these images as well as their impact on exercise behavior were born.

The Content of Exercise Imagery

Consistent with imagery use among athletes, exercisers employ imagery for cognitive and motivational purposes. Technique imagery is a cognitive type of exercise imagery in which exercisers imagine engaging in the elemental aspects of an exercise task (Hausenblas et al., 1999). For example, exercisers may imagine lifting weights with proper form or following a series of steps in an aerobic class.[1] Exercisers also report using imagery for a number of motivational functions. Appearance imagery involves imagining being toned, losing weight, or achieving some other type of body ideal and is the type of imagery typically employed most frequently among exercisers (Hausenblas et al., 1999; Gammage et al., 2000; Wilson, Rodgers, Hall, & Gammage, 2003; Giacobbi, Hausenblas, & Penfield, 2005; Cumming, 2008; Cumming & Stanley, 2009; Hall et al., 2010; Thogersen-Ntoumani, Cumming, Ntoumanis, & Nikitaras, 2012; Stanley, Cumming, Standage, & Duda, 2012; Munroe-Chandler, Kim, & Gammage, 2004). Exercisers use energy imagery to help them feel in control of their arousal levels (e.g., imagine using exercise to help relieve stress, or imagine getting psyched-up to do a workout). Other types of motivational imagery are related to fitness and health (i.e., imagine feeling more fit or healthy; Giacobbi, Hausenblas, Fallon, & Hall, 2003), emotions and feelings (i.e., imagine feeling accomplished and proud; Giacobbi et al., 2003), and self-efficacy and confidence (i.e., imagine persevering through a difficult workout; Giacobbi et al., 2003; Kim & Giacobbi, 2009). Finally, exercisers also imagine the context in which they exercise (i.e., imagining the physical space, the weight machines, the steps, the pool, etc.; Giacobbi et al., 2003) as well as plans and strategies related to exercising (Kim & Giacobbi, 2009).

Who Uses Exercise Imagery?

It is clear that imagery is used widely among exercisers. Thus, imagery may prove to be an effective intervention technique for improving rates of exercise behavior in the population. To determine how imagery interventions might be tailored to suit the needs of particular sub-groups within the population it is important to consider how these different groups use exercise imagery naturally.

Exercise frequency. Individuals who exercise more often also tend to use all types of exercise imagery more often (Hall et al., 2010; Gammage et al., 2000; Gammage, Hall, & Martin Ginis, 2004; Giacobbi, 2007).

Age. Some researchers have demonstrated that the age of an exerciser may also be related to their use of exercise imagery. For example, Giacobbi (2007) demonstrated that appearance/health imagery and technique imagery were used more frequently by younger individuals than by their older counterparts. Indeed, Kim and Giacobbi (2009) demonstrated that the content of exercise imagery among middle-aged adults is somewhat different from that of younger adults. Specifically, older adults use imagery related to exercise plans and strategies whereas this was not described as a function of imagery among younger adults (Kim & Giacobbi, 2009). Understanding the specific types of images that are endorsed by adults of different ages may help practitioners determine the optimal content for exercise imagery interventions.

Gender. Comparisons of imagery use by gender have been relatively unexplored in the exercise-imagery literature. In the few studies that have examined gender differences in exercise imagery use, both genders reported using appearance imagery the most frequently followed by technique and energy imagery, respectively (Gammage et al., 2000). Men have been found, however, to use more technique imagery than women, and women use more appearance imagery than men (Cumming, 2008; Gammage et al., 2000). Additionally, among individuals who exercise at a very high frequency, men use more energy imagery than women (Hausenblas & Symons Downs, 2002). Compared to women, men also report better imagery ability with respect to technique imagery (Cumming, 2008). Although a few studies have found gender differences in imagery use, Hall and his colleagues (2010) found that men and women did not differ in their use of the various imagery functions.

Measurement of Exercise Imagery

There are two questionnaires that have been developed to measure the frequency with which exercisers use different types of imagery. The Exercise Imagery Questionnaire (EIQ; Hausenblas et al., 1999; Gammage et al., 2000) includes nine items which assess technique (e.g., "When I think about exercising I imagine perfecting my technique"; n = 3), appearance (e.g., "I imagine a 'firmer-me' from exercising"; n = 3), and energy (e.g., "To get me energized, I imagine exercising"; n = 3) imagery. Each item is measured on a 9-point scale which ranges from 1 (*never*) to 9 (*always*).

The Exercise Imagery Inventory (EII; Giacobbi et al., 2005) is a 19-item, self-report scale which assesses four exercise imagery factors: Appearance-health imagery (e.g., "I imagine a 'fitter-me' from exercising"; n = 8), exercise technique imagery (e.g., "When I think about exercising, I imagine my form and body position"; n = 4), exercise self-efficacy (e.g., "I imagine having the confidence to exercise"; k = 3), and exercise feelings (e.g., "I imagine reducing my stress from exercising"; n = 4). Each item is measured on a 7-point scale ranging from 1 (*rarely*) to 7 (*often*).

Applied Model of Imagery Use in Exercise

Given the correlational evidence linking exercise imagery use to exercise-related cognitions and behavior, and the need to intervene to increase exercise behavior among individuals who do not exercise enough, an applied model of exercise imagery was developed by Munroe-Chandler and Gammage (2005) and is shown in Figure 6–2. Loosely based on an applied model of imagery use in sports (Martin et al., 1999), the applied model of imagery use in exercise provides a foundation for the development of exercise imagery interventions. The applied model of imagery use in exercise demonstrates the potential role of the various imagery functions on cognitive and behavioral outcomes as well as potential mediators and moderators of these relationships. The model provides a foundation for the development of exercise imagery interventions and identifies relationships that are worthy of investigation within the domain of exercise imagery.

Imagery Ability in Exercise

Individual differences in imagery ability influence the learning and performance of motor skills (Goss et al., 1986; Hall, Buckolz, & Fishburne, 1989). In the applied model of imagery use in exercise, imagery ability is proposed as a potential moderator of the relationship between imagery use and exercise-related outcomes (i.e., cognitive and behavioral; Munroe-Chandler & Gammage, 2005); however, this proposition has received little research attention and is emerging as a new area of investigation within

FIGURE 6–2 An Applied Model of Imagery Use In Exercise

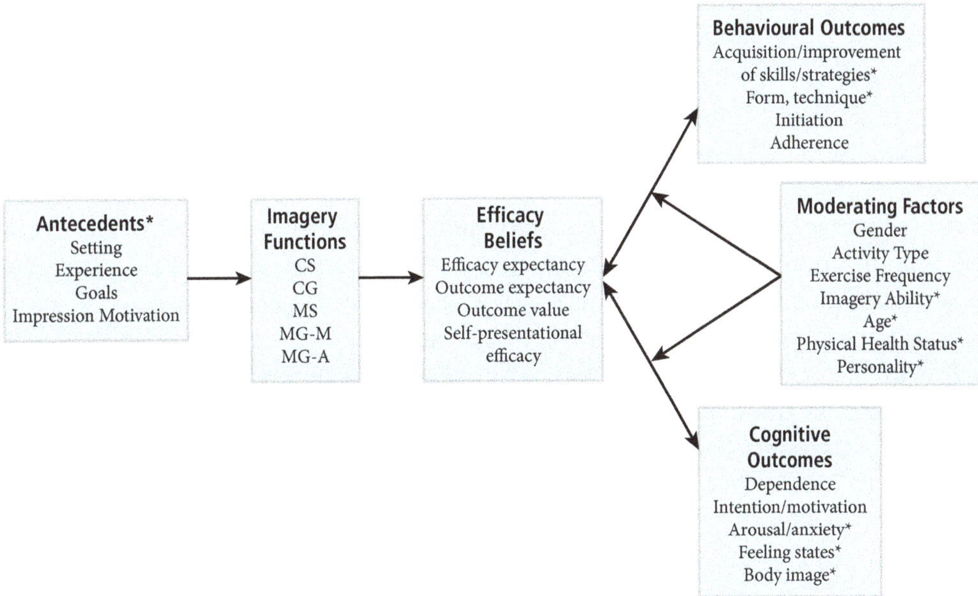

(Reprinted from Munroe-Chandler, K. J. and Gammage, K. L. (2005). Now see this: A new vision of exercise imagery. *Exercise and Sport Sciences Reviews, 33*(4), 201–205. ©2005 by the American College of Sports Medicine.)

the exercise imagery literature. To date, 'ease of imaging' has been assessed using companion scales that are administered along with the EIQ or the EII. For each item on the EIQ or EII, participants are asked to indicate how easy it is for them to see (i.e., picture in their mind) or feel (i.e., feel what it would be like in real life) the content of the item. The ease of imaging items are rated on a 7-point scale ranging from 1 (*very hard to see/feel*) to 7 (*very easy to see/feel*) and are averaged to form ease of imaging subscales for each imagery type.

To date, only one study has used these companion scales to test if imagery ability moderates the relationships between imagery use and exercise-related outcomes. Cumming (2008) found that only imagery ability related to appearance/health imagery (and not other types of imagery) moderated the relationship between appearance/health imagery use and leisure-time exercise, coping efficacy, and scheduling efficacy. Additional tests of this proposed path within the applied model should be pursued.

Imagery and Motivation for Exercise

It is clear that individuals employ images to serve a variety of functions in the exercise domain. Researchers have begun to examine these images in the context of self-determination theory (Deci & Ryan, 1985) to help explain exercise imagery from a motivational perspective. In a cross-sectional study examining motivation for exercise and imagery use among female university students, Wilson et al. (2003) found that introjected regulation (a type of controlling motive that represents self-imposed pressure such as feelings of guilt associated with not exercising) was strongly related to appearance imagery. Identified regulation and intrinsic motivation were also related to appearance and technique imagery. This was the first study to demonstrate that the various functions of imagery were differentially associated with different types of motivation. The findings from this study suggest that, perhaps, using specific types of imagery may result in increases in different types of motivation. Given that researchers have found more self-determined motives to be more strongly associated with exercise adherence, it is possible that imagery could result in increases in exercise behavior through its impact on motivation. Experimental research is needed to substantiate this suggestion.

Stanley et al. (2012) also examined the use of different types of imagery among regular exercisers and found that the use of technique imagery and enjoyment imagery are positively related to autonomous motivation, whereas the use of appearance imagery is positively associated with controlled motivation. Given that autonomous motivation is more highly correlated with exercise behavior, it may be the case that imagery interventions aimed at helping participants initiate, increase, or maintain regular exercise behavior will be more effective if they employ technique imagery and energy imagery and avoid appearance imagery. It should be noted, however, that the study conducted by Stanley et al. (2012) was correlational; thus, it is speculative to suggest that increasing the use of energy and technique imagery will result in increases in autonomous motivation.

Further investigations into the associations between imagery use and exercise motivation were conducted by Hall et al. (2010). In addition to investigating these associations among regular exercisers only, Hall et al. also looked at the patterns of associations between imagery and motivation for non-exercisers who intended to begin exercising regularly (intenders) and non-exercisers who did not intend to begin exercising regularly (non-intenders). Interestingly, the pattern of motives reported by the regular exercisers and the intenders did not differ; however, the pattern of motives for the non-intenders did differ from that of the other two groups. The associations between imagery use and motivation also differed between groups. Overall, among regular exercisers and non-exercisers who intend to begin exercising, imagery use was associated with more self-determined motivation but unrelated to amotivation and external regulation. Among non-intenders, however, the use of appearance imagery had strong correlations with all forms of motivation, the use of energy imagery related to all forms except amotivation, and the use of technique imagery was related to all forms except external. These findings suggested that if imagery were to be used as an intervention strategy for increasing exercise behavior among non-exercisers, tailoring the intervention to the participants' intentions may be necessary.

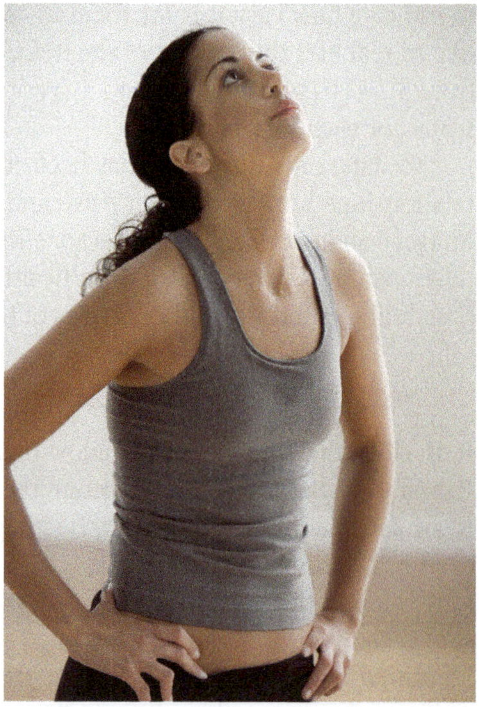

Given the correlational links between imagery use and motivation for exercise, in addition to an observation that integrated regulation among exercisers far exceeds the levels of integration reported by non-exercisers, Duncan, Hall, Wilson, and Rodgers (2012) sought to test the impact of an imagery intervention on the motivation of female, non-exercisers (N = 102) as they initiated and maintained an 8-week cardiovascular exercise program. All of the women visited the study facility to exercise three times per week. The women were also assigned randomly to listen to an audio-recorded imagery script that targeted the development of integrated regulation or to an attention control script that provided information about the health benefits of exercise. At the conclusion of the 8-week intervention, the women assigned to the imagery intervention reported greater increases in integration than women in the control condition. Because the exercise program was standardized and assigned to women in both conditions, the researchers were not able to extend their analyses to examine the impact of the intervention on behavior. Further research is needed to determine if exercise behavior can be increased among exercise initiates by increasing their use of specific types of imagery.

Imagery and Self-Efficacy for Exercise

There is considerable evidence for the role of self-efficacy in the initiation and maintenance of regular exercise (McAuley, Pena, & Jerome, 2001). Individuals who have higher levels of self-efficacy tend to engage in more frequent exercise or physical activity (e.g., Bandura, 1997; McAuley & Jacobson, 1991; Rodgers & Gauvin, 1998; Rodgers & Sullivan, 2001). According to Bandura (1997), imagery can be a source of self-efficacy by providing people with a sense of performance accomplishment as well as vicarious experience. It is not surprising then, that self-efficacy-related imagery is frequently used by exercisers. Importantly, however, different types of self-efficacy have been found to play different roles in the initiation and maintenance of behavior. For example, an exerciser may feel confident in her ability to go for a 30-minute jog, but have little confidence that she could still do it if it were raining outside. Thus, the exerciser is high in self-efficacy related to the actual task (jogging for 30 minutes) but lower in her self-efficacy for overcoming a barrier to doing this on a regular basis (weather conditions). The implications of this are that interventions aimed at increasing one type of self-efficacy may not be effective for increasing the other types. Additionally, individuals may only be in need of an intervention that targets one type of self-efficacy. Therefore, understanding the ways in which different types of imagery relate to different types of self-efficacy may point to effective targets for exercise imagery interventions.

Although this line of research is relatively new, researchers have begun to identify clear links between the various imagery functions and different types of self-efficacy for exercise. Not surprisingly, use of the imagery functions is associated with specific types of self-efficacy in a very intuitive fashion. For example, individuals who more frequently use technique imagery, in which they imagine engaging in specific exercise tasks, tend to have greater task-related self-efficacy (Cumming, 2008). Energy imagery is also linked to task self-efficacy (Wesch, Milne, Burke, & Hall, 2006). Given that task self-efficacy may involve confidence for things like completing a workout with vigor and enthusiasm, and energy imagery may involve imagining completing a workout with vigor and enthusiasm, this link is intuitive. Thus, it seems clear that the content of exercise imagery is associated strongly with related types of self-efficacy.

Because of the strength of the relationships between imagery and self-efficacy, researchers have begun testing the hypothesis that imagery interventions may be used to increase self-efficacy for exercise which, in turn, will lead to actual engagement in exercise behavior.

In one study, sedentary women who wanted to begin a routine of regular exercise were assigned to one of three imagery intervention groups or to an attention-control group (Duncan, Rodgers, Hall, & Wilson, 2011). Each of the three imagery groups involved imagery related to a different type of self-efficacy for exercise (task, coping, and scheduling). In the task imagery group, participants imagined confidently engaging in the exercises and completing a session of moderate-intensity cardiovascular exercise. In the coping group, the participants imagined successfully overcoming some of the common barriers to regular exercise, such as exercising even if they were tired, stiff, or sore. In the scheduling group, women imagined successfully incorporating exercise into their daily and weekly routines. The findings from this study showed that as the participants began and maintained an exercise program, their self-efficacy increased in all three of these areas; but, in each group, the specific type of self-efficacy that they used in the imagery sessions increased the most. These findings showed that imagery can be used to increase self-efficacy for exercise and is thus an effective intervention tool in the exercise domain.

A second study looking at the impact of an imagery intervention on self-efficacy on exercise behavior involved a possible-selves imagery intervention (Murru & Martin Ginis, 2010). The participants in this study were university students who did not meet the guidelines for regular physical activity. The participants were asked to imagine either a hoped for possible-self or a feared possible self; or they were assigned to a control condition in which they completed a quiz about physical activity. The results showed that participants who engaged in the possible-selves imagery (both types), had significantly higher subsequent ratings of planning and barriers self-efficacy compared to participants in the control group. The participants in the imagery conditions also reported engaging in more minutes of physical activity during the four weeks following the intervention; however, this finding was non-significant. The results of this study suggest that imagery may increase self-efficacy and trigger the use of self-regulatory skills needed for engagement in exercise behavior. This study provided the first evidence supporting the possible impact of an imagery intervention on exercise behavior.

Imagery and Affect During and After Exercise

Although some people report that they enjoy exercising, most people do not find exercise to be inherently fun. Enjoyment of exercise, however, is associated with increased exercise participation. It has been suggested that imagery may be one way to increase perceptions of enjoyment related to exercise (Munroe-Chandler & Gammage, 2005). To test whether enjoyment of exercise could be enhanced using exercise imagery, Stanley and Cumming (2010) recruited 75 individuals to engage in one of three imagery conditions (enjoyment imagery, energy imagery, or technique imagery) while riding a stationary bike at a moderate intensity for 20 minutes. Controlling for pre-exercise affect, the researchers found that the enjoyment imagery group reported significantly more post-exercise enjoyment compared to the other two groups. This finding was corroborated by a second study in which 88 participants were assigned engaged in 20 minutes of moderate-intensity stationary cycling and either one of three imagery conditions (enjoyment imagery, energy imagery, technique imagery) or to a no-imagery control group. During the exercise bout, the participants in the enjoyment and energy imagery conditions reported more positive affect compared to the participants in the no-imagery control group. Participants in the enjoyment imagery and energy imagery conditions also reported greater changes in positive affect from pre- to post-exercise. Taken together, these two studies suggest that exercise imagery may indeed be useful for increasing affect during and after exercise.

Some initial evidence has also been presented for the utility of a guided imagery intervention that targeted intrinsic motivation (i.e., enjoyment of exercise) for increasing self-reported exercise behavior over a two-week period (Andersson & Moss, 2011). In this study, participants were assigned to engage in a single session of one of four conditions (guided imagery, implementation intentions, relaxation, or control). After two weeks, individuals in the guided imagery and implementation intention interventions reported having engaged in more exercise (as measured by exercise diaries) than participants in the other two groups. Thus, engaging imagery aimed at increasing intrinsic motivation may result in actual changes in exercise behavior. More research is needed to determine if these changes will persist over the long-term and contribute to an optimal pattern of exercise behavior.

Some General Recommendations

Although exercisers use both cognitive and motivational imagery, correlational studies show that the latter is used to a much greater extent. Because the many common barriers to regular exercise are motivational (e.g., Reichert, Barros, Domingues, & Hallal, 2007), using motivational imagery to encourage regular exercise may be ideal. Although no experimental studies have tested the optimal amount of exercise imagery, findings from correlational and experimental studies suggest that the more imagery that is used, the better the motivational and behavioral outcomes will be. Thus, both frequent and infrequent exercisers alike should be encouraged to frequently use exercise imagery.

Some other recommendations for imagery interventions are:

- Imagery can be used before or during an exercise session. The intervention research that has been conducted to date indicates that imagery can have a positive impact on motivational outcomes when it is employed before (Duncan et al., 2011; 2012) or during (Stanley & Cumming, 2010) an exercise session.
- Tailor imagery to the preferences of the individual exerciser. Some research has shown that subgroups of the population differentially endorse the imagery functions (e.g., Kim & Giacobbi, 2009). Ensuring that individuals utilize specific types of imagery that they buy into and that feel most natural for them, may result in better outcomes.
- Match the type of imagery used to the desired outcome of the imagery intervention. As suggested in the applied model of imagery use in exercise (Munroe-Chandler & Gammage, 2005), the type of imagery employed in an intervention should align with cognitive or motivational outcome that is targeted by the intervention.

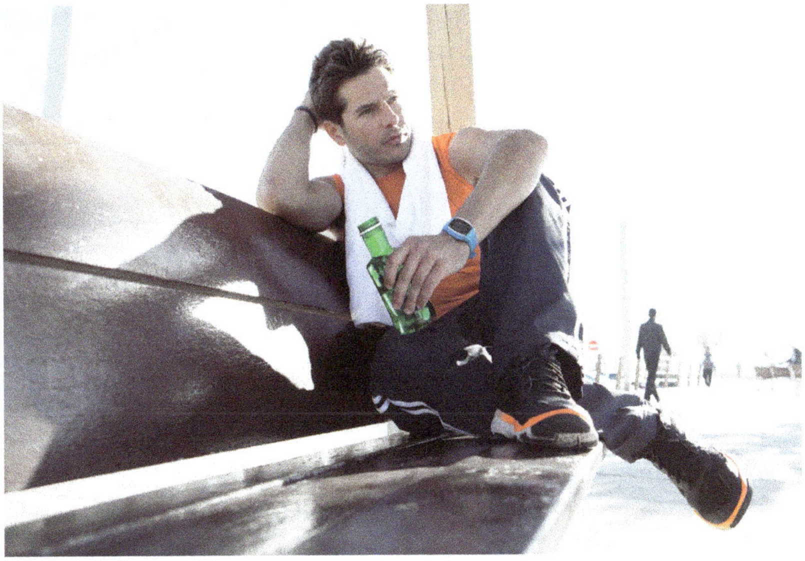

Image © MJTH, 2014. Used under license from Shutterstock, Inc.

Imagery in Sport Injury Rehabilitation

In the sport injury rehabilitation setting, imagery can serve a number of functions. Although athletes tend to use imagery less during rehabilitation than they do in training and competition, it is used for similar cognitive and motivational purposes. Athletes use imagery techniques to cope with the pain and stress of their injuries, to promote healing, and to enhance their motivation to adhere to rehabilitation programs (Brewer, Jeffers, Petitpas, & van Raalte, 1994; Evans, Hardy, & Fleming, 2000; Lynch, 1988; Porter & Foster, 1986; Rotella & Heyman, 1993; Singer & Johnson, 1987).

During rehabilitation, imagery is often used in conjunction with one or more additional psychological techniques, such as progressive relaxation, positive self-talk, or goal setting. Yet, whether it is used alone or as part of a more comprehensive psychological strategy, those who use imagery as part of their treatment program generally report less pain, faster recovery, and significantly better overall mood as rehabilitation progresses (Christakou & Zervas, 2007; Ievleva & Orlick, 1991; Johnson, 2000).

Athletes who use imagery during rehabilitation typically rely heavily on cognitive and motivational imagery, but also use healing and pain management imagery intermittently as they recover. Visual and auditory imagery modalities are used occasionally, but kinesthetic imagery is used most frequently because of its connection to not only the rehearsal of rehabilitation exercises, but to the mental practice of sport-specific skills as well (Driediger, Hall, & Callow, 2006). Athletes who regularly employ imagery report using it less during rehabilitation than they do in training and competition (Sordoni, Hall, & Forwell, 2000).

Cognitive Imagery Interventions

In the rehabilitation setting, CS imagery is primarily used to learn and perform therapeutic exercises properly. It is typically initiated immediately before and during each exercise at a therapy appointment. CS imagery is also used to re-learn previously automated skills. For example, a runner who has experienced prolonged recovery after a knee injury might use imagery to regain his or her normal gait pattern (Driediger et al., 2006). CS imagery has also been shown to significantly predict self-efficacy in rehabilitations settings. Milne, Hall, and Forwell (2005) surveyed 270 injured athletes to explore the relationship between imagery use, self-efficacy, and adherence to rehabilitation programs. They found that cognitive imagery accounted for 1.8% of the variance in task self-efficacy, which in turn significantly predicted exercise quality.

CG imagery is not used for purposes directly related to rehabilitation, but can help injured athletes maintain their strategic abilities in their sport. This type of imagery allows athletes to mentally practice strategies and tactics related to performance while they are unable to do so physically. Injured athletes who still attend team practices may use this type of imagery to practice drills that their teammates are working on in real time, giving them some ability to stay current with their training.

Motivational Imagery Interventions

Motivational imagery is widely used in conjunction with rehabilitation, and is arguably the most important function of imagery in this setting. Broadly, it is used for goal setting and to enhance mental toughness, maintain concentration, and foster positive attitudes through the difficulties of recovery. MS imagery targets process and outcome goals related to rehabilitation. Athletes use this to motivate themselves to perform rehabilitation exercises. For example, an athlete might imagine that each exercise repetition is a step toward a treatment goal or milestone, like being able to move from basic range of motion exercises to resistance training. Athletes also use MS imagery to motivate themselves toward specific outcome goals such as being fully recovered, returning to their training schedule, or ultimately winning a major competition. Importantly, research evidence suggests that motivational imagery has only a weak to moderate relationship with rehabilitation adherence (Scherzer, Brewer, Cornelius, van Raalte, Petitpas, Sklar et al., 2001). Wesch and colleagues (2011) conducted a prospective observational study of 90 injured athletes receiving treatment through outpatient physiotherapy clinics to investigate the relationship between motivational imagery use and treatment adherence. They found that motivational imagery had weak associations with exercise frequency and duration, but these associations became reciprocal in nature toward the end (weeks 6–8) of the rehab program. That is, greater use of imagery increased adherence, and increased adherence promoted more imagery use (Wesch, Hall, Prapavessis, Maddison, Bassett, Foley et al., 2011). Achieving positive treatment outcomes is a more powerful motivator than simply imaging positive outcomes, but motivational imagery may improve adherence as rehabilitation progresses and therefore lead to better overall recovery.

MG imagery performs two functions in rehabilitation (Driediger et al., 2006). Firstly, it is used to modulate arousal (i.e., MG-A imagery). Athletes can employ calming images to control the stress associated with their injury and being unable to play, or they may use energizing images to facilitate stress and get "fired up" to complete their rehabilitation sessions. Secondly, it performs a mastery-based function (i.e., MG-M imagery). In this scenario, it is used to maintain focus during rehabilitation and to motivate the athlete to get through difficult or painful situations. Although MG imagery is related to self-efficacy in training and competition, it is not often used to increase confidence or maintain a positive attitude during rehabilitation.

Healing Imagery Interventions

Healing imagery is unique to the injury rehabilitation setting, and can take the form of either positive images of internal physiological processes (e.g., a fractured bone knitting back together) or external recovery images (e.g., regaining quadriceps strength after knee surgery) (Lynch, 1988; Rotella & Heyman, 1993). It is generally used during sedentary physiotherapy activities like icing, and before going to sleep (Driediger et al., 2006).

Healing imagery has been associated with faster recovery times for injured athletes. Ievleva and Orlick (1991) divided 32 recovered ankle or knee injury patients into three groups (fast, moderate, and slow healers, based on recovery times) and collected information about their healing imagery use during rehabilitation. The results demonstrated that the use of healing imagery was significantly associated with faster recovery. There have also been medium to large treatment effects of healing imagery on pain (Christakou & Zervas, 2007; Cupal & Brewer, 2001), edema (Christakou & Zervas, 2007), muscular endurance during rehabilitation exercises (Christakou, Zervas, & Lavallee, 2007), muscular strength (Cupal & Brewer, 2001), and re-injury anxiety (Cupal & Brewer, 2001).

Pain Management Imagery Interventions

Athletes use pain management imagery specifically to prepare for expected pain, provide a distraction during painful situations, and to block or disperse pain (Driediger et al., 2006). Athletes may use techniques such as focusing on their pain-free future selves, "shutting off" their minds, using cold images to dull pain, or visualizing discomfort dispersing slowly in order to cope with pain from their injury itself, or during treatment. There has been limited research in this area, but evidence supports the effectiveness of pain management imagery during injury rehabilitation, particularly following surgical procedures (Ross & Berger, 1996). Cupal and Brewer (2001) conducted a randomized controlled trial in which an intervention group (n = 10) received 10 guided imagery sessions following anterior cruciate ligament reconstruction. At 24 weeks post-surgery, the intervention group reported significantly greater knee strength and significantly less re-injury anxiety and pain compared to the placebo and control groups. Pain management imagery may therefore be a useful addition to post-operative treatment, although more research is needed in this area.

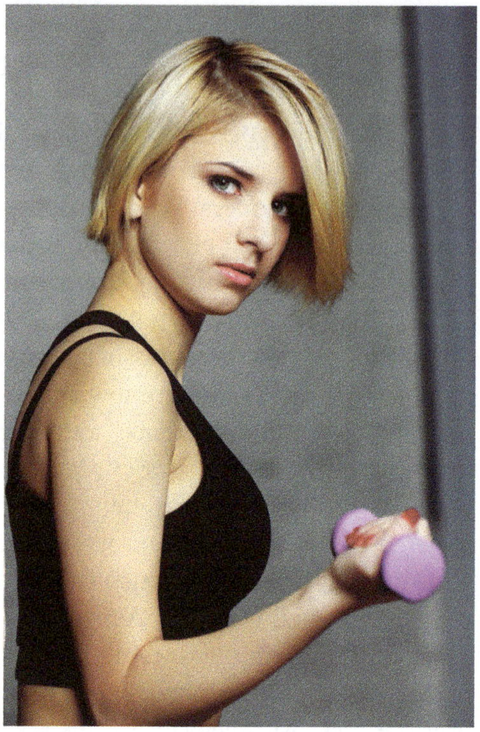

Special Considerations in Injury Rehabilitation

When athletes use imagery during injury rehabilitation, they report using it most frequently during physiotherapy appointments (Driediger et al., 2006). The thirty seconds just before performing an exercise provides an opportunity for the athlete to mentally rehearse the movements and to prepare for any anticipated discomfort. Imagery also serves pain management and motivational purposes, but in different proportions at certain stages of recovery.

Early rehabilitation phase. The period immediately after sustaining an injury is often characterized by feelings of distress, particularly for elite level athletes. While coping with intense negative emotions during this time, athletes may not be ready to fully engage in their rehabilitation, so the use of psychological skills like imagery may not be helpful in the first few treatment sessions. Athletes have also reported being unable to control their images in the days or weeks after injury, experiencing spontaneous negative flashbacks of the injury event (Evans, Hare, & Mullen, 2006).

To focus imagery in a constructive way, it is important that physicians and therapists provide detailed injury information to the athlete. This can facilitate imagery by giving the athlete specific understanding of the anatomical structures and physiological processes underlying recovery (Green, 1992; Heil, 1993). Having visual reference material, such as x-rays or surgical videos, can help the athlete produce clear, vivid images. Additionally, athletes should be given an outline of their rehabilitation program, including general timelines, recovery expectations, and the evaluation criteria that the medical team will use to assess progress. This will help the athlete to set goals and match his or her imagery to the current stage of rehabilitation. It may also be helpful to have the athlete speak with a peer who has undergone rehabilitation for the same injury in order to develop imagery clarity and vividness. Asking the athlete to describe the sensations and emotions associated with the injury, then using those descriptive words in imagery scripts, can help make imagery more personal and effective.

In the early stages, imagery is used to foster a positive attitude toward rehabilitation, to build the athlete's confidence to perform exercises, and to encourage healing. It also serves a pain management function. Greater use of pain-focused imagery has been observed at the beginning of rehabilitation programs than later in recovery. Kinesthetic imagery may be more vivid than other forms of imagery at this stage, due to the physical sensations associated with the injury itself, and the emphasis on movement and control while learning to perform therapeutic exercises (Hare, Evans, & Callow, 2008).

Mid-rehabilitation phase. Imagery use typically increases as recovery progresses because athletes gain familiarity with the use of imagery in the rehabilitation setting and the routine of rehabilitation activities becomes more comfortable. For those who are unaccustomed to using imagery in training and competition, new exercises may take additional effort to image successfully. Setting aside time to practice imagery skills can be a valuable part of the rehabilitation program for these individuals (Hare et al., 2008).

Generally, imagery during the mid-rehabilitation phase is more positive than during early rehabilitation (Evans et al., 2006). It continues to serve healing and pain management functions, and is increasingly used as a motivation tool to promote rehabilitation adherence (Evans et al., 2006). Importantly, adherence motivation may be linked to rehabilitation progression (Hare et al., 2008). Athletes who perceive that they are not healing as quickly as they should be, or who feel as though they have reached a plateau in their recovery, often have difficulty persevering in their rehabilitation program. It is therefore crucial to ensure that imagery accurately reflects rehabilitation goals and realistically depicts the individual's recovery trajectory.

As rehabilitation continues, athletes begin to use CS imagery to rehearse sport performance skills. This allows them to maintain their training to some extent by mentally running drills and executing plays. This may be particularly important for those with prolonged recovery times after severe injury. Imagining themselves executing specific skills can help keep athletes feeling engaged with their sport, preventing impressions of falling hopelessly behind in their training. As athletes begin looking ahead to returning to sport, feeling as though they have been able to practice some aspect of performance while injured can be a powerful motivator to get through the later stages of rehabilitation.

End of rehabilitation/return to sport phase. When athletes are close to recovery and approaching a return to sport, the motivation function of imagery is largely gone, replaced with an emphasis on skill rehearsal and performance confidence. CS and, to a lesser extent CG imagery, are used to build confidence in the athlete's ability to overcome the potential loss of skill or fitness associated with time away from training, doubts about performance, and re-injury fears (Evans et al., 2006). Athletes typically do not use imagery for healing or pain management purposes at this point in rehabilitation.

Although the focus tends to be on positive future-self images, some unintentional negative images may arise as return to sport approaches. Athletes may be distracted by thoughts of the worst possible outcomes, like re-injury or poor performance (Monsma, Mensch, & Farroll, 2009). These images can sometimes be created on purpose, however, to motivate the athlete to increase his or her effort through the end of rehabilitation in order to avoid such negative events (Driediger et al., 2006). This illustrates the combination of automatic and deliberate imagery that exists during this stage of recovery, marking the transition back to performance-oriented imagery applications (Hare et al., 2008).

One of the greatest barriers to implementing an imagery intervention during rehabilitation is the fact that therapists may not see the benefit of using it (Francis, Andersen, & Maley, 2000; Wiese, Weiss, & Yukelson, 1991). In some cases, these individuals may simply have too little experience with imagery to understand its effects, or others may not believe in its efficacy (Green, 1992). Wiese et al. (1991) administered a questionnaire to 115 Athletic Trainers to investigate the use of psychological strategies with injured athletes. They found that athletes' understanding of imagery was rated much lower in importance during rehabilitation than other factors including interpersonal communication by the trainer, coach support, and a focus on short-term treatment goals. In the same survey, trainers' understanding of imagery was rated as much less important than their ability to enhance patient self-confidence, understand motivation, or set realistic goals. This is not to say that therapists have negative attitudes toward psychological interventions in general, merely that imagery and other techniques are typically viewed as less influential than other treatment factors.

There is some indication that athletic therapists tend to have more positive views of imagery than physiotherapists (Hamson-Utley, Martin, & Walters, 2008). This is likely due to the level of familiarity with psychological interventions that athletic therapists gain through their proximity to athletes during training and competition. Regardless of their level of awareness, however, therapists may have limited competence to deal with psychological issues in rehabilitation (Gordon, Milios, & Grove, 1991). Athletes with previous injury experience, especially those who have used imagery during rehabilitation before, may be able to manage this aspect of their treatment independently (Hare et al., 2008). In other cases, enlisting the services of a sport psychology consultant during rehabilitation can improve treatment outcomes.

Patient acceptance of treatment may have a powerful influence on the recovery process. If athletes believe that imagery is efficacious, they are more likely to use it and to experience its benefits. Brewer and colleagues (1994) conducted a series of studies to examine perceptions of psychological interventions and found high mean ratings for imagery intervention acceptability amongst a small sample of sport medicine patients. Moreover, there is evidence that athletes receiving physiotherapy believe imagery can serve cognitive, motivational, and healing purposes (Driediger et al., 2006). Fostering these beliefs can encourage athletes to use imagery more frequently and with greater quality during injury rehabilitation.

How It Is Measured

The Athletic Injury Imagery Questionnaire-2 (AIIQ-2) was developed specifically to assess imagery use during injury rehabilitation. It is a 12-item questionnaire with an equal number of questions examining the cognitive, motivational, and healing functions of imagery. Example items include: "Prior to performing a rehabilitation exercise, I am able to imagine myself completing it perfectly" (cognitive); "I imagine myself achieving my treatment goals" (motivational); and "I imagine my body repairing itself" (healing). Imagery use is rated on a 9-point Likert scale from 1 "never" to 9 "always" (Sordoni, Hall, & Forwell, 2002). It has been used extensively in the literature, and has been shown to be valid and reliable in a number of study populations (Driediger et al., 2006; Hare et al., 2008; Milne et al., 2005; Wesch et al., 2011; Sordoni et al., 2002).

Why It Works

There are a number of hypotheses to explain why imagery helps athletes during injury rehabilitation, although there has been very little research in this area. In this setting imagery is often considered to be mental rehearsal for physical skills, used to re-establish fine and gross motor movements (Green, 1992). To account for its effect on muscle activation, psychoneuromuscular theory suggests that vivid imagined events elicit neuromuscular responses similar to those produced by actual physical execution of the movements (Jacobson, 1930; Hale, 1982; Harris & Robinson, 1986; Christakou, Zervas, & Lavallee, 2007). Conversely, the neural training hypothesis states that imagery leads to adaptive changes in the same central processes that are responsible for increasing muscle activation during muscle training (Enoka & Fuglevand, 1993; Jeannerod, 1995; Ranganathan, Siemionow, Liu, Sahgal, & Yue, 2003; Rieser, 2005). Although there is some evidence in support of both theories, the mechanism underlying the effect of imagery on muscle activation is still unclear.

In terms of pain management, it has been proposed that imagery practice leads to a state of hypoarousal, whereby sympathetic nervous system activation is attenuated, resulting in decreased pain and greater overall relaxation (Christakou & Zervas, 2007; Jacobs, Benson, & Friedman, 1996; Lazar, Bush, Gollub, Fricchione, Khalsa, & Benson, 2000). Gate control theory postulates that imagery may block thoughts of pain, which decreases perceptions of pain and ultimately reduces the amount of painful stimuli transmitted to the brain (Christakou & Zervas, 2007; Melzack, 1999; 2001). A third hypothesis is that imagery causes a release of endorphins, which diminish the sensation of pain through inhibition of afferent neurons projecting to the brain (Christakou & Zervas, 2007; Ganong, 2003; Rosenzweig, Leiman, & Breedlove, 1999). Unfortunately, however, there is a paucity of research support for any one individual theory and future studies will be needed to explain the effect of imagery on pain.

Some General Recommendations

Imagery is not a stand-alone intervention in injury rehabilitation. There is no substitute for physical therapy, so imagery should be used as adjunct to established treatment protocols. Structured rehabilitation that includes imagery has been shown to be more effective than standard treatment alone (Brewer et al., 1994; Cupal, 1998; Faris, 1985; Ievleva & Orlick, 1991). Indeed, athletes who use imagery report increased satisfaction with their rehabilitation experience compared to those who do not (Law, Driediger, Hall, & Forwell, 2006).

Furthermore, it is important for injured athletes to feel like active agents in their own recovery (Durso-Cupal, 1996; Cupal & Brewer, 2001). For individuals who are accustomed to having mastery over their physical performance, passively undergoing treatment can be frustrating and demoralizing. Even when the athlete has limited control over the healing process, using imagery can help him or her feel involved and able to actively work toward a positive rehabilitation outcome.

Some other recommendations for imagery interventions are:

- Explain to the athlete the additional benefits of using imagery during rehabilitation, to make sure he or she has realistic expectations about the added value of imagery in the treatment program.

- Even athletes who use imagery regularly in training and competition may find the rehabilitation setting challenging; unfamiliar movements may be difficult to visualize, or negative emotional responses to treatment setbacks might interfere with successful imaging.
- Make sure imagery timing and content is situation appropriate, because imagery that is matched to appropriate goals during recovery will increase imagery quality and motivation to continue using it (Evans et al., 2006).

CHAPTER SUMMARY

Mental imagery plays an important role in sport, exercise, and injury rehabilitation. It serves both cognitive and motivational functions, although the extent to which these types of imagery are used depends on the setting. The cognitive function of imagery in sport is related to rehearsing skills and strategies associated with sport performance. Similarly, the role of cognitive imagery in exercise and injury rehabilitation is primarily to support techniques associated with performing specific exercises. Differences begin to emerge, however, when examining the motivational role of imagery. In sport, motivational imagery is used to support cognitions related to goal achievement, arousal regulation, and self-confidence. In exercise it is also used for purposes related to energy and self-efficacy, but can be used for motivations associated with appearance, fitness and health, and emotional control as well. In rehabilitation, motivational imagery is largely associated with goal setting, arousal regulation, and maintaining mental focus, and is often used in conjunction with healing and pain control imagery.

Imagery has been shown to have powerful effects on behavior, self-confidence, and a number of other cognitions, but it is a skill and requires deliberate practice to be used successfully. As an intervention, imagery techniques show promise for applications ranging from improving tactical performance in sport, to maintaining regular exercise behavior, to speeding recovery times after orthopaedic surgery. Although much additional research is needed, there is evidence that including imagery as part of sport and exercise routines can lead to better overall outcomes for individual athletes and exercisers.

ENDNOTE

1. Some researchers have made a distinction between two types of technique imagery (Giacobbi et al., 2003). Specifically, Giacobbi et al. (2003) describe exercise technique imagery as being distinct from aerobic routines.

REVIEW QUESTIONS

1. Identify the types of cognitive and motivational imagery used by athletes.
2. What have cognitive imagery interventions with athletes shown?
3. What are the general findings from MGM imagery interventions implemented with athletes?
4. Which imagery function is used most frequently by exercisers?
5. How might imagery ability impact the behavioral or cognitive outcomes of an exercise imagery intervention?
6. Discuss how imagery can be used during exercise to impact motivational outcomes.

7. How is CG imagery used during injury rehabilitation?
8. What are the two functions of MG imagery during rehabilitation?
9. Identify some of the barriers to implementing an imagery intervention during rehabilitation, and describe how you would overcome these.

SUGGESTED READINGS

Blair, A., Hall, C., & Leyshon, G. (1993). Imagery effects on the performance of skilled and novice soccer players. *Journal of Sports Sciences, 11*, 95–101.

Callow, N., Hardy, L., & Hall, C. (2001). The effects of a motivational general-mastery imagery intervention on the sport confidence of high-level badminton players. *Research Quarterly for Exercise and Sport, 72*(4), 389–400.

Cumming, J., Olphin, T., & Law, M. (2007). Self-reported psychological states and physiological responses to different types of motivational general imagery. *Journal of Sport & Exercise Psychology, 29*, 629–644.

Cupal, D. D., & Brewer, B. W. (2001). Effects of relaxation and guided imagery on knee strength, reinjury anxiety, and pain following anterior cruciate ligament reconstruction. *Rehabilitation Psychology, 46*(1) 28–43.

Driediger, M., Hall, C., Callow, N. (2006). Imagery use by injured athletes: A qualitative analysis. *Journal of Sports Sciences 24*(3), 261–271.

Duncan, L. R., Hall, C. R., Wilson, P. M., & Rodgers, W. M. (2012). The use of a mental imagery intervention to enhance integrated regulation for exercise among women commencing an exercise program. *Motivation and Emotion, 36*, 452–464.

REFERENCES

Andersson, E. K., & Moss, T. P. (2011). Imagery and implementation intention: A randomized controlled trial of interventions to increase exercise behaviour in the general population. *Psychology of Sport and Exercise, 12*, 63–70.

Annett, J. (1995). On knowing how to do things: A theory of motor imagery. *Cognitive Brain Research, 3*, 65–69.

Bandura, A. (1997). *Self-efficacy: The exercise of control.* New York: W.H. Freeman.

Betts, G. H. (1909). *The distribution and functions of mental imagery.* New York, NY: Columbia University, Teachers College.

Blair, A., Hall, C., & Leyshon, G. (1993). Imagery effects on the performance of skilled and novice soccer players. *Journal of Sports Sciences, 11*, 95–101.

Brewer, B. W., Jeffers, K. E., Petitpas, A. J., & van Raalte, J. L. (1994). Perceptions of psychological interventions in the context of sport injury rehabilitation. *The Sport Psychologist, 8*, 176–188.

Bull, S. J., Albinson, J. G., & Shambrook, J. (1996). *The mental game plan: Getting psyched for sport.* Brighton, UK: Sports Dynamic.

Callow, N., Hardy, L., & Hall, C. (2001). The effects of a motivational general-mastery imagery intervention on the sport confidence of high-level badminton players. *Research Quarterly for Exercise and Sport, 72*(4), 389–400.

Christakou, A., & Zervas, Y. (2007). The effectiveness of imagery on pain, edema, and range of motion in athletes with a grade II ankle sprain. *Physical Therapy in Sport 8,* 130–140.

Christakou, A., Zervas, Y., & Lavallee, D. (2007). The adjunctive role of imagery on the functional rehabilitation of a grade II ankle sprain. *Human Movement Science 26,* 141–154.

Clark, L. V. (1960). Effect of mental practice on the development of a certain motor skill. *Research Quarterly, 31*, 560–569.

Cogan, K. D., & Petrie, T. A. (1995). Sport consultation: An evaluation of a season-long intervention with female collegiate gymnasts. *The Sport Psychologist, 9*, 282–296.

Cumming, J. (2008). Investigating the relationship between exercise imagery, leisure-time exercise behavior, and self-efficacy. *Journal of Applied Sport Psychology, 20,* 184–198.

Cumming, J., & Hall, C. (2002). Deliberate imagery practice: The development of imagery skills in competitive athletes. *Journal of Sport Sciences, 20*, 137–145.

Cumming, J., Olphin, T., & Law, M. (2007). Self-reported psychological states and physiological responses to different types of motivational general imagery. *Journal of Sport & Exercise Psychology, 29*, 629–644.

Cumming, J., & Stanley, D. M. (2009). Are images of exercising related to feeling states? *Journal of Imagery Research in Sport and Physical Activity, 4,* 1–20.

Cupal, D. D. (1998). Psychological interventions in sport injury prevention and rehabilitation. *Journal of Applied Sport Psychology, 10,* 103–123.

Cupal, D. D., & Brewer, B. W. (2001). Effects of relaxation and guided imagery on knee strength, reinjury anxiety, and pain following anterior cruciate ligament reconstruction. *Rehabilitation Psychology, 46*(1) 28–43.

Deci, E. L., & Ryan, R. M. (1985). *Intrinsic motivation and self-determination in human behaviour.* New York, NY: Plenum Press.

Denis, M. (1985). Visual imagery and the use of mental practice in the development of motor skills. *Canadian Journal of Applied Sport Sciences, 10*, 4S–16S.

Driediger, M., Hall, C., & Callow, N. (2006). Imagery use by injured athletes: A qualitative analysis. *Journal of Sports Sciences 24*, 261–271.

Duncan, L. R., Hall, C. R., Wilson, P. M., & Rodgers, W. M. (2012). The use of a mental imagery intervention to enhance integrated regulation for exercise among women commencing an exercise program. *Motivation and Emotion, 36,* 452–464.

Duncan, L. R., Rodgers, W. M., Hall, C. R., & Wilson, P. M. (2011). Using imagery to enhance three types of exercise self-efficacy among sedentary women. *Applied Psychology: Health and Well-Being, 3,* 107–126.

Durand, M., Hall, C., & Haslam, I. R. (1997). The effects of combining mental and physical practice on motor skill acquisition: A review of the literature and some practical implications. *The Hong Kong Journal of Sports Medicine and Sports Science, 4,* 36–41.

Durso-Cupal, D. D. (1996). The efficacy of guided imagery on recovery for individuals with anterior cruciate ligament (ACL) replacement. (Unpublished doctoral dissertation.) Utah State University, Logan, UT, USA.

Enoka, R. M., & Fuglevand, A. J. (1993). Neuromuscular basis of maximum voluntary force capacity of muscle. In M. D. Grabiner (Ed.), *Current issues in biomechanics* (pp. 215–235). Champaign, IL: Human Kinetics.

Evans, L., Hardy, L., & Fleming, S. (2000). Intervention strategies with injured athletes: An action research study. *The Sport Psychologist, 14,* 188–206.

Evans, L., Hare, R., & Mullen, R. (2006). Imagery use during rehabilitation from injury. *Journal of Imagery Research in Sport and Physical Activity 1,* 1–19.

Faris, G. J. (1985). Psychological aspects of athletic rehabilitation. *Clinics in Sports Medicine, 4,* 545–551.

Francis, S. R., Andersen, M. B., & Maley, P. (2000). Physiotherapists' and male professional athletes' views on psychological skills for rehabilitation. *Journal of Science and Medicine in Sport 3*(1) 17–29.

Gammage, K. L., Hall, C. R., & Martin Ginis, K. A. (2004). Self-presentation in exercise contexts: Differences between high and low frequency exercisers. *Journal of Applied Social Psychology, 34,* 1638–1651.

Gammage, K. L., Hall, C. R., & Rodgers, W. M. (2000). More about exercise imagery. *The Sport Psychologist, 34,* 348–359.

Ganong, W. F. (2003). *Review of medical physiology.* New York: Lange Medical Books, McGraw-Hill.

Giacobbi, P. R. Jr. (2007). Age and activity-level differences in the use of exercise imagery. *Journal of Applied Sport Psychology, 19,* 487–493.

Giacobbi, P., Hausenblas, H., Fallon, E., & Hall, C. (2003). Even more about exercise imagery: A grounded theory of exercise imagery. *Journal of Applied Sport Psychology, 15,* 160–175.

Giacobbi, P. R. Jr., Hausenblas, H. A., & Penfield, R. D. (2005). Further refinements in the measurement of exercise imagery: The Exercise Imagery Inventory. *Measurement in Physical Education and Exercise Science, 9,* 251–266.

Gordon, S., Milios, D. & Grove, J. R. (1991). Psychological aspects of the recovery process from sport physiotherapists. *Australian Journal of Science and Medicine in Sport, 23,* 53–60.

Goss, S., Hall, C., Buckolz, E., & Fishburne, G. (1986). Imagery ability and the acquisition and retention of movements. *Memory & Cognition, 14,* 469–477.

Green, L. B. (1992). The use of imagery in the rehabilitation of injured athletes. *The Sport Psychologist, 6,* 416–428.

Gregg, M., Hall, C., & Hanton, S. (2007). Perceived effectiveness of mental imagery. *Journal of Sport Behavior, 30,* 398–414.

Gregg, M., Hall, C., & Nederhof, E. (2005). The imagery ability, imagery use and performance relationship. *The Sport Psychologist, 19,* 93–99.

Guillot, A., Nadrowska, E., & Collet, C. (2009). Using motor imagery to learn tactical movements in basketball. *Journal of Sport Behavior, 32*(2), 189–206.

Hale, B. D. (1982). The effects of internal and external imagery on muscular and ocular concomitants. *Journal of Sport Psychology, 4,* 379–387.

Hall, C. R. (1995). The motivational function of mental imagery for participation in sport and exercise. In J. Annett, B. Cripps, & H. Steinberg (Eds.), *Exercise addiction: Motivation for participation in sport and exercise* (pp. 15–21). Leicester, UK: British Psychological Society.

Hall, C. R. (2001). Imagery in sport and exercise. In R. N. Singer, H. A. Hausenblas, & C. M. Janelle (Eds.), *Handbook of sport psychology* (2nd ed., pp. 529–549). New York: John Wiley & Sons.

Hall, C. R., Buckolz, E., & Fishburne, G. J. (1989). Searching for a relationship between imagery ability and memory of movements. *Journal of Human Movement Studies, 17,* 89–100.

Hall, C. R., Mack, D. E., Paivio, A., & Hausenblas, H. A. (1998). Imagery use by athletes: Development of the sport imagery questionnaire. *International Journal of Sport Psychology, 29,* 73–89.

Hall, C. R., Munroe-Chandler, K. J., Fishburne, G. J., & Hall, N. D. (2009). The Sport Imagery Questionnaire for Children (SIQ-C). *Measurement in Physical Education and Exercise Science, 13,* 93–107.

Hall, C. R., Rodgers, W. M., Wilson, P. M., & Norman, P. (2010). Imagery use and self-determined motivations in a community sample of exercisers and non-exercisers. *Journal of Applied Social Psychology, 40,* 135–152.

Hall, C. R., Stevens, D. E., & Paivio, A. (2005). *The Sport Imagery Questionnaire: Test manual.* Morgantown, WV: Fitness Information Technology.

Hamson-Utley, J. J., Martin, S., & Walters, J. (2008). Athletic trainers' and physical therapists' perceptions of the effectiveness of psychological skills within sport injury rehabilitation programs. *Journal of Athletic Training 43*(3), 258–264.

Hare, R., Evans, L., & Callow, N. (2008). Imagery use during rehabilitation from injury: A case study of an elite athlete. *The Sport Psychologist, 22,* 405–422.

Harris, D. V., & Robinson, W. J. (1986). The effects of skill level on EMG activity during internal and external imagery. *Journal of Sport Psychology, 8,* 105–111.

Hausenblas, H. A., Hall, C. R., Rodgers, W. M., & Munroe, K. J. (1999). Exercise imagery: Its nature and measurement. *Journal of Applied Sport Psychology, 11,* 171–180.

Hausenblas, H. A., & Symons Downs, D. (2002). Relationship among sex, imagery, and exercise dependence symptoms. *Psychology of Addictive Behaviors, 16,* 169–172.

Heil, J. (1993). Mental training in injury management. In J. Heil (Ed.), *Psychology of sport injury* (pp. 151–174). Champaign, IL: Human Kinetics.

Holmes, P. S., & Collins, D. J. (2001). The PETTLEP approach to motor imagery: A functional equivalence model for sport psychologists. *Journal of Applied Sport Psychology, 13,* 60–83.

Ievleva, L., & Orlick, T. (1991). Mental links to enhanced healing: An exploratory study. *The Sport Psychologist, 5,* 25–40.

Jacobs, G. D., Benson, H., & Friedman, R. (1996). Topographic EEG mapping of the relaxation response. *Biofeedback and Self Regulation, 21,* 121–129.

Jacobson, E. (1930). Electrical measurements of neuromuscular states during mental activities. *American Journal of Physiology, 94,* 22–34.

Jeannerod, M. (1995). Mental imagery in the motor context. *Neuropsychologia 33,* 1419–1432.

Johnson, E. L., & Lutgendorf, S. K. (2002). Contributions of imagery ability to stress and relaxation. *Annals of Behavioral Medicine, 23,* 273–281.

Johnson, U. (2000). Short-term psychological intervention: a study of long-term injured competitive athletes. *Journal of Sport Rehabilitation, 9,* 207–218.

Kim, B. H., & Giacobbi, P. R. Jr. (2009). The use of exercise-related mental imagery by middle-aged adults. *Journal of Imagery Research in Sport and Physical Activity, 4,* 1–38.

Law, B., Driediger, M., Hall, C., & Forwell, L. (2006). Imagery use, perceived pain, limb functioning and satisfaction in athletic injury rehabilitation. *New Zealand Journal of Physiotherapy, 34*(1), 10–16.

Lazar, S. W., Bush, G., Gollub, R. L., Fricchione, G. L., Khalsa, G., & Benson, H. (2000). Functional brain mapping of the relaxation response and meditation. *Neuroreport, 11,* 1581–1585.

Lynch, G. P. (1988). Athletic injuries and the practicing sport psychologist: Practical guidelines for assisting athletes. *The Sport Psychologist, 2,* 161–167.

Martin, K. A., Moritz, S. E., & Hall, C. R. (1999). Imagery use in sport: A literature review and applied model. *The Sport Psychologist, 13,* 245–268.

McAuley, E., & Jacobson, L. (1991). Self-efficacy and exercise participation in sedentary adult females. *American Journal of Health Promotion, 5,* 185–207.

McAuley, E., Pena, M. M., & Jerome, G. J. (2001). Self-efficacy as a determinant and an outcome of exercise. In G. C. Roberts (Ed.), *Advances in motivation in sport and exercise* (pp. 235–261). Champaign, IL: Human Kinetics.

Melzack, R. (1999). From the gate to the neuromatrix. *Pain Supplement 6,* S121–126.

Melzack, R. (2001). Pain and the neuromatrix in the brain. *Journal of Dental Education 65,* 1378–1382.

Milne, M., Hall, C., & Forwell, L. (2005). Self-efficacy, imagery use, and adherence to rehabilitation by injured athletes. *Journal of Sport Rehabilitation, 14,* 150–167.

Monsma, E., Mensch, J., & Farroll, J. (2009). Keeping your head in the game: Sport-specific imagery and anxiety among injured athletes. *Journal of Athletic Training 44*(4), 410–417.

Morris, T., Spittle, M., & Watt, A. P. (2005). *Imagery in sport.* Champaign, IL: Human Kinetics.

Munroe, K. J., Hall, C. R., Simms, S., & Weinberg, R. (1998). The influence of type of sport and time of season on athletes' use of imagery. *The Sport Psychologist, 12,* 440–449.

Munroe-Chandler, K. J., & Gammage, K. L. (2005). Now see this: A new vision of exercise imagery. *Exercise and Sport Science Reviews, 33,* 201–205.

Munroe-Chandler, K. J., Hall, C. R., Fishburne, G. J., & Shannon, V. (2005). Using cognitive general imagery to improve soccer strategies. *European Journal of Sport Science, 5*(1), 41–49.

Munroe-Chandler, K. J., Hall, C., Fishburne, G., & Strachan, L. (2007). Where, when and why athletes use imagery: An examination of developmental differences. *Research Quarterly for Sport and Exercise, 78*(2), 103–116.

Munroe-Chandler, K. J., Kim, A. J., & Gammage, K. L. (2004). Using imagery to predict weightlifting dependency in men. *International Journal of Men's Health, 3,* 129–139.

Murru, E. C., & Martin Ginis, K. A. (2010). Imagining the possibilities: The effects of a possible selves intervention on self-regulatory efficacy and exercise behavior. *Journal of Sport and Exercise Psychology, 32,* 537–554.

Paivio, A. (1985). Cognitive and motivational functions of imagery in human performance. *Canadian Journal of Applied Sport Science, 10,* 22–28.

Paivio, A. (1986). *Mental representations: a dual coding approach.* Oxford. England: Oxford University Press.

Perry, C., & Morris, T. (1995). Mental imagery in sport. In T. Morris & J. Summers (Eds.), *Sport psychology: Theory, applications and issues* (pp. 339–385). Brisbane, Australia: Wiley.

Pham, L. E., & Taylor, S. E. (1999). From thought to action: Effects of process-versus outcome-based mental simulations on performance. *Personality and Social Psychology Bulletin, 25,* 250–260.

Porter, K., & Foster, J. (1986). *The mental athlete: Inner training for peak performance.* New York: Ballantine Books.

Ranganathan, V. K., Siemionow, V., Liu, Z. J, Sahgal, V., & Yue, G. H. (2003). From mental power to muscle power—gaining strength by using the mind. *Neuropsychologia, 42,* 944–956.

Rawlings, E. I., Rawlings, I. L., Chen, S. S., & Yilk, D. (1972). The facilitating effects of mental rehearsal in the acquisition of pursuit tracking. *Psychonomic Science, 26,* 71–73.

Reichert, F. F., Barros, A. J. D., Domingues, M. R., & Hallal, P. C. (2007). The role of perceived personal barriers to engagement in leisure-time physical activity. *American Journal of Public Health, 97,* 515–519.

Richardson, P. A., & Latuda, L. M. (1995). Therapeutic imagery and athletic injuries. *Journal of Athletic Training 30*(1) 10–12.

Rieser, M. (2005). Strength gains by motor imagery of maximal contractions. *Zeitschrift Fur Sport Psychologie, 12,* 11–21.

Rodgers, W. M., & Gauvin, L. (1998). Heterogeneity of incentives for physical activity and self-efficacy in highly active and moderately active women exercisers. *Journal of Applied Social Psychology, 29,* 1016–1029.

Rodgers, W. M., & Sullivan, M. J. L. (2001). Task, coping and scheduling self-efficacy in relation to frequency of physical activity. *Journal of Applied Social Psychology, 31,* 741–753.

Rosenweig, M. R., Leiman, A. L., & Breedlove, S. M. (1999). *Biological Psychology: An introduction to behavioral, cognitive and clinical neuroscience* (2nd ed.). Sunderlande, MA: Sinauer Associates.

Ross, M. J., & Berger, R. S. (1996). Effects of stress inoculation training on athletes' postsurgical pain and rehabilitation after orthopedic injury. *Journal of Consulting and Clinical Psychology, 64*(2), 406–410.

Rotella, R. J., & Heyman, S. R. (1993). Stress, injury, and the psychological rehabilitation of athletes. In J. M. Williams (Ed.). *Applied sport psychology: Personal growth to peak performance* (2nd ed.) (pp. 338–355). Mountain View, CA: Mayfield.

Scherzer, C. B., Brewer, B. W., Cornelius, A. E., van Raalte, J. L., Petitpas, A. J., Sklar, J. H., et al. (2001). Psychological skills and adherence to rehabilitation after reconstruction of the anterior cruciate ligament. *Journal of Sport Rehabilitation, 10,* 165–172.

Short, S. E., Ross-Stewart, L., & Monsma, E. V. (2006). Onwards with the evolution of imagery research in sport psychology. *Athletic Insight, 8*(3), 47–63.

Singer, R. N., & Johnson, P. J. (1987). Strategies to cope with pain associated with sport-related injuries. *Athletic Training, 22,* 100–103.

Sordoni, C., Hall, C., & Forwell, L. (2000). The use of imagery by athletes during injury rehabilitation. *Journal of Sport Rehabilitation, 9,* 329–338.

Sordoni, C., Hall, C., & Forwell, L. (2002). The use of imagery in athletic injury rehabilitation and its relationship to self-efficacy. *Physiotherapy Canada, 54,* 177–185.

Stanley, D. M., & Cumming, J. (2010). Are we having fun yet? Testing the effects of imagery use on the affective and enjoyment responses to acute moderate exercise. *Psychology of Sport and Exercise, 11,* 582–590.

Stanley, D. M., & Cumming, J. (2010). Not just how one feels, but what one images? The effects of imagery use on affective responses to moderate exercise. *International Journal of Sport and Exercise Psychology, 8,* 343–359.

Stanley, D. M., Cumming, J., Standage, M., & Duda, J. L. (2012). Images of exercising: Exploring the links between exercise imagery use, autonomous and controlled motivation to exercise, and exercise intention and behavior. *Psychology of Sport and Exercise, 13,* 133–141.

Start, K. B., & Richardson, A. (1964). Imagery and mental practice. *British Journal of Educational Psychology, 34,* 280–284.

Taylor, S. E., Pham, L. B., Rivkin, I. D., & Armor, D. A. (1998). Harnessing the imagination: Mental simulation, self-regulation, and coping. *American Psychologist, 53,* 429–439. *Psychology, 7,* 174–194.

Taylor, S. E., & Schneider, S. K. (1989). Coping and the simulation of events. *Social Cognition, 7,* 174–194.

Thogersen-Ntoumani, C., Cumming, J., Ntoumanis, N., & Nikitaras, N. (2012). Exercise imagery and its correlates in older adults. *Psychology of Sport and Exercise, 13,* 19–25.

Wesch, N., Hall, C., Prapavessis, H., Maddison, R., Bassett, S., Foley, L., et al. (2011). Self-efficacy, imagery use, and adherence during injury rehabilitation. Scandinavian Journal of Medicine & Science in Sports, doi: 10.1111/j.1600-0838.2011.01304.x.

Wesch, N. N., Milne, M. I., Burke, S. M., & Hall, C. R. (2006). Self-efficacy and imagery use in older adult exercisers. *European Journal of Sport Science, 6,* 197–203.

Westlund, N., Pope, P., & Tobin, D. (2012). Cognitive general imagery: The forgotten imagery function? *Journal of Imagery Research in Sport and Physical Activity, 7.* doi: 10.1515/1932-0191.1075

White, A., & Hardy, L. (1998). An in-depth analysis of the use of imagery by high level slalom canoeists and artistic gymnasts. *The Sport Psychologist, 12,* 387–403.

Wiese, D. M., Weiss, M. R., & Yukelson, D. P. (1991). Sport psychology in the training room: A survey of athletic trainers. *The Sport Psychologist, 5,* 15–24.

Wilson, P. M., Rodgers, W. M., Hall, C. R., & Gammage, K. L. (2003). Do autonomous exercise regulations underpin different types of exercise imagery? *Journal of Applied Sport Psychology, 15,* 294–306.

Chapter 7

Self-Talk

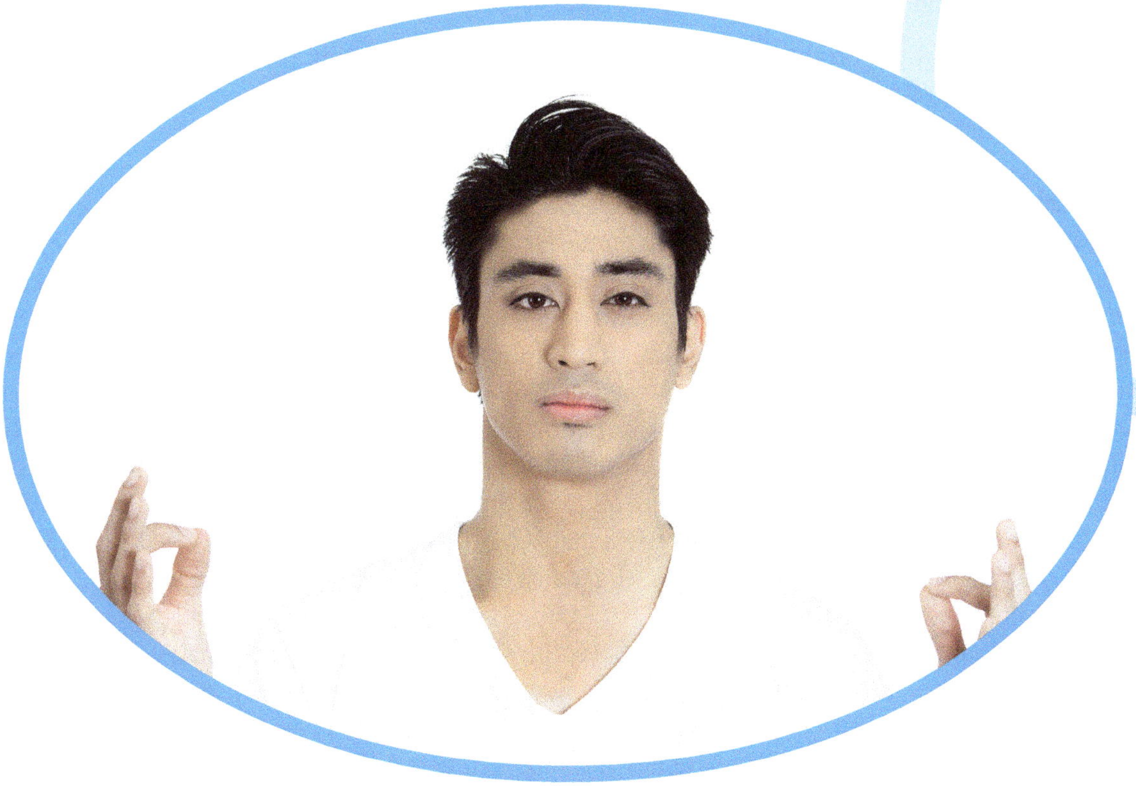

Introduction

We all hold internal conversations as we go about our lives. Psychologists have labeled one important type of these inner monologues as "self-talk," in which you give opinions and evaluations on what you're doing as you're doing it. Thus, self-talk is a form of self-regulation. Theodorakis, Weinberg, Natsis, Douma, and Kazakas (2000) defined self-talk as "what people say to themselves either out loud or as a small voice inside their head" (p. 254). Two important aspects of self-talk are included in this definition: (a) self-talk can be said either overtly or covertly, and (b) self-talk is comprised of statements that are addressed to oneself and not to others. Hardy (2006) has argued that this definition is probably a little simplistic, failing to identify the potential uses of self-talk. Hardy defined self-talk as:

> (a) verbalizations or statements addressed to the self; (b) multidimensional in nature; (c) having interpretive elements associated with the content of statements employed; (d) is somewhat dynamic; and (e) serving at least two functions; instructional and motivational. (p. 84).

This definition elaborates on the one by Theodorakis et al. by indicating that self-talk is multidimensional, can be interpreted in various ways, and serves more than one function.

More specifically, Hardy (2006) discusses six dimensions that comprise the nature of self-talk and offers some clarity about what exactly self-talk is. The first dimension is valence and is concerned with whether self-talk is positive or negative. Research has mainly focused on this dimension by examining the effects of positive versus negative self-talk on performance levels. When your self-talk is upbeat and self-validating, the results generally are positive; you tend be more motivated and are more likely to achieve your goals. When the voice is critical and harsh, however, the effect can be very crippling. Your mind tends to be less free to roam through creative solutions for the problems you face. Yet, a review of the research (Tod, Hardy, & Oliver, 2011) showed that although negative self-talk is commonly thought to have detrimental effects on motor skill performance, this may not be the case. Some researchers (e.g., Hardy, Hall, & Alexander, 2001; Van Raalte, Brewer, Rivera, & Petitpas, 1994) have posed a possible explanation for why negative self-talk is not debilitative to performance, namely, that some individuals may interpret their negative self-talk as motivational. Also, this finding for negative self-talk questions the value of thought-stopping interventions, which aim to reduce the amount of negative self-talk said by performers (Tod et al.).

The second dimension is overtness. Self-talk can be covert (i.e., said using a small voice inside one's head, and so cannot be heard by another individual), or can be overt, which is also called external self-talk. In the case of overt self-talk, another individual can hear what you said to yourself even though your speech is not directed at them. There has yet to be a direct comparison between the effectiveness of overt and covert self-talk in physical activity settings. The third dimension of self-talk is concerned with the degree to which self-talk statements are self-determined. Self-talk can be conceptualized as 'assigned' and 'freely chosen' (Hardy, 2006). The former signifies self-statements generated with absolutely no self-determined control over them, such as when a sport psychologist or coach gives athletes words or phrases to say to themselves. The latter represents self-talk that is completely determined by the individual, and consequently occurs in a natural manner.

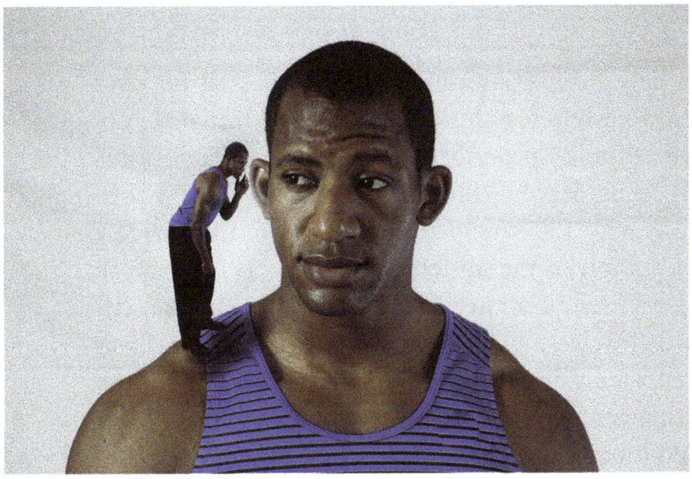

The fourth dimension is motivational interpretation and entails whether individuals view their self-talk as motivating or de-motivating. In their review of the research literature, Tod et al. (2011) concluded that motivational self-talk generally has a positive influence on performance. The functions that self-talk can serve is the fifth dimension. The functions are the reasons why an individual might employ self-talk. Two broad categories have been proposed: instructional and motivational (Theodorakis et al., 2000). Moreover, Theodorakis and his colleagues have suggested that the effects of instructional and motivational self-talk on performance might depend on the type of task being performed. As the execution of precision-based tasks can be aided through increased attentional focus on pertinent technical components, instructional self-talk, which focuses on technical, tactical, and kinesthetic aspects of movements, was thought to be more effective than motivational self-talk for the execution of such tasks. In contrast, motivational self-talk was predicted to be more effective for the execution of conditioning-based tasks characterized by strength and endurance, as motivational self-talk is used to increase effort, foster self-confidence, and create positive moods. In their review of the research conducted to date, Tod et al. found a lack of support for differential effects of instructional and motivational self-talk. Instructional self-talk was not consistently more effective than motivational self-talk for the execution of precision-oriented tasks. Moreover, motivational self-talk was not more effective than instructional self-talk for conditioning-based tasks in most studies conducted to date.

The final self-talk dimension is frequency, which is concerned with how often an individual employs self-talk. Research suggests that successful athletes may use more self-talk than unsuccessful athletes (Mahoney & Avener, 1977). Also, Hardy, Hall, and Hardy (2004) found that the frequency with which athletes employ self-talk increases across phases of the season (i.e., off-season to early competitive-season to late competitive-season), suggesting that there is a dynamic aspect to self-talk.

Self-talk is often included as an integral component of psychological interventions. Furthermore, many people (e.g., athletes, coaches) believe self-talk interventions can enhance performance and psychological states such as self-confidence. It is only recently that sufficient research has been conducted to determine whether this belief is justified, and much of this research has been conducted in sport. Let's see what the research has to say.

Self-Talk in Sport

Although investigators have been examining self-talk in sport for over three decades, most of the early research focused on the effectiveness of positive versus negative self-talk on performance. To expand upon this rather narrow research focus, Hardy, Gammage, and Hall (2001) conducted a qualitative study with 150 varsity athletes in order to provide a relatively complete description of the athletes' self-talk. To accomplish this they asked the athletes four questions: *where* and *when* they use self-talk, *what* they say to themselves, and *why* they use it. Overall, it was revealed that athletes reported using self-talk in a variety of settings both at and away from sporting venues. They used it before, during, and after both practice and competition. The content of their self-talk was multidimensional, as were the reasons why athletes employed self-talk. Two general reasons (functions) emerged: instruction and motivation.

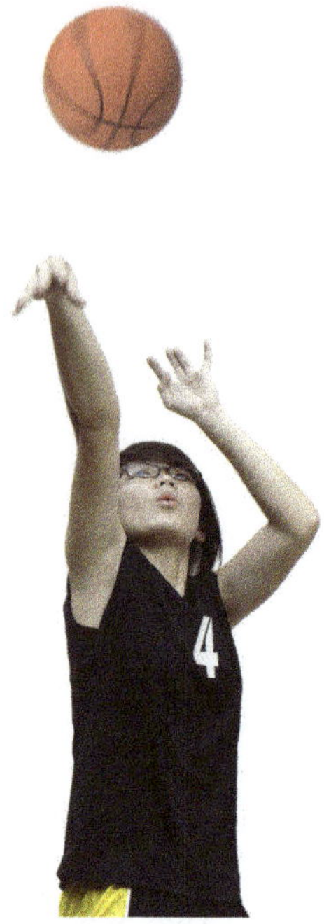

In a follow-up study (Hardy, Hall, & Hardy, 2005), quantitative data were generated that supported the findings of Hardy et al. (2001). In addition, individual and team sport athletes were found to differ in the content of their self-talk. Specifically, team sport athletes reported more negative and overt self-talk than individual sport athletes. No differences in the content of self-talk (what athletes say to themselves) were revealed across sex or skill level. Athletes were found to employ self-talk more frequently in conjunction with the competition setting than the practice setting. Moreover, athletes reported using self-talk most frequently during practice and competition (rather than before or after). With respect to why athletes used self-talk, increased use of nearly all the functions of self-talk was found in association with competition as opposed to practice. Although sex and skill level differences were not found for the use of the functions of self-talk, sport type differences did emerge. Individual sport athletes reported a greater use of self-talk compared to team sport athletes.

In another study, Hardy et al. (2004) investigated how athletes use self-talk. It was found that the majority of athletes reported that they increasingly employed self-talk as the year progressed from the off-season through the early competitive season to the late competitive season. The extent to which athletes of different sex, sport type, and skill level differed in how they utilized self-talk was also considered. Significant effects for sport type and skill level were found. In general, individual sport and skilled athletes used self-talk more frequently than team sport and less skilled athletes, respectively.

Given the work of James Hardy and his colleagues, we presently have a good understanding of athletes' use of self-talk. We can now consider self-talk interventions that have been conducted to influence performance and cognitions. Because there is considerable evidence that the type of self-talk is important with respect to performance outcomes, we will discuss interventions comparing positive and negative self-talk, and those comparing instructional and motivational self-talk. Then we will consider interventions that have examined the influence of self-talk on cognitions such as attention and self-confidence.

Positive vs. Negative Self-Talk

Van Raalte, Brewer, Lewis, Linder, Wildman, and Kozimor (1995) tested 45 male undergraduate students on a novel dart throwing task. Participants were given 15 practice throws with the objective being to hit the center of the bull's eye. Performance accuracy was assessed as distance from the bull's eye. Participants were divided into three groups before completing 15 experimental (real) trials. The positive self-talk group was asked to say "you can do it" before each throw. The negative self-talk group was asked to say "you cannot do it" before each throw, and the control group was given no self-talk instructions. The positive self-talk group significantly outperformed the negative self-talk group and the control group, which did not significantly differ from each other (see Figure 7–1).

More recently, Hamilton, Scott, and MacDougall (2007) examined the effect of positive and negative self-talk on performance on a cycling ergometer task. More specifically, the researchers investigated the impact of self-regulated positive self-talk, assisted positive self-talk, and assisted negative self-talk on performance. In the self-regulated self-talk condition, cyclists were introduced to positive self-talk and encouraged to use it. In the assisted positive and assisted negative self-talk conditions cyclists were audibly provided with self-talk. The assisted self-talk conditions were not unlike a coach cueing the cyclists as to which thoughts may be most appropriate at different points of the performance session. Employing a single-subject multiple-baseline design, nine university students volunteered for the study. They all were familiar with cycling on a stationary bike, although none of the participants reported cycling at a competitive level. Three participants were assigned to each of the three experimental conditions. The dependent variable was the total amount of work by each cyclist over a 20-minute session. Total work (kpm/20 minutes) was the product of rotations per minute (rpm) and resistance. Each participant completed a 20-minute cycling ergometer workout twice a week with workouts being spaced at least one day apart. The cyclists were able to view an output reading of their rpm as well as the ergometer resistance during each 20-minute workout. They were able to alter both rpm and resistance throughout the workout to optimize their control over their level of work. In addition, the researchers told the cyclists every two minutes about the amount of time remaining in the workout.

FIGURE 7–1 Results

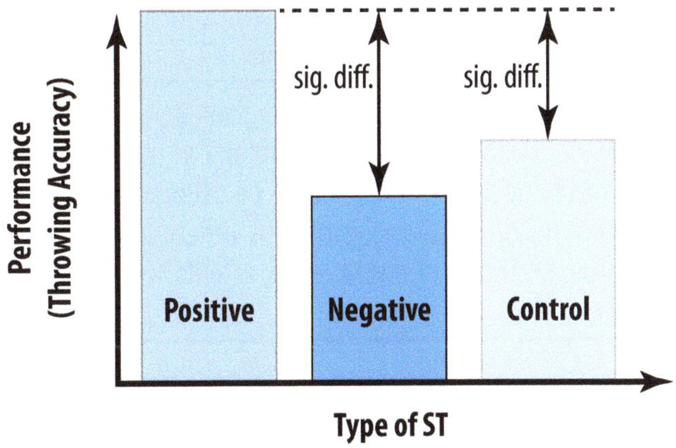

Van Raalte et al. (1995)

A baseline phase was followed by an intervention phase with the total number of workouts for each participant being 10. The self-talk interventions given to each of the three groups are outlined in Table 7–1.

It was found that positive self-talk, whether self-regulated or assisted, improved endurance performance. The finding that assisted positive self-talk facilitated performance gains may be especially important when a coach or sport psychologist is working with an athlete who has little or no experience with the use of mental skills. The researchers argued that by helping the athlete in the early skill acquisition stage through an assisted positive self-talk intervention, the athlete may be likely to learn the skill more rapidly, develop self-confidence earlier, stay motivated longer, and experience performance increases sooner.

In addition, it was shown that two of the three cyclists who received the assisted negative self-talk intervention improved their performance. Although this finding suggests that negative self-talk can actually enhance performance, when Tod et al. (2011) reviewed all the studies examining negative self-talk, the conclusion was that negative self-talk probably does not help performance but it also does not have a detrimental effect on performance.

TABLE 7–1 **Self-Talk Interventions Employed**
1. **Self-regulated positive self-talk group:** Participants in this group were given an introduction to positive self-talk. They were instructed in how to use positive statements to increase confidence, prolong persistence, and increase effort. Participants in this group were given a sheet with examples of statements, which they could use or modify, prior to the beginning of each intervention session. Examples of positive statements were: "My legs are strong and powerful" and "I can maintain this pace."
2. **Assisted positive self-talk group:** Participants were given the same introduction as those participants in the self-regulated positive self-talk group. However, participants in this group were then advised that they would be listening to an audiotape as they cycled. The tape contained positive statements which participants were encouraged to internalize and elaborate. The script for the tape was identical to the list given to participants in the self-regulated positive self-talk group.
3. **Assisted negative self-talk group:** Participants were given an introduction to self-talk. However, they were then advised that they would be listening to an audiotape as they cycled. The tape contained negative comments and participants were advised that they would be listening to this tape for the remainder of the intervention sessions. The script for this tape consisted of a variety of negative statements that the participants were asked to internalize. Examples of negative statements were: "My legs are weak and lethargic" and "I can't maintain this pace."
Hamilton et al. (2007)

Instructional vs. Motivational Self-Talk

One of the first studies to compare instructional and motivational self-talk was conducted by Theodorakis et al. (2000). They examined the effectiveness of these two types of self-talk on increasing performance in different motor tasks. Specifically, four laboratory experiments were conducted including a soccer accuracy test, a badminton service test, a sit-up test, and a knee extension task on an isokinetic dynamometer. In each experiment there were three groups. The instructional self-talk group was asked to use an instructional phrase (e.g., "I see the target") before each performance attempt. The motivational self-talk group said "I can" before each performance attempt. The control group was given no self-talk instructions. Results of the soccer and badminton experiments indicated that the instructional self-talk group improved their performance significantly more than the motivational self-talk and control groups. Results of the sit-up experiment indicated no significant differences between the three groups, although all groups showed improvements across trials. Results of the knee extension task experiment showed a significant improvement for both the motivational and instructional groups compared to the control group. It was concluded that when the task requires fine motor movements, instructional self-talk is more effective, whereas when the task requires predominantly strength and endurance, both motivational and instructional self-talk are effective.

Theodorakis and his colleagues (Hatzigeorgiadis, Theodorakis, & Zourbanos, 2004) again investigated instructional and motivational self-talk, this time on the performance on two water polo tasks. In the first experiment, participants in three groups (i.e., instructional self-talk, motivational self-talk, control) threw a water polo ball at a target. The second experiment involved throwing a water polo ball for distance and the same three groups were employed. In each experiment the participants were 60 swimming class students (30 males and 30 females, different students in each experiment) with no prior experience in water polo. The participants in both experiments had a mean age of about 21 years.

The same experimental design was employed in both experiments. Participants were tested twice, at baseline and intervention. When they arrived for baseline testing they were allowed five minutes to warm up in the swimming pool. After the warm-up they were given instructions regarding the throwing technique. Then they made 10 throws either at a target or for distance and an average score was calculated for the 10 attempts. The intervention testing took place two weeks after the baseline testing and during that period participants did not have the chance to practice. The control group repeated the procedures followed in the baseline testing. The self-talk groups were told that in order to examine the effectiveness of a learning strategy they would have to use key words before each throw. In order to ensure that the key words were actually said, participants were instructed to speak audibly. The key words were used immediately before each throw. In order to get familiar with the use of self-talk, participants were asked to use the key words for four practice throws. One experimental group used motivational self-talk ("I can"), and the other used instructional self-talk ("ball-target" in experiment one and "elbow-hand" in experiment two). Then, the self-talk participants made 10 throws either at a target or for distance and again an average score was calculated for the 10 attempts.

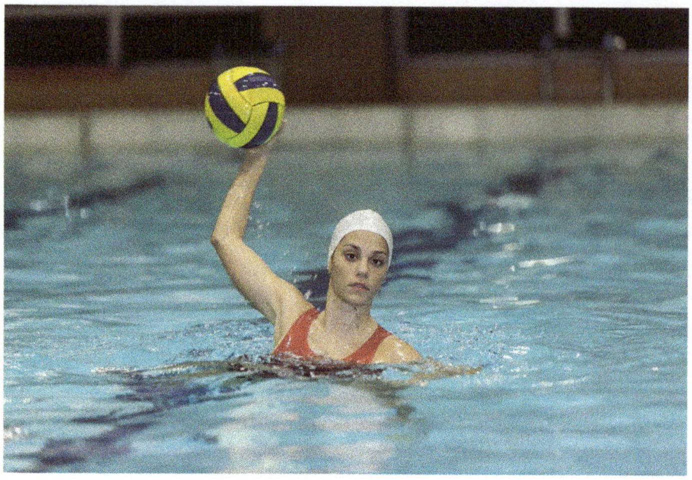

For throwing at a target (the first experiment), both self-talk groups improved their performance in comparison to the baseline measure, with participants using instructional self-talk improving more. The control group had no change in performance. For throwing for distance (the second experiment), only the motivational self-talk group improved its performance significantly from baseline to intervention testing. The researchers concluded that their results provide further support for the effectiveness of self-talk on improving motor skill performance, and emphasized the importance of matching self-talk with the demands of the task to be performed, precision (throwing at a target) or power (throwing for distance). In their review of the literature, however, Tod et al. (2011) concluded that overall there was little support for such a matching approach. That is, there is a lack of support for the differential effects of instructional and motivational self-talk.

Influence of Self-Talk on Cognitions

Research examining the effects of self-talk on cognitions is somewhat limited. Bell and Hardy (2009) employed self-talk as a means of directing athletes' attentional focus. The purpose of their study was to determine the effects of three attentional foci on the performance of skilled golfers. Thirty-three skilled male golfers were assigned to one of three attentional focus groups. Participants in the internal focus group were instructed to focus on the motion of the arms during the swing and specifically to maintain the hinge in the wrists through impact. These golfers were also asked to repeat the phrase *wrist hinge* prior to shot execution to promote an internal focus. Golfers in the proximal external focus group were instructed to focus on the position of the clubface through the swing, in particular, keeping the clubface square through impact. These participants were asked to use the phrase *square face* prior to shot execution. Golfers assigned to the distal external focus group were instructed to focus explicitly on the flight of the ball after it had left the clubface and in particular the direction in which they intended to play the ball. These participants were asked to repeat the phrase *straight flight* immediately prior to shot execution.

Golf performance was assessed in both a neutral condition and one intended to provoke anxiety. Anxiety was induced via a combination of social evaluation and financial incentives. In each condition, the golfers completed three blocks of ten shots. After each block the golfers were given the opportunity for a short break and reminded of their assigned self-talk and the importance of using it prior to every shot. Performance was measured according to the distance (i.e., short or long) the ball finished from the hole.

It was found that performance was significantly more accurate for the distal external focus group in comparison to both the proximal external focus group and internal focus group under both the neutral and anxiety conditions. In addition, the proximal external focus group displayed superior performance compared to the internal focus group, again under both conditions. The researchers concluded that their results were consistent with previous work (e.g., McNevin, Shea, & Wulf, 2003); however, they cautioned that self-talk strategies alone may not be sufficient as a mechanism to direct attentional focus. It would be relatively easy to combine self-talk strategies with imagery or process goals to direct attentional focus.

In another study, Hatzigeorgiadis, Zourbanos, Mpoumpaki, and Theodorakis (2009) examined the effects of motivational self-talk on self-confidence, anxiety, and task performance in tennis players. It was hypothesized that the use of motivational self-talk would increase self-confidence, reduce anxiety, and enhance forehand drive performance. Both self-confidence and anxiety were assessed using the Competitive State Anxiety Inventory-2 revised (Cox, Martens, & Russell, 2003). The participants were 72 (36 males and 36 females) competitive young tennis players (mean age 13.47 ± 1.78). The study was conducted in five sessions: baseline assessment, three training sessions, and final assessment.

The baseline assessment initially entailed informing the players that for the following five sessions they were going to participate in a program aimed at assessing their tennis abilities. The objective was to raise players' anxiety to levels comparable to a sport competition, so that the hypothesized impact of self-talk could be detected. Importantly, players were told that the whole procedure was going to be recorded, that the results were to be made public, that performance of individuals was going to be compared, and that awards (tennis goods) would be given to the top three players. Next, the players performed three sets of 10 forehand drives. The first set was used for purposes of familiarization (not assessed), whereas the two following sets were assessed. Upon completion of the third set, players' self-confidence and anxiety were measured.

Following the baseline assessment, participants were randomly assigned to either a self-talk group or a control group. The two groups followed similar training protocols for the next three training sessions. In addition, all players received additional training as part of their participation in the program. For the training phase, the backhand drive was used, so that players did not practice the stroke that was to be evaluated in the final assessment. Players in the self-talk group were introduced to the use of self-talk and were informed that they were going to use this strategy for their training. The instructor explained and showed them how to use self-talk. Players in the control group spent the same time receiving a short lecture on tactical aspects of the shot. All participants performed four sets of eight drives.

Players in the self-talk group used one cue for each set. These cue words were provided by the instructor and were both instructional (e.g., shoulder, low, deep) and motivational (e.g., go, I can, strong). The rationale for using instructional and motivational cues for the training phase was to have players practicing, understanding, and learning how to use the self-talk technique thoroughly. The players were told that they could repeat the cue aloud or in their head, according to their preference.

For the final assessment the testing procedure employed in the baseline assessment was repeated. Players were reminded of the stressful instructions. With regard to the awards, to keep all players' involvement high irrespective of their scores in the initial assessment, it was announced that the awards would be given to players showing the most improvement compared to their initial test. In addition, to maintain stress levels, an individual was introduced to the players as a member of the tennis federation who had come to watch their test. As in the baseline assessment, all players performed three sets of 10 drives, with the first set used for familiarization. Players in the self-talk group were asked to choose and state a motivational cue of their preference that they would use before each forehand drive. Upon completion of drive performance, self-confidence and anxiety were assessed.

The self-talk and control groups did not significantly differ at baseline with respect to forehand drive performance, self-confidence, and anxiety. Following the intervention, task performance improved for the self-talk group and remained stable for the control group. Moreover, self-confidence increased and anxiety decreased for the self-talk group, whereas no changes were observed for the control group. Correlation analysis demonstrated that changes in forehand drive performance were moderately related to changes in self-confidence. The researchers concluded that self-talk can enhance self-confidence and reduce cognitive anxiety, and that increases in self-confidence may be one mechanism explaining the facilitating effects of self-talk on performance.

Some General Recommendations

After reviewing the research, Tod et al. (2011) concluded that there is support for self-talk as a psychological intervention in sport; however, they questioned whether self-talk is effective due to the specific education involved in teaching athletes to use verbal cues, or because of some less specific factors such as hope, expectation, or practitioner allegiance. Regardless, there certainly are some general recommendations that can be made:

- While practitioners would be well advised to promote the use of positive self-talk by athletes, they should not be concerned if athletes use some negative self-talk. The existing research indicates that negative self-talk does not impede performance (Tod et al., 2011).
- Athletes should be encouraged to employ both instructional and motivational self-talk to enhance performance. The literature does not support differential effects for instructional and motivational self-talk (Tod et al., 2011).
- Practitioners should encourage athletes to use self-talk to increase self-confidence and reduce anxiety.
- Used in conjunction with other psychological techniques such as goal setting and imagery, self-talk may be helpful in directing athletes' attentional focus.

Self-Talk in Exercise

Given the evidence that has been acquired over the past few decades showing the influence of self-talk on motivation and performance in sport, a natural extension was to examine the role of self-talk in exercise. Self-talk has been found to have an influence on cognitions, emotions, and motivation, all of which

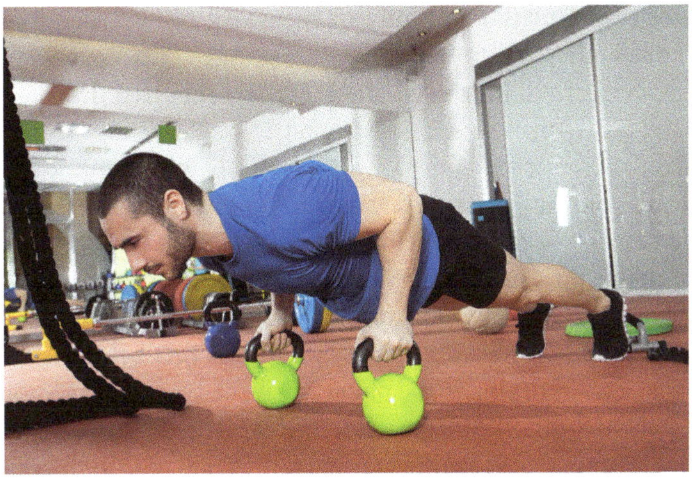

contribute to initiation and maintenance of exercise behavior. Indeed, initial studies have demonstrated that most exercisers (up to 95% in a study conducted by Gammage, Hardy, and Hall [2001]) report using self-talk. Research examining the influence of self-talk in exercise is new. To our knowledge, no studies conducted to date have tested the effects of a self-talk intervention on exercise behavior. The studies that have been conducted in this area, however, provide (a) an important descriptive picture of how self-talk is used naturally by exercisers and (b) implications for the development of interventions in the future.

Characteristics of Exercise Self-Talk

One of the first studies to look at the use of self-talk among exercisers was conducted by Gammage et al. (2001). Following a framework that had proven useful for examining the characteristics of exercise imagery, Gammage et al. conducted a qualitative study among 164 exercisers to explore the "4 Ws" of self-talk in exercise: where they use it, when they use it, what they say, and why they use it. We present an overview of their findings in combination with findings from other researchers, according to each "W", below:

Where. The most common setting in which exercisers reported using self-talk was at the workout location (e.g., the field, the gym, etc.). Exercisers also reported using self-talk outside of the workout environment, for example, at home or at work; however, this was much less common.

When. The exercisers in this study reported using self-talk most often during their exercise. More specifically, they used self-talk to motivate themselves when the workout got tough, when they started to feel tired, or when they felt they needed an extra push to the end. Although much less frequent, the exercisers also reported using self-talk before and after their workouts and during other miscellaneous times throughout the day.

What. The "what" component of the "4 Ws" describes the structure, nature, and content of the self-talk. With regard to structure, it seems that exercisers prefer short statements; although exercisers reported using cue words (e.g., "focus") and full sentences (e.g., "I will feel proud of myself once I am finished with this workout"), they reported using short phrases (e.g., "you can do it") most often. In addition, although both perspectives were used, the exercisers reported that their statements were typically in the second person rather than in the first person.

The nature of self-talk can be positive, negative, or neutral. To determine the nature of self-talk use in exercise, Gammage et al. (2001) asked the exercisers to list their self-talk statements and the researchers coded whether the statements seemed positive, negative, or neutral. The researchers found that more of the statements were positive than negative; however, the majority of the statements were neutral. One limitation to the approach that Gammage et al. took to determining the valence of self-talk was that the researchers were not able to determine the exercisers' perceptions behind some of the neutral statements; the exercisers may use self-talk that appears neutral to an outside observer but actually is intended to be positive (or negative). More research is needed to elucidate the benefits and consequences of using positive, negative, and neutral self-talk.

Finally, the "what" category of the "4 Ws" also describes what exercisers say to themselves. Gammage et al. (2001) demonstrated that the self-talk of exercisers covers a wide variety of topics including: (a) general task instructions such as "breathe," specific task instructions such as "remember to use your legs to help pull the bike pedal up"; (b) the results that will be achieved from exercising (e.g., "this will help me look and feel my best"); (c) workout details such as the amount of time remaining; and (d) reminders of their goals. In addition to the findings reported by Gammage et al., St. Clair Gibson and Foster (2007) demonstrated that the "what" of self-talk during exercise changes as a function of the exercise intensity. Specifically, when people are exercising at a low intensity, their self-talk tends to be dissociative. That is, their self-talk is conversational and may not actually be related to the exercise itself. In contrast, when the exercise intensity is high, exercisers tend to use more associative self-talk which involves self-statements about the physiological experience of exercising, task instructions, and pace control.

Why. The final "W" describes why exercisers use self-talk. Just as athletes do, exercisers report using self-talk for both instructional and motivational purposes. Exercisers describe using self-talk to assist them with specific tasks such as a sequence of steps in an aerobics class or with more general strategies such as remembering to breathe. From the motivational perspective, exercisers use self-statements related to arousal (e.g., getting energized to do a workout), mastery (e.g., staying confident when a workout is challenging), and drive (e.g., maintaining the motivation to exercise).

These findings reported by Gammage et al. (2001) describe the way in which exercisers use self-talk naturally. To date, there have been no formal tests of certain elements or styles of self-talk against others. More research is needed before we can make firm recommendations regarding best practices for the where, when, what, and why of self-talk in exercise. The natural use of self-talk by exercisers, however, does provide preliminary insight into some self-talk strategies that may prove useful for future self-talk interventions in the exercise domain.

Who Uses Exercise Self-Talk

As we have mentioned previously, Gammage et al. (2001) found that in a sample of college-aged exercisers, 95% reported using self-talk. With regard to gender, it appears that both men and women apply self-talk to a similar degree and that the 4 Ws of self-talk may not differ dramatically by gender. Further evidence was provided by O'Brien Cousins and Gillis (2005) who conducted a qualitative study of the exercise-related self-talk of middle-aged and older men and women. The design and the relatively small sample size of this study prohibits us from drawing firm conclusions about the use of self-talk across genders and age groups; however, the findings suggest that age may be a more important moderator of self-talk use than gender. Specifically, it appears that younger men and women (aged 40 to 55 years) tend to use general self-statements such as "just do it" and don't use as many specific instructional or motivational statements. In comparison, older men and women (aged 56 years and older) use more specific statements about the safety, benefits, consequences of exercising, and actually are more likely to talk themselves out of exercising.

Another factor that may have an influence on self-talk use is an exerciser's stage of change. According to the Transtheoretical Model (Prochaska & Velicer, 1997), individuals who are not regularly active but are thinking about becoming more active are in the ***contemplation stage***. Individuals who have taken exercise adoption one step further and begun to make tracks toward actually becoming more active are in the ***action stage***, and individuals who exercise regularly and are no longer making changes in their exercise routine are in the ***maintenance stage***. O'Brien Cousins and Gillis (2005) interviewed individuals who varied in their stage of change for exercise and found that the stage may dictate the type of self-talk that is employed most frequently. In this study, O'Brien Cousins and Gillis found evidence that people who were in the contemplation stage were more likely to use self-talk to talk themselves out of exercising. These people, particularly those in the older age group, tended to question the safety of exercise or to accept a small amount of exercise as being enough for one week. In contrast, people in the action stage reported using quite a bit of self-talk (i.e., more than individuals in other stages of change) and used it primarily for motivational purposes. Finally, individuals who were in the maintenance stage tended to use general types of self-talk such as "just do it" rather than more specific motivational or instructional statements. These participants actually reported that using more specific statements would cause them to over-think their exercise and could actually be a deterrent. These findings indicate that the stage of change of an exerciser may impact the frequency, nature, and content of self-talk.

Measurement of Self-Talk in Exercise

As we discussed earlier in the chapter, measurement of self-talk (across all domains) is typically conducted via questionnaire, although some studies on athletes' overt self-talk also have been conducted. Whereas assessing overt self-talk potentially provides for a more objective assessment, it does not allow researchers to determine how an individual perceives their own self-statements. Recall that when Gammage et al. (2001) used a coding scheme to classify exerciser self-statements as positive, negative, or neutral, a great deal of self-talk was classified as neutral despite the fact that the exercisers may have attached a positive or negative valence to the statement. To account for this limitation, it would be possible to have exercisers rate the valence of their own self-talk statements. For example, Hardy, Hall, and Alexander (2001) had athletes indicate their typical self-talk statements and rate the valence of each statement. In doing this Hardy et al. (2001) found that a much greater percentage of the self-talk was rated as positive, suggesting that self-report assessments of self-talk valence may be more accurate.

To date, there are no validated self-report questionnaires available to assess self-talk in an exercise context. Therefore, an important future direction for self-talk research would be to develop and validate

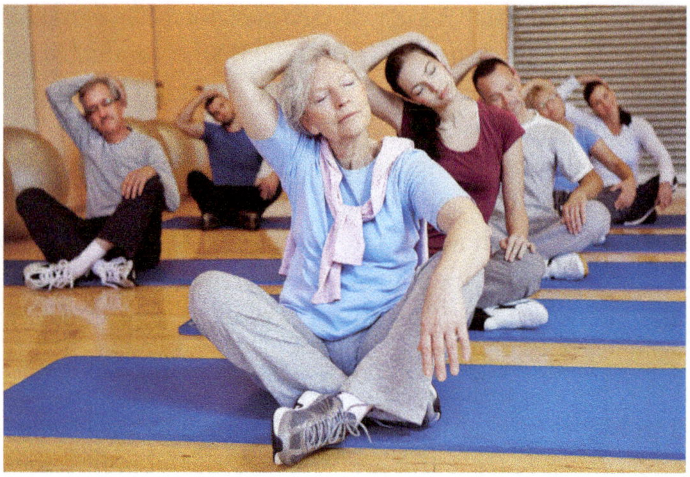

a questionnaire that can reliably assess the use of self-talk among exercisers. Establishing such a tool will be critical for the assessment of self-talk interventions in the exercise context to determine from pre- to post-intervention whether the overall use of self-talk had changed or whether certain characteristics of the self-talk had changed in response to the intervention. We suggest that researchers who wish to develop a tool for assessing self-talk in exercise borrow a questionnaire from the sport psychology literature (e.g., the Self Talk Use Questionnaire; Hardy, Hall, & Hardy, 2005) and use the 4 Ws described by Gammage et al. (2001) to adapt it for exercise.

How Self-Talk in Exercise Works

Given the relatively few studies that have examined self-talk in exercise, we cannot even be sure that self-talk is an effective intervention approach let alone draw conclusions about why it works. We can, however, consider potential hypotheses regarding the influence of self-talk in exercise which may, in turn, point to research questions for subsequent study. Below we discuss four potential mechanisms by which self-talk may influence cognitions, motivation, and behavior in the exercise domain.

Attentional focus. Hardy (2006), in a review of the self-talk literature in sport and exercise, identified the potential for self-talk to assist in attentional focus as a potential explanation for its impact on performance. Nideffer (1976) described attentional focus as having two dimensions: width, which can be either broad or narrow, and direction, which can be either internal or external. When these dimensions are combined they form four possible categories describing how attention can be focused: broad-internal, broad-external, narrow-internal, and narrow-external. The situation dictates which type of focus is advantageous at any given time. It has been suggested that self-talk can be used to help shift attention between categories. Self-talk as a means to shift attentional focus may prove to be helpful in the exercise context. Consider a situation in which an exerciser, out for a 10 km jog on a local recreation trail, finds himself breathless and uncomfortable as he makes his way up a steep hill. If his focus is narrow and internal, he may focus exclusively on the discomfort he is feeling in his lungs. Using self-talk statements such as "relax," or "adjust your pace," the exerciser may be able to shift his focus to a broad-internal focus which could help him regulate his running and experience less discomfort. In the same scenario he also could use a self-statement like "it's nice to be running outside" which may trigger a shift to a broad-external focus and allow him to realize that the discomfort he feels will only last for a few seconds of an otherwise flat and pleasant run.

Information processing. Another mechanism by which self-talk may be helpful for exercisers is through its impact on information processing. Landin (1994) suggested that self-talk can have a powerful influence on how information is processed. For example, using cue words throughout an aerobics routine may help a participant keep up with the steps and experience stronger feelings of mastery during her workout.

Another way in which self-talk may impact on information processing is by influencing the depth at which information is processed. According to Petty and Cacioppo (1986), information that is processed deeply can have a stronger influence on attitudes. Developing positive attitudes toward exercise is an important antecedent to being motivated to exercise and to actually engaging in exercise; thus, if self-talk could influence the depth at which information related to exercise is processed, it stands to reason that it could have an influence on subsequent motivation and behavior. Indeed, Noar, Benac, and Harris (2007) have indicated that when information is tailored to the individual receiving the information, it is processed more deeply, increasing the impact of the information on subsequent attitudes, intentions, or behavior. Information that is repeated to oneself is inherently personalized (i.e., tailored), thus, it is possible that self-talk statements may be processed deeply and will be more likely to be endorsed by the individual.

Baldwin, Rothman, Vander Weg, and Christensen (2013) explored the relationship between self-talk and information processing in a study of 76 college students who were assigned randomly to respond to either self-generated arguments (i.e., a proxy for self-talk) or other-generated arguments about the benefits of exercise. The researchers asked the participants to (a) list the thoughts they had when reading either of the arguments, (b) rate the persuasiveness of the arguments, and (c) indicate their attitudes toward exercise and their intentions to exercise in the next month. The results showed a non-significant trend in which the participants listed more positive thoughts about the arguments that were self-generated. The findings also showed that self-generated arguments were rated as significantly more persuasive and led to more positive attitudes and intentions toward exercise. These findings suggest that we are biased in our cognitive processing toward self-generated thoughts. Although this bias may be limiting in certain social conditions, it does suggest one reason that self-talk may be effective.

Motivation. A third reason that self-talk may be effective for changing behavior in an exercise context is through its impact on motivation. One central tenet of self-determination theory (Deci & Ryan, 1985) is that we tend to persist at a behavior when our motivation to engage in that behavior is self-determined. When exercisers use self-talk they are reinforcing ideas and beliefs that come from within themselves and creating a personal state of being that is consistent with persistence with exercise.

Self-efficacy. As we have discussed in previous chapters, self-efficacy plays an important role in exercise behavior. Bandura (1986) specified four sources of self-efficacy; one of which is verbal persuasion. Although this source of self-efficacy is proposed to have a less powerful influence on self-perceptions than past experience and vicarious experiences, it can still affect self-efficacy in a meaningful way, particularly when the source is credible. As Baldwin et al. (2013) found in their study of self- versus other-generated arguments for exercise, we tend to be biased toward ourselves, believing ourselves to be credible sources of information. As such, self-talk may be an effective way to bolster self-efficacy for exercise.

Although self-talk does have the potential to be a powerful source of self-efficacy, there is some evidence that it may only be minimally effective in the absence of previous mastery experiences. For example, O'Brien Cousins (2003) conducted a qualitative study of the self-talk of active and inactive older adults. In this study O'Brien Cousins showed that whereas active individuals reported using both negative and positive self-talk but were able to balance the negative with the positive self-talk based on positive past experiences, the self-talk of inactive adults was dominated by negative statements. Given that positive self-talk seems to be more adaptive and more strongly related to engagement in exercise behavior, it is possible that self-talk alone may not be an effective strategy for increasing self-efficacy and exercise behavior among individuals without past mastery experiences.

Some General Recommendations

Although there is a paucity of research examining self-talk in the exercise domain, the few studies that have been conducted, in addition to evidence from sport psychology, point to some important implications for the use of self-talk as an intervention strategy in exercise.

- The use of positive self-talk should be encouraged. Although studies testing the use of positive self-talk versus negative self-talk have yet to be conducted, descriptive evidence collected to date suggests that positive self-talk (and not negative self-talk) should be encouraged in the exercise domain.
- Exercisers should use self-generated statements. As we saw in the study conducted by Baldwin et al. (2013), self-generated statements may be more credible than statements generated by others. By using self-generated statements the exerciser may process the statement deeply and come to strongly endorse its message, perceive it as a credible source of persuasion from which self-efficacy can be enhanced, or perceive it as a reminder that they personally endorse exercise, reinforcing their motivation to be active. As interventionists, exercisers often look to us to provide them with the solutions. A more effective approach, as suggested by the literature, would be to help an exerciser develop a list of his or her own self-talk statements.
- Self-talk should be aligned with characteristics of the exerciser or the situation. The description of self-talk in exercise provided by Gammage et al. (2001) points to a vast array of circumstances in which self-talk can be used, as well as numerous characteristics that the self-talk statement might take. Research presented by O'Brien Cousins and Gillis (2005) indicated that individual characteristics of an exerciser, such as their stage of change, may dictate the type of self-talk that would be most effective. Although no intervention studies have tested this idea, it is not without merit. Individuals who have just begun to exercise by swimming laps a couple of times per week may need to focus on specific instructional self-talk to the proper stroke technique whereas people who have been maintaining exercise for months or years may benefit more from general motivational statements such as "stick with it!". Much more research is needed to determine the optimal type of self-talk to be used under varying conditions.

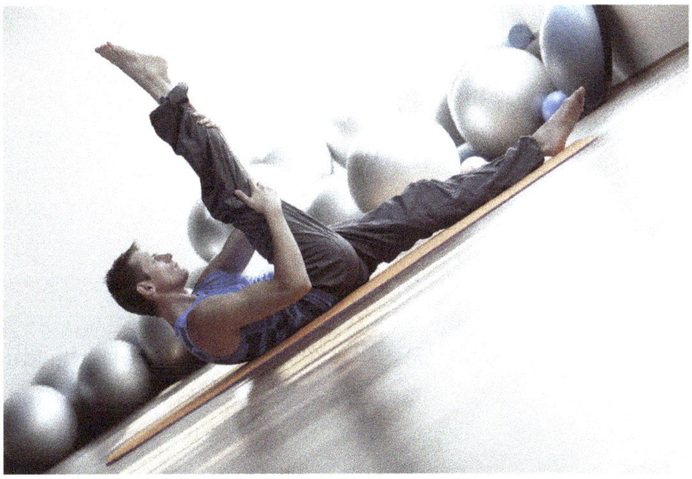

Self-Talk in Injury Rehabilitation

Positive and Negative Self-Talk

It is easy to imagine the types of things that an injured athlete might say to himself or herself, relating to both the injury experience and the challenges faced during treatment. The valence of self-talk is clearly of particular importance in this setting. Negative self-talk can prolong the duration of distressful emotions, such as anxiety, fear, or rumination, which have a tendency to negatively affect behavior during a rehabilitation program (Williams & Roepke, 1993). Positive self-talk, however, can help the athlete overcome these negative emotional states. It can promote better attentional focus, assist in building confidence, create positive mood, trigger desired actions, increase effort, and control anxiety (Hardy, Jones, & Gould, 1996).

In the hours and days immediately following an injury, many athletes experience anger, frustration, and feelings of hopelessness. These feelings can result in, among other things, lowered self-efficacy and reduced effort during rehabilitation sessions. It has been demonstrated, however, that positive self-talk can be used to overcome negative or irrational thoughts post-injury (Nippert & Smith, 2008).

Theodorakis and colleagues (1998) specifically examined the effects of positive self-talk on performance and anxiety during rehabilitation. They recruited 30 athletes (aged 18–23 years) who had undergone a knee arthroscopy at least six weeks prior to inclusion. Participants were randomized into experimental ($n = 16$) and control ($n = 14$) groups. Both groups were prescribed the same rehabilitation protocol, consisting mainly of quadriceps strengthening exercises, to be completed three times per week for two weeks. Those in the experimental condition were also primed with positive messages during their rehabilitation sessions, both before and during each set of exercises. Participants were instructed to repeat these messages either aloud or in their heads as they performed the movements. Quadriceps strength was recorded for both groups using a CYBEX machine at the first, third, and sixth (final) session. Anxiety was measured using a revised version of the Mental Readiness Form anxiety scale. The researchers found significantly greater performance improvement in the experimental group compared to the control group, but there was no decrease in anxiety associated with the self-talk intervention (Theodorakis, Beneca, Goudas, Antoniou, & Malliou, 1998).

The Theodorakis et al. (1998) study illustrates two important aspects of self-talk interventions. First, self-talk statements in the experimental group were not self-determined. When researchers or practitioners prime participants with specific messages, some individuals may relate to them while others do not. They may also fail to have the intended effect if the individual interprets the statement as de-motivating. This may account for the lack of effect of the self-talk intervention on anxiety in this study. Moreover, the null effect may be attributed in part to the intervention length. Two weeks is a relatively short time in which to achieve significant change, especially when self-talk is directed specifically at exercise performance. It is necessary to also address the negative emotional reactions the athlete may be experiencing during his or her time away from the rehabilitation setting to ensure that progress made during treatment is not offset by negative self-talk occurring in other aspects of the individual's life.

Instructional and Motivational Self-Talk

Self-talk is a valuable learning tool. It promotes selective attention to the appropriate features of a skill, blocks out distractions, and helps an individual focus on feedback for error detection and reinforcement. Instructional self-talk, in particular, can facilitate knowledge retention and can foster self-reliance and confidence (Anderson, 2013). When an athlete is faced with having to perform rehabilitation exercises, which often rely on accurate and effortful movement, instructional self-talk can be extremely helpful in achieving desired outcomes. Individuals can talk themselves through the different components of an exercise, or provide themselves with constant feedback on technique, allowing for more efficient use of treatment time, and an easier transition from in-clinic to at-home programs.

For example, consider a patient who is undergoing rehabilitation following shoulder surgery. One of the exercises that she is prescribed involves walking her fingers up a wall to regain range of motion. The exercise is progressive in nature, with its goal being the ability to extend the arm vertically overhead. With only a few degrees of movement in the shoulder joint at the beginning of rehabilitation, the patient might give herself general instructions while doing the exercise, such as "relax my neck while I extend my arm," or "breathe out as I walk my fingers up the wall." More specific self-talk may focus on the technical aspects of the exercise as range of motion increases: "maintain good posture to ensure my shoulder muscles are doing the work," or "do not let my arm supinate as I extend it up the wall." The degree of specificity in one's self-talk can be quite unique to the individual, but it can be effective provided that it contains the cues or key words that trigger the desired behavioral response.

Aside from such straightforward applications of instructional self-talk, this technique can also be a useful strategy for overcoming the stress associated with recovery. Cue-instructional self-talk, or the use of self-instruction to trigger adaptive behaviors and replace interfering or useless thoughts, can be employed to manage negative or de-motivating emotions (Ahern & Lohr, 1997). These messages include instructions like "don't do this, do this instead" or "stop thinking about that, focus on this." These types of self-talk are associated with two common psychological intervention methods: ***attention refocusing*** (e.g., focusing on an external cue instead of negative self-talk) and *cognitive restructuring* (e.g., pointing out the irrationality of thoughts and restructuring them to match reality; Ahern & Lohr, 1997).

It has also been shown that cognitive stress management techniques, including self-talk, can improve healing. In their seminal study, Ievleva and Orlick (1991) demonstrated that, after knee or ankle injury, fast healers used highly positive self-talk, whereas slow healers used self-talk that was totally negative and unforgiving. Those who healed at the average rate exhibited a combination of self-talk styles. Positive messages, such as "I can do it" appear to facilitate recovery, whereas negative messages, such as "Why me?" seem to have an inhibitory effect (Ievleva & Orlick, 1991). This may be attributed to the behavior elicited by these messages. Those with an optimistic outlook are more likely to put in the effort required for successful recovery, but those with self-talk that reinforces the negative aspects run a much higher risk of low self-efficacy and decreased motivation (Carver, Scheier, & Segerstrom, 2010). Positive emotion may also be involved in the biological process of healing (Gouin & Kiecolt-Glaser, 2011). Additional research is therefore needed to explore the underlying mechanisms of self-talk's effect on recovery after a variety of injury types, both from behavioral and biological perspectives.

Motivational self-talk is also crucial during rehabilitation. Maintaining focus and effort can be a challenge as recovery progresses, and the dialogue a patient has with himself or herself can play a large role in sustaining progress. Although there has been very little research into the motivational function of self-talk during rehabilitation, it is intuitive that motivational messages will facilitate positive outcomes. It must be noted, however, that not all motivational self-talk need be positive in valence. Many athletes will interpret negative self-talk (e.g., "That's not good enough," or "That technique is all wrong," or "You won't ever get better doing it that way") as motivational (Hardy, Hall, & Alexander, 2001; Van Raalte et al., 1994).

Adherence

Related to its motivational function, it is possible that self-talk could lead to better rehabilitation adherence. One study examined this relationship in a group of 54 patients following ACL reconstruction (Scherzer, Brewer, Cornelius, van Raalte, Petitpas, Sklar, et al., 2001). Measures of adherence were taken at each postoperative therapy appointment, and included recorded attendance at rehabilitation sessions, the practitioner-rated Sport Injury Rehabilitation Adherence Scale, and self-rated adherence to home-based exercises in the previous week. The findings indicated that positive self-talk was associated with home exercise completion ($r = .52$, $p < 0.05$), but no correlation existed between self-talk and home cryotherapy, adherence scale ratings, or attendance at rehabilitation appointments. Interestingly, most patients in the study denied using self-talk, suggesting that this process may occur without conscious control for some individuals (Scherzer et al., 2001). This single study does not constitute a significant amount of research in this area, however, and its results should be interpreted with caution due to the small sample size. Future studies are recommended to further investigate the effect of self-talk on rehabilitation adherence.

Injury Prevention

One unique approach to understanding the role of self-talk in sport injury has been to investigate its effect on return to sport and the prevention of re-injury. Chase and colleagues (2005) interviewed 10 female gymnasts (aged 12–17 years), all of whom had been injured previously, to assess fear of injury and psychological strategies used to overcome this fear. Two predominant injury fears existed in this group, namely the difficulty of returning to competition after injury and being unable to participate because of injury. The gymnasts also expressed a significant fear of incurring a serious injury while performing a difficult skill (Chase, Magyar, & Drake, 2005).

Participants reported using self-talk (e.g., "Just go for it") as a thought-stopping strategy when they felt that their fear was preventing them from performing a specific skill or portion of a routine. Positive self-communication was believed to reinforce self-confidence for performing difficult or scary skills, and helped the gymnasts overcome avoidance and rumination related to previous injuries sustained under similar circumstances. They used self-talk for cognitive restructuring and refocusing to minimize carryover from previous injury experiences (Chase et al., 2005).

How It Is Measured

Theodorakis, Hatzigeorgiadis, and Chroni (2008) have recently developed the Functions of Self-Talk Questionnaire, a 25-item instrument that assesses five dimensions of self-talk: confidence, automaticity, cognitive and emotional control, attention, and effort. Although it was not developed for use in rehabilitation settings explicitly, it may be useful to assess patient's self-talk practice. The positive self-talk subscale of the Sport Injury Survey (Ievleva & Orlick, 1991) has been used to assess self-talk specifically during rehabilitation (Scherzer et al., 2001). This subscale consists of a single question ("Do you find yourself 'talking' to yourself about your injury?"), with a follow-up item for those who answer affirmatively ("To what extent is this self-talk positive in comparison to negative?").

Some General Recommendations

Self-talk, whether for instructional or motivational purposes, positively contributes to injury recovery (Cupal, 2008). Practitioners generally have positive attitudes toward self-talk (Hamson-Utley, Martin, & Walters, 2008), and rate methods for encouraging positive self-thoughts as important for athlete recovery (Wiese, Weiss, & Yukelson, 1991). Considering current demand for psychological training for rehabilitation personnel, including self-talk guidance (Gordon, Potter, & Ford, 1998), there are a few recommendations for those intending to employ a self-talk intervention:

- Injured individuals may not be aware of the extent to which they are using negative self-talk, or how it might affect their recovery. Practitioners can help these individuals to positively reframe messages, or encourage patients to self-talk out loud to promote greater attention to the content of the messages.
- Self-talk can be very important when returning to sport or exercise after injury, especially for those with lingering re-injury fear. Motivational forms of self-talk should be encouraged at this stage.

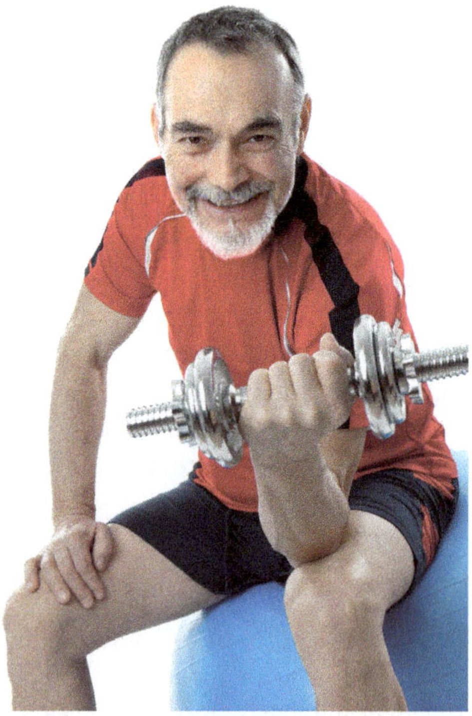

Image © Alexander Raths, 2014. Used under license from Shutterstock, Inc.

CHAPTER SUMMARY

Across the domains of sport, exercise, and injury rehabilitation, researchers have demonstrated that self-talk can be a useful tool. Although there have not been any formal tests of self-talk interventions among exercisers, researchers have shown that self-talk is used naturally by individuals in all three domains to serve both instructional and motivational purposes. Generally, empirical evidence suggests that although negative self-talk can be motivating for some individuals, practitioners should advocate for the use of positive self-talk. In certain cases, in order to use positive self-talk, athletes or exercisers will need to employ a thought-stopping or cognitive-restructuring technique in which they inhibit a negative self-talk statement and replace it with a positive one. Another important conclusion that can be drawn from the self-talk literature is the role of the practitioner in helping to establish self-talk statements. Practitioners have the knowledge to help create a plan for the 4 Ws of self-talk use by athletes (i.e., *where* and *when* and *why* they should use it, and *what* they should say to themselves). In this chapter, however, we have shown how important it is for athletes and exercisers to personally endorse their self-talk statements. Thus, coaches, trainers, and therapists should work with their athletes and exercisers to ensure that they believe in the self-talk statements. Further research is needed to test specific components of self-talk against one another to determine best practices for self-talk interventions.

REVIEW QUESTIONS

1. List the six dimensions of self-talk.
2. In sport, what types of self-talk interventions have proven to be effective?
3. In what setting is self-talk most frequently used by exercisers?
4. In this chapter we discussed four mechanisms by which self-talk may influence cognitions, motivation, or behavior in an exercise context. Pick one of these proposed mechanisms and describe, in detail, how it may explain the effects of self-talk.
5. Explain how self-talk can lead to both *positive* and *negative* moods during injury rehabilitation.
6. How can instructional self-talk be used to enhance injury rehabilitation outcomes?
7. Describe two ways in which self-talk might improve injury rehabilitation adherence.

SUGGESTED READINGS

Gammage, K. L., Hardy, J., & Hall, C. R. (2001). A description of self-talk in exercise. *Psychology of Sport and Exercise, 2,* 233–247.

Hamilton, R. A., Scott, D., & MacDougall, M. P. (2007). Assessing the effectiveness of self-talk interventions on endurance performance. *Journal of Applied Sport Psychology, 19,* 226–239.

Scherzer, C. B., Brewer, B. W., Cornelius, A. E., van Raalte, J. L., Petitpas, A. J., Sklar, J. H., et al. (2001). Psychological skills and adherence to rehabilitation after reconstruction of the anterior cruciate ligament. *Journal of Sport Rehabilitation, 10,* 165–172.

Theodorakis, Y., Beneca, A., Goudas, M., Antoniou, P., & Malliou, P. (1998). The effect of self-talk on injury rehabilitation. *European Yearbook of Sport Psychology, 2*, 124–135.

Tod, D., Hardy, J., & Oliver, E. (2011). Effects of self-talk: A systematic review. *Journal of Sport & Exercise Psychology, 33*, 666–687.

REFERENCES

Ahern, D. K., & Lohr, B. A. (1997). Psychosocial factors in sports injury rehabilitation. *Clinics in Sports Medicine, 16*(4), 755–768.

Anderson, A. (2013). Learning strategies in physical education: Self-talk, imagery, and goal setting. *Journal of Physical Education, Recreation & Dance, 68*(1), 30–35.

Baldwin, A. S., Rothman, A. J., Vander Weg, M. W., & Christensen, A. J. (2013). Examining causal components and a mediating process underlying self-generated health arguments for exercise and smoking cessation. *Health Psychology, 32*(12), 1209–1217.

Bandura, A. (1986). *Social foundations of thought and action.* Englewood Cliffs, NJ: Prentice-Hall.

Bell, J. J., & Hardy, J. (2009). Effects of attentional focus on skilled performance in golf. *Journal of Applied Sport Psychology, 21*, 163–177.

Carver, C. S., Scheier, M. F., & Segerstrom, S. C. (2010). Optimism. *Clinical Psychology Review, 30*(7), 879–889.

Chase, M. A., Magyar, T. M., & Drake, B. M. (2005). Fear of injury in gymnastics: Self-efficacy and psychological strategies to keep on tumbling. *Journal of Sports Sciences, 23*(5), 465–475.

Cox, R. H., Martens, M. P., & Russel, W. D. (2003). Measuring anxiety in athletics: the revised Competitive State Anxiety Inventory-2. *Journal of Sport and Exercise Psychology, 25*, 519–533.

Cupal, D. D. (2008). Psychological interventions in sport injury prevention and rehabilitation. *Journal of Applied Sport Psychology, 10*(1), 103–123.

Deci, E. L., & Ryan, R. M. (1985). *Intrinsic motivation and self determination in human behaviour.* New York: Plenum Press.

Gammage, K. L., Hardy, J., & Hall, C. R. (2001). A description of self-talk in exercise. *Psychology of Sport and Exercise, 2*, 233–247.

Gordon, S., Potter, M., & Ford, I. W. (1998). Toward a psychoeducational curriculum for training sport-injury rehabilitation personnel. *Journal of Applied Sport Psychology, 10*(1), 140–156.

Gouin, J. P., & Kiecolt-Glaser, J. K. (2011). The impact of psychological stress on wound healing: Methods and mechanisms. *Immunology and Allergy Clinics of North America, 31*, 81–93.

Hamilton, R. A., Scott, D., & MacDougall, M. P. (2007). Assessing the effectiveness of self-talk interventions on endurance performance. *Journal of Applied Sport Psychology, 19*, 226–239.

Hamson-Utley, J. J., Martin, S., & Walters, J. (2008). Athletic Trainers' and Physical Therapists' perceptions of the effectiveness of psychological skills within sport injury rehabilitation programs. *Journal of Athletic Training, 43*(3), 258–264.

Hardy, J. (2006). Speaking clearly: A critical review of the self-talk literature. *Psychology of Sport and Exercise, 7,* 81–97.

Hardy, J., Gammage, K., & Hall, C. R. (2001). A description of athlete self-talk. *The Sport Psychologist, 15,* 306–318.

Hardy, J., Hall, C. R., & Alexander, M. R. (2001). Exploring self-talk and affective states in sport. *Journal of Sports Sciences, 19,* 469–475.

Hardy, J., Hall, C. R., & Hardy, L. (2004). A note on athletes' use of self-talk. *Journal of Applied Sport Psychology, 16,* 251–257.

Hardy, J., Hall, C. R., & Hardy, L. (2005). Quantifying athletes' self-talk. *Journal of Sport Sciences, 23,* 905–917.

Hardy, L., Jones, G., & Gould, D. (1996). *Understanding psychological preparation for sport.* Chichester: John Wiley.

Hatzigeorgiadis, A., Theodorakis, Y., & Zourbanos, N. (2004). Self-talk in the swimming pool: The effects of self-talk on thought content and performance on water-polo tasks. *Journal of Applied Sport Psychology, 16,* 138–150.

Hatzigeorgiadis, A., Zourbanos, N., Mpoumpaki, S., & Theodorakis, Y. (2009). Mechanisms underlying the self-talk–performance relationship: The effects of motivational self-talk on self-confidence and anxiety. *Psychology of Sport and Exercise, 10,* 186–192.

Ieveleva, L., & Orlick, T. (1991). Mental links to enhanced healing: An exploratory study. *The Sport Psychologist, 5,* 25–40.

Landin, D. (1994). The role of verbal cues in skill learning. *Quest, 46,* 299–313.

Mahoney, M. J., & Avener, M. (1977). Psychology of the elite athlete: An exploratory study. *Cognitive Therapy and Research, 1,* 135–141.

McNevin, N. H., Shea, C. H., & Wulf, G. (2003). Increasing the distance of an external focus of attention enhances learning. *Psychological Research, 67,* 22–29.

Nideffer, R. M. (1976). Test of attentional and interpersonal style. *Journal of Personality and Social Psychology, 34,* 394–404.

Nippert, A. H., & Smith, A. M. (2008). Psychologic stress related to injury and impact on sport performance. *Physical Medicine and Rehabilitation Clinics of North America, 19,* 399–418.

Noar, S. M., Benac, C. N., & Harris, M. S. (2007). Does tailoring matter? Meta-analytic review of tailored print health behavior change interventions. *Psychological Bulletin, 133,* 673–693.

O'Brien Cousins (2003). A self-referent thinking model: How older adults may talk themselves out of being physically active. *Health Promotion Practice, 4,* 439–448.

O'Brien Cousins, S., & Gillis, M. M. (2005). "Just do it … before you talk yourself out of it": The self-talk of adults thinking about physical activity. *Psychology of Sport and Exercise, 6,* 313–334.

Petty, R. E., & Cacioppo, J. T. (1986). The elaboration likelihood model of persuasion. In *Communication and Persuasion* (pp. 1–24). New York: Springer.

Prochaska, J. O., & Velicer, W. F. (1997). The transtheoretical model of behaviour change. *American Journal of Health Promotion, 12,* 38–48.

Scherzer, C. B., Brewer, B. W., Cornelius, A. E., van Raalte, J. L., Petitpas, A. J., Sklar, J. H., et al. (2001). Psychological skills and adherence to rehabilitation after reconstruction of the anterior cruciate ligament. *Journal of Sport Rehabilitation, 10*, 165–172.

St. Clair Gibson, A., & Foster, C. (2007). The role of self-talk in the awareness of physiological state and physical performance. *Sports Medicine, 37*(12), 1029–1044.

Theodorakis, Y., Beneca, A., Goudas, M., Antoniou, P., & Malliou, P. (1998). The effect of self-talk on injury rehabilitation. *European Yearbook of Sport Psychology, 2*, 124–135.

Theodorakis, Y., Hatzigeorgiadis, A., & Chroni, S. (2008). Self-talk: It works, but how? Development and preliminary validation of the Functions of Self-Talk Questionnaire. *Measurement in Physical Education and Exercise Science, 12*(1), 10–30.

Theodorakis, Y., Weinberg, R., Natsis, P., Douma, I., & Kazakas, P. (2000). The effects of motivational versus instructional self-talk on improving motor performance. *The Sport Psychologist, 14*, 253–272.

Tod, D., Hardy, J., & Oliver, E. (2011). Effects of self-talk: A systematic review. *Journal of Sport & Exercise Psychology, 33*, 666–687.

Van Raalte, J. L., Brewer, B. W., Lewis, B. P., Linder, D. E., Wildman, G., & Kozimor, J. (1995). Cork! The effects of positive and negative self-talk on dart throwing performance. *Journal of Sport Behavior, 18*, 50–57.

Van Raalte, J. L., Brewer, B. W., Rivera, P. M., & Petitpas, A. J. (1994). The relationship between observable self-talk and competitive junior tennis players' match performances. *Journal of Sport & Exercise Psychology, 16*, 400–415.

Wiese, D., Weiss, M., & Yukelson, D. (1991). Sport psychology in the training room. A survey of athletic trainers. *The Sport Psychologist, 5*, 15–24.

Williams, J. & Roepke, N. (1993). Psychology of injury and injury rehabilitation. In R. N. Singer, M. Murphy, & L. K. Tennant (Eds), *Handbook of research on sport psychology* (pp. 815–839). New York: Macmillan.

Chapter 8

Biofeedback

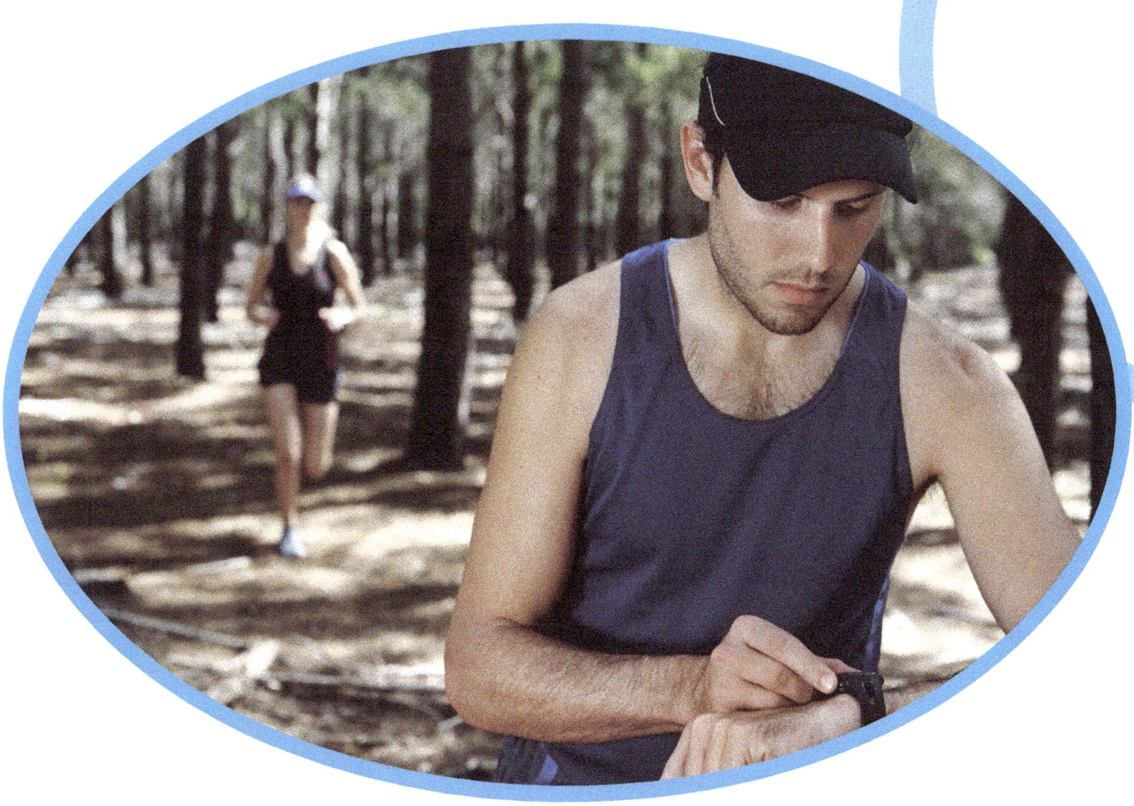

Introduction

Chances are you have taken your temperature or stepped on a scale. The thermometer indicates whether you're running a fever, the scale whether you have gained weight. Both devices provide 'feedback' about your body's condition. Once you have this information, you can take steps if necessary to improve this condition. When you are running a fever, you go to bed and drink plenty of fluids. When you have gained weight, you can eat less and be more physically active. Biofeedback is the process of gaining greater awareness of various physiological functions by using instruments that provide information on the activity of those same functions, with a goal of being able to manipulate them at will. Three organizations, the Association for Applied Psychophysiology and Biofeedback, the Biofeedback Certification International Alliance, and the International Society for Neurofeedback and Research, developed a consensus definition of biofeedback in 2008:

> 'Biofeedback is a process that enables an individual to learn how to change physiological activity for the purposes of improving health and performance. Precise instruments measure physiological activity such as brainwaves, heart function, breathing, muscle activity, and skin temperature. These instruments rapidly and accurately 'feed back' information to the user. The presentation of this information—often in conjunction with changes in thinking, emotions, and behavior—supports desired physiological changes. Over time, these changes can endure without continued use of an instrument.'
>
> (AAPB, 2013)

Biofeedback is often considered a type of complementary and alternative medicine. It is designed to enable you to use your thoughts to control your body. It is based on the idea that people have the innate potential to influence with their minds many of the automatic, involuntary functions of their bodies. In the early stages of biofeedback research, some investigators thought that we might be able to 'will' ourselves to be more creative by changing the patterns of our brainwaves. Others thought that biofeedback might make it possible to do away with drug treatments that often cause uncomfortable side effects in patients with conditions such as high blood pressure. While most researchers today agree that such high hopes were not realistic, biofeedback, sometimes called biofeedback training, is used to help manage many physical and mental health issues, including:

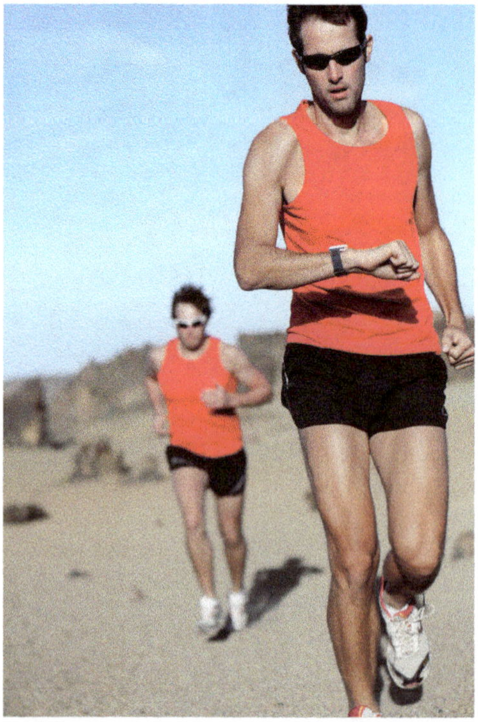

- Anxiety or stress
- Asthma
- Backaches
- Chemotherapy side effects

- Chronic pain
- Constipation
- Headaches
- High blood pressure
- Incontinence
- Irritable bowel syndrome
- Phobias
- Raynaud's disease
- Stuttering

Moreover, it has been demonstrated that we have more control over so-called involuntary bodily functions than we once thought possible. It has also been shown however, that nature limits the control we can exert.

With biofeedback the individual's goal is to learn to control involuntary functions such as heart rate, blood pressure, breathing, skin temperature, and muscle tension. For example, a woman may monitor an auditory signal of her own heart and attempts through using different thoughts, feelings, and sensations to slow her heart rate. Once she learns the feelings associated with the reduction of her heart rate, the biofeedback instrument providing the auditory signal is removed and she tries to control her heart rate without it. Thus, the biofeedback therapist teaches the patient how to affect a particular function specific to a problem through mental or physical exercises.

The provision of biofeedback requires the appropriate instrumentation. Heart rate is one of the more commonly measured physiological functions, and others are described in Table 8–1. Some biofeedback measurement techniques such as an electroencephalograph (EEG) can be relatively expensive while others (e.g., measurement of skin temperature) are quite affordable. As biofeedback devices

TABLE 8–1 Biofeedback Devices

Brain activity—Electroencephalogram (EEG) monitors the activity of brain waves linked to different mental states, such as wakefulness, relaxation, calmness, light sleep, and deep sleep.	**Muscle tension—**An Electromyogram (EMG) uses electrodes or other types of sensors to measure muscle tension. By the EMG alerting you to muscle tension, you can learn to recognize the feeling early on and try to control the tension right away.
Skin temperature—Sensors attached to your fingers or feet measure your skin temperature. Because your temperature often drops when you're under stress, a low reading can prompt you to begin relaxation techniques.	**Sweat gland activity—**Sensors measure the activity of your sweat glands and the amount of perspiration on your skin, alerting you to anxiety.

become less costly and more portable, the use of biofeedback in sport, exercise, and injury rehabilitation will undoubtedly increase. In general, biofeedback appeals to people for a variety of reasons:

- It is noninvasive
- It may enhance performance
- It helps people take charge of their health
- It may be an option when other treatments have not worked well

Biofeedback Challenges

- Biofeedback stands and falls on the measurement devices selected.
- Devices can be costly and require precise set up and calibration.
- Biofeedback provides information on the response being tested but without a trained professional offers no guidance to interpreting and changing this response.
- Technical advances offer an increasing range of psychological indices to detect.

Biofeedback in Sport

In the 1980s biofeedback was already viewed by sport psychology as having significant potential for athletic performance enhancement. A review of studies investigating the effect of biofeedback training on sports performance by Zaichkowsky and Fuchs in 1988 reported that 83% of the 42 studies examined found biofeedback training to be helpful in facilitating performance. Some sports have made more use of biofeedback than others, with rifle shooting being an example of a sport in which the use of biofeedback became widely accepted. A study conducted by Daniels and Landers (1981) is an example of research conducted in this sport. Participants were high level junior shooters aged 18–20 years. The shooters were divided into two groups, verbal instruction (control) and respiratory/HR biofeedback. This type of biofeedback was provided because in shooting it is extremely important to keep all body functions as calm as possible in order to prevent the body from moving or wobbling. The dependent measure was amount of error (absolute error) from center of target to the center of the bullet hole for each shot. Measurements were taken pre-training and post-training and the biofeedback training consisted of five sessions of 40 shots each. As can be seen in Table 8–2, the biofeedback group significantly reduced their error scores while the control group showed basically no change.

TABLE 8–2 Results

Group	Pre		Post
Biofeedback	2.98	↓	2.37
Verbal Instruction	2.95	↔	3.01
AE in cm			

Daniels & Landers (1981)

Research (Blumenstein, 2002; Zaichkowsky & Fuchs, 1988) has shown that biofeedback training can reduce performance anxiety, increase muscle strength, reduce pain and fatigue, increase flexibility, and regulate heart rate. Of course, there has been considerable interest in whether biofeedback training can enhance athletic performance. Positive findings have been reported in a number of performance-based settings including archery (Ren, 1995), golf (Crews, 1991), long-distance running (Caird, McKenzie, & Sleivert, 1999), and karate (Collins, 1995).

To provide structure and guidance in the application of biofeedback interventions, Blumenstein, Bar-Eli, and Tenenbaum (1997) developed a protocol termed the Wingate five-step approach. They developed this protocol because biofeedback devices are not typically designed for use during competitions, but rather to train athletes to gain greater control of their psychological functions. Often this training takes place in laboratory settings. The Wingate five-step approach consists of: (1) introduction (i.e., learning various self-regulation techniques); (2) identification (i.e., identifying and strengthening the most efficient biofeedback response modality); (3) simulation (i.e., biofeedback training with simulated competitive stress); (4) transformation (i.e., transformation of the biofeedback training to practice); and (5) realization (i.e., using the biofeedback training during competition). These steps are shown in Figure 8–1.

Bar-Eli, Dreshman, Blumenstein, and Weinstein (2002) used an adapted version of the Wingate five-step approach to enhance the performance of 11–14-year-old swimmers. One of the main purposes in the training of child swimmers is the acquisition of technical skills. In order to apply the Wingate five-step approach for this purpose, it was believed that the first three steps of the approach would be sufficient, namely, introduction, identification, and simulation. These steps are connected more to the instructional process, whereas transformation and realization (i.e., the last two steps) are more appropriate for athletes preparing for competition.

Participants were 38 male (n = 31) and female (n = 7) swimmers who had trained regularly for at least two years and participated in 3–4 competitions a year. The swimmers were randomly assigned to the biofeedback group or the control group. The groups met 38 times each over the course of 14 weeks. In the first session (baseline), each of the participants was requested to swim 50 m freestyle as fast as he or she could. The swimmers were evaluated by three coaches on their swimming technique. In addition, the participants' swimming time was measured.

Figure 8–1 Wingate Five-step Approach

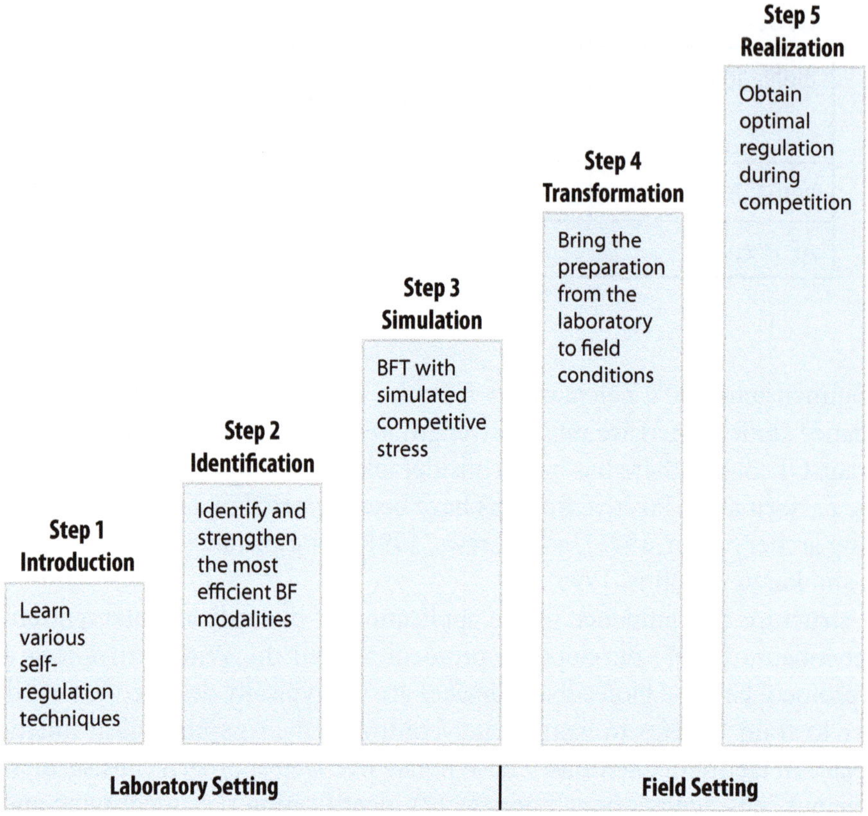

Note: BF = biofeedback; BFT = biofeedback training. Adapted from Blumenstein & Weinstein (2011). Biofeedback training: Enhancing athletic performance. *Biofeedback, 39,* 101–104.

In sessions 2–17, which took place during weeks 2–7 of the study, the biofeedback group underwent step 1 (i.e., introduction) of the treatment. In this step the athletes were taught various self-regulation techniques, such as autogenic training, imagery, and biofeedback training. Each session lasted for about 35 minutes and was given to the biofeedback group in addition to their regular training sessions. During this period (sessions 2–17), the control group underwent identical regular training sessions to prevent any potential influence of different training environments. However, to exclude the "Hawthorne Effect" as a potential explanation for any possible performance improvements in the biofeedback group, the control group also had sessions lasting about 35 minutes but they involved various relaxing activities such as listening to quiet music, observing nature movies, and playing table games.

In session 18, both groups were measured in a procedure which was identical to the one they underwent during the baseline session. In sessions 19–37, which took place during weeks 7–13 of the study, the biofeedback group underwent steps 2 (i.e., identification) and 3 (i.e., simulation) of the Wingate five-step approach. The athletes in step 2 identified and strengthened their most efficient biofeedback training response modality, which was either heart rate (HR), electromyography (EMG), or galvanic skin response (GSR). In step 3, the simulation consisted of listening to original (competitive) noise recorded during a high-level international swimming contest. During sessions 19–37, the control group continued to engage in relaxing activities. In session 38, both groups were measured again in a procedure which was identical to the baseline session.

The results for the evaluation scores revealed a significant Group × Measurement Time interaction which was attributed to the greater rate of progress obtained by the biofeedback group throughout the study, in comparison to the control group. As indicated in Table 8–3, there were increasing differences between the two groups at each measurement time, from the non-significant difference at baseline, to the largest difference obtained at the third measurement. Corresponding results were found for swimming times. Again there was a significant Group × Measurement Time interaction. As can be seen in Table 8–4, the biofeedback group decreased their swimming times over the three measurements while the swimming times for the control group remained relatively stable.

TABLE 8–3 Means and Standard Deviations for Evaluation Scores by Measurements

Group	Measurement		
	1 (Baseline)	2	3
Biofeedback Group			
M	2.97	3.55	4.42
SD	0.32	0.27	0.23
Control Group			
M	2.90	3.31	3.75
SD	0.38	0.28	0.40

TABLE 8–4 Means and Standard Deviations for Swimming Times (in sec.) by Measurements

Group	Measurement		
	1 (Baseline)	2	3
Biofeedback Group			
M	33.36	32.10	30.99
SD	2.87	2.81	2.48
Control Group			
M	38.29	38.37	37.61
SD	4.04	4.07	4.26

Bar-Eli and colleagues concluded that the results from both the evaluation scores and the swimming times indicated that participants in the biofeedback group consistently exhibited the greatest improvements. In other words, using regular training plus biofeedback training will lead to better results than using regular training only. Moreover, these results demonstrate that the superiority of the Wingate approach increases over time (measurements). Other studies have also supported using the Wingate five-step approach (e.g., Bar-Eli & Blumenstein, 2004; Edmonds, Tenenbaum, Mann, Johnson, & Kamata, 2008).

More recently, researchers have integrated biofeedback training within a comprehensive psychological skills training program. For example, Beauchamp, Harvey, and Beauchamp (2012) developed and implemented a multifaceted psychological skills training program for the Canadian National Short Track Speedskating team over a 3-year period leading up to the Vancouver 2010 Olympic Games. The skaters were 10 male and 10 female athletes recruited from the National Training Center in Montreal, Canada. The intervention was periodized over three years with the Speedskating Canada yearly training plan. The intervention consisted of seven phases conducted over the three years: (1) orientation/observation, (2) sport analysis, (3) individual/team assessment, (4) concept utilization, (5) psychological skills training intervention strategies, (6) implementation, and (7) evaluation.

The psychological skills incorporated in the intervention included relaxation, imagery, self-talk, and focusing, as well as biofeedback training. The biofeedback measures were heart rate, respiration rate, heart rate variability (HVR), muscle activity, skin temperature, skin conductance, and neurofeedback (EEG). Biofeedback sessions were conducted on a weekly basis in phases 3 and 4 until automaticity was established for each measure. In phases 5 and 6, a schedule of four to six sessions per measure was implemented, except because HRV was considered a core element in the biofeedback training program, on average six to ten sessions were conducted for HRV.

Overall, the intervention was considered a success. The goal of the intervention was to prepare the skaters to perform their best under the pressure of the Olympic Games. This was achieved from both a team perspective and an individual perspective. The team won two gold medals, two silver medals, and a bronze medal. Moreover, 14 of the skaters were finalists in their events. Finally, the International Skating Union's overall ranking for both the team and individuals improved over the course of the intervention.

Some General Recommendations

Biofeedback training should only be considered if the athlete is willing to invest the time and effort required to achieve results. For example, while the steps in the Wingate five-step approach have flexible time-limit sessions that can be individualized (Bar-Eli & Blumenstein, 2004), a minimum of about 10 sessions for each of the first four steps is recommended with each session lasting up to 60 minutes (Blumenstein & Weinstein, 2011). Other recommendations are:

- The type of biofeedback utilized should be tailored to a combination of the athlete and the sport.
- Biofeedback effectiveness can be enhanced when it is combined with other psychological skills such as imagery and self-talk.

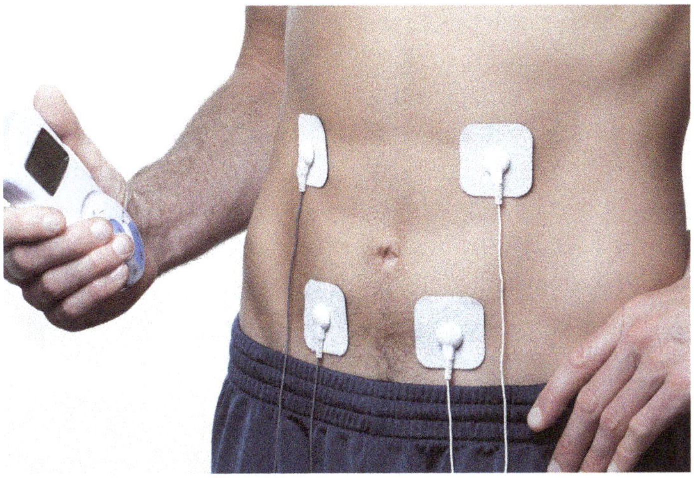

Biofeedback in Exercise

As it does in the realm of sports, biofeedback can have important implications in the exercise domain as well. Controlling physiological responses such as heart rate and blood pressure can help reduce the load that exercise places on the body, allowing a person to exercise at higher intensities or for a longer duration at a decreased metabolic cost (Petruzello, Landers, & Salazar, 1991). Additionally, using instruments to acquire feedback about our physiological responses to exercise may help motivate subsequent behavior. Consider the phenomenon of the "weekend warrior"—the person who is too busy with work, family, and other commitments during the week to engage in physical activity so he packs all of his exercise into the weekends, often overdoing it in terms of intensity or duration. Indeed, regulating the intensity at which we exercise is often a challenge. Whereas some people exercise infrequently and at an intensity unnecessarily high to achieve health benefits (and often suffer sore muscles as a consequence), many people do not exercise at an intensity that is high enough. Biofeedback is one way for these exercisers to learn how to self-regulate in order to achieve optimal exercise intensity.

In the domain of exercise, biofeedback occurs largely by heart rate monitoring, although, as we will see, some studies have been conducted using muscle EMGs. Also, advances in technology have led to improvements in commercial heart rate monitoring technology and the development of products like the fitbit, the Nike + iPod, and the adidas miCoach which provide biofeedback information to recreational exercisers. Thus, whereas biofeedback training was once quite costly, it is becoming increasingly affordable and prominent within recreational exercise settings.

Biofeedback of Aerobic Exercise

The most common type of biofeedback training in the exercise domain involves training heart rate during aerobic exercise. Numerous studies have demonstrated that in both healthy and clinical populations, providing heart rate feedback during aerobic exercise (traditionally during treadmill or cycle ergometer tests) can result in attenuated heart rate response. For example, Perski and Engel (1980) demonstrated that among ten young (mean age = 23.9 years), healthy, untrained participants, the five participants who were randomly assigned to receive heart rate feedback while cycling on an ergometer at 50 percent of their maximum heart rate were able to maintain heart rates 20% lower than the five participants who did not receive feedback. In a subsequent study, Fredrikson and Engel (1985) found similar results among patients with borderline hypertension. In this study, over 5 days (and 25 training trials), six patients who received beat-to-beat heart rate feedback were able to maintain a heart rate approximately ten beats per minute lower than six patients who did not receive heart rate feedback. Researchers have also reported that reducing heart rate during exercise can lead to significantly lower systolic blood pressure and other measures of physiological stress (Goldstein, Ross, & Brady, 1977). Taken together, these findings demonstrated that heart rate can be brought under voluntary control during physical exercise. Among patients with cardiovascular diseases, these findings are particularly important given the obvious benefits of reducing the workload placed on the heart while also engaging in health-enhancing exercise behavior.

One interesting finding with potentially important practical implications relates to the modality by which heart rate feedback is delivered. Specifically, Moleiro and Cid (2001) randomly assigned 35 participants to receive either heart rate feedback via biofeedback techniques (i.e., participants could view a graph of their heart rate patterns in real time in addition to an electronic display of their beats per minute) or via verbal prompts to reduce their heart rate while exercising. After five experimental sessions, Moleiro and Cid found that participants trained using the biofeedback technique had significantly greater attenuation of heart rate increases than participants trained using verbal feedback. Incorporating these findings into actual practice may be achievable through the use of some of the new commercial heart rate monitoring devices, fitness assistant products such as the fitbit, and mobile phone applications. These technologies allow exercisers to carry their biofeedback devices with them at all times and access this information regularly.

Whereas heart rate monitoring is the most common formal intervention modality for biofeedback of aerobic exercise, regulating exercise intensity through mindfulness of physiological exertion has promise as well. Requiring no equipment, training exercisers to be mindful of their physiological exertion, using a validated scale such as the Borg Ratings of Perceived Exertion (RPE) scale (see Table 8–5), and to adjust their exercise intensity accordingly could easily be implemented across large numbers of people. Dunbar and Kalinski (2004) tested this idea among six post-menopausal women as they participated in a 20-week aerobic exercise program. Before the program began, the women were given explicit descriptions about each of the categories on the Borg RPE scale. Then, in each week of the program the researchers gave them verbal descriptions of which RPE category to aim for. The program was designed such that the women would exercise at low intensity for relatively short duration (i.e., 40% of maximum heart rate for 15 minutes) at the beginning of the program, increase to higher intensity and longer duration (i.e., 60% of maximum heart rate for 30 minutes) by the end of the first five weeks, and maintain this higher intensity until the end of the program. During each exercise session the researchers gave the participants a verbal description of the intensity to which they should aim, rather than any specific feedback. The findings showed that at low intensities (i.e., 40–50% of maximum heart rate), the women were easily able to achieve the target exercise intensity; however, when instructed to exercise in higher categories of RPE, they initially failed to achieve the desired intensities. Interestingly, this failure to achieve the target heart rate range based on RPE did not last for the remainder of the program; over time, the women became acclimatized to using RPE to regulate the intensity of their exercise and were able to achieve the target heart rate ranges. Overall, Dunbar and Kalinski concluded that, although it

TABLE 8–5 Borg Ratings of Perceived Exertion

How you might describe your exertion	Borg rating of your exertion	Examples (for most adults <65 years old)
None	6	Reading a book, watching television
Very, very light	7 to 8	Tying shoes
Very light	9 to 10	Chores like folding clothes that seem to take little effort
Fairly light	11 to 12	Walking through the grocery store or other activities that require some effort but not enough to speed up your breathing
Somewhat hard	13 to 14	Brisk walking or other activities that require moderate effort and speed your heart rate and breathing but don't make you out of breath
Hard	15 to 16	Bicycling, swimming, or other activities that take vigorous effort and get the heart pounding and make breathing very fast
Very hard	17 to 18	The highest level of activity you can sustain
Very, very hard	19 to 20	A finishing kick in a race or other burst of activity that you can't maintain for long

Source: Borg, G. A. (1982). Psychophysical bases of perceived exertion. *Medicine and Science in Sports and Exercise, 14,* 377–381.

may take time to develop skills for using RPE to regulate exercise intensity at higher levels of exertion, this could be a safe and effective way to help exercisers achieve the exercise intensities necessary to accrue health benefits.

Biofeedback of Strengthening Activities

The effects of strengthening exercises can also be improved with biofeedback training. Whereas heart rate training is the typical biofeedback strategy employed in the context of aerobic exercise, electromyography (EMG) can be used to improve self-regulation of strengthening exercises. For example, Lucca and Recchiuti (1983) enrolled 30 female undergraduate students into either an isometric exercise group, an isometric exercise plus biofeedback group, or a control group that did not do any isometric exercise training. To provide biofeedback they used a Cyborg J-33 unit with electrodes connected to the exercised leg that provided auditory feedback (i.e., beeps) to the participants as they attempted to extend their leg in an isometric contraction for 6 seconds. The participants in both exercise training groups performed five contractions with rest periods of 25 seconds between them. After 19 days of training, the group that received biofeedback in addition to the exercise training produced significantly greater gains in peak torque than the other two groups.

Biofeedback Training to Increase Physical Activity among Children

In recent decades, concern about the amount of physical activity being achieved by children across the developed world has been growing. Researchers and practitioners have been seeking creative and engaging ways to teach children about the benefits of physical activity and to increase activity levels in this population. Could biofeedback be used as a means to keep children engaged in monitoring and regulating their own physical activity levels? McManus, Masters, Laukkanen, Yu, Sit, and Ling (2008) sought to answer this question among 210 primary school students from three schools in Hong Kong. At one school, the children received an educational program about heart rate monitoring, physical activity, and health and engaged in heart rate monitoring with feedback (for two weeks) and without feedback (for an additional two weeks). At the second school, the children engaged in heart rate monitoring with and without feedback (as above) but did not receive an educational intervention or any information about interpreting heart rates. The third school served as a control and did not engage in any educational intervention or heart rate feedback. The findings showed that, regardless of whether or not they received an educational program, both groups who received heart rate feedback increased their total daily physical activity by an average of 24% over the short-term (i.e., during the one-month period they wore the heart rate monitors). Both groups also increased their vigorous physical activity by an average of 6% over this period. At a six-month follow-up, after heart rate monitoring had been discontinued, differences in physical activity (at all intensities) between the heart rate biofeedback groups and the control group were no longer apparent. Although McManus et al. showed that biofeedback was useful for increasing physical activity among children, one important component of biofeedback—that over time, changes can endure without the use of instrumentation (AAPB, 2013)—was not achieved. Therefore, more research is needed to determine how to sustain the effects of a biofeedback intervention among children.

Biofeedback Using Modern Technology

As mentioned previously, with the development of new heart rate monitoring technology and mobile phone applications, the potential for biofeedback to be used widely among exercisers is growing. To date, most of these technologies allow simply for self-monitoring among exercisers; however, more recent technology is beginning to incorporate mechanisms for delivering feedback to exercisers and changing the motivational climate. For example, van der Vlist, Bartneck, and Maueler (2011) have reported on a device called the MoBeat, which measures exercise pace and intensity and then adjusts the music tempo to indicate to the exerciser if they should speed up or slow down. When the appropriate intensity is reached, the MoBeat rewards the exerciser by playing richer-sounding music. A within-subjects pilot test among 26 participants comparing the MoBeat to a commercially-available heart rate monitor indicated that the MoBeat was just as effective for keeping participants exercising at a desired

RPE but also increased intrinsic motivation and attentional focus. Although these findings are preliminary, they represent an emerging area in the field of exercise biofeedback and a potential means of making this intervention strategy accessible to the general public.

Some General Recommendations

Whereas biofeedback in an exercise setting was initially limited to laboratory settings with advanced monitoring equipment, this intervention strategy is becoming increasingly common in real-world exercise settings. Although technological advances in biofeedback allow for light-weight and portable instrumentation, the goal of biofeedback to train exercisers to self-regulate in the absence of instrumentation should not be lost. Practitioners should make an effort to increase the mindfulness of exercisers who use instrumentation for biofeedback to ensure that they are developing an awareness of the physiological experience of exercising and could self-regulate if the instrumentation were removed. Other general recommendations include:

- Consider the means by which feedback is delivered to exercisers. Whereas some studies show that exercisers respond best to numeric or graphical feedback from the biofeedback instruments (Moleiro & Cid, 2001), other researchers find that verbal feedback is sufficient for training exercisers to achieve optimal exercise intensities (Dunbar & Kalinski, 2004).
- The specific instrumentation used to provide biofeedback should align with the goals of the intervention. Exercisers needing a boost in intensity may benefit from biofeedback instruments that are combined with motivational tools such as the MoBeat (van der Vlist et al., 2011). Among clinical populations, however, where the goal is to decrease heart rate, blood pressure, or other physiological responses to exercise, simpler heart rate monitoring tools may be more appropriate.
- Combining biofeedback interventions with educational interventions that teach exercisers about the information that is fed back to them and the health implications of achieving desired exercise levels may be one way to increase mindfulness and self-regulation of exercise.

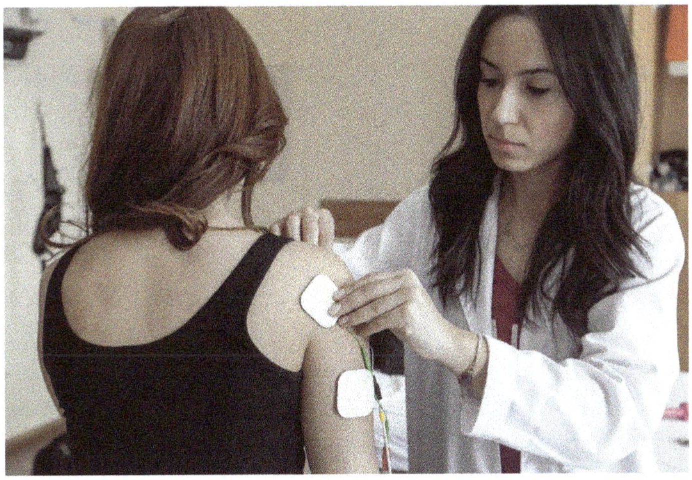

Biofeedback in Injury Rehabilitation

After an injury a number of issues must be overcome, including decreased muscle function, reflex inhibition, reduced receptor activity leading to proprioceptive difficulties, and pain. Biofeedback can be a helpful adjunct to standard rehabilitation programs by specifically addressing these concerns. The benefits of biofeedback, regardless of the modality, can be attributed to its effect on motor learning and its ability to enhance physical training (e.g., support muscle strengthening), but perhaps its greatest advantage is its role in maximizing the athlete's effort. For example, traditional electrical stimulation is a routine part of physiotherapy and acts by eliciting muscular contractions through artificial means. When applied to a muscle during therapy, this external stimulation can trigger and sustain a contraction in the absence of any voluntary input from the patient. This can be helpful from a physical recovery standpoint, but has limited effect on retraining neuromuscular control. Biofeedback, on the other hand, requires conscious interpretation of visual, auditory, or tactile information, and corresponding voluntary action by the patient. In other words, biofeedback influences the underlying processes of muscle activation by linking physiological and psychological functions.

While athletes are rehabilitating injuries, or receiving care after surgery, they spend a lot of time in physiotherapy clinics or other treatment settings. Having regularly scheduled appointments and set routines is ideal for implementing a biofeedback intervention, and patients are typically willing to put in the effort necessary for the intervention to be successful. Additionally, the relationship between biofeedback techniques and recovery can be less abstract than in sport or exercise settings, as the equipment used for biofeedback is often the same as what a therapist would use to treat the individual (e.g., electromyography machines, heart rate monitors). For these reasons, there has been a long history of research in this area and biofeedback is a widely accepted intervention in injured populations (see Giggins, Persson, & Caulfield, 2013, for a review).

Knee Injuries

Much of the biofeedback research has been conducted with patients recovering from knee surgery. These individuals are usually characterized by inhibited muscle function, reduced neuromuscular control, and atypical gait patterns in the postoperative period, making them prime candidates for biofeedback interventions. EMG biofeedback is the most commonly used technique in this population (Giggins et al., 2013). This type of system consists of electrodes or needles that are attached to the patient and a sensitive voltmeter that converts the electrical signals associated with muscle activity into visual or audible signals. Therapists are able to use this system to monitor how well athletes are recovering, and can be alerted to any lingering deficits in muscular control or activation. This information can also be used to help the patient identify the feelings associated with suboptimal performance, thereby enhancing the outcomes of rehabilitation exercises.

EMG biofeedback is generally regarded as a helpful method of addressing muscle inhibition after many types of knee surgery (Levitt, Deisinger, Wall, Ford, & Cassisi, 1995; Neblett & Perez, 2010). In fact, some clinicians recognize biofeedback as an integral part of postoperative rehabilitation for anterior cruciate ligament (ACL) reconstruction (Wilk, Macrina, Cain, Dugas, & Andrews, 2012). Yet, there are limitations to its effectiveness. For example, Boucher et al. (2009) found that biofeedback resulted in improved active range of motion, but had no effect on overall function or strength in patients post-arthroscopy (Boucher, Wang, Trudelle-Jackson, & Olson, 2009). In a recent review of four randomized controlled trials examining the effect of biofeedback for patients either receiving treatment for patellafemoral pain syndrome (PFPS) or recovering after arthroscopic meniscectomy, Silkman and McKeon (2010) found conflicting evidence. Two studies reported that EMG biofeedback was effective at improving muscle activation and quadriceps function when combined with a conventional therapeutic exercise program, compared to a conventional program alone (Kirnap, Calis, Turgut, Halici, & Tuncel, 2005; Ng, Zang, & Li, 2006). The other two studies found that EMG did not improve outcomes when combined with a standard program (Dursun, Dursun, & Kilic, 2001; Yip & Ng, 2006). Identifying the most effective biofeedback intervention in a given patient population is therefore still a major research and clinical focus.

Several studies have focused on the use of EMG biofeedback following meniscal repair (Krebs, 1981; Sprenger, Carlson, & Wessman, 1979). There is some evidence that EMG potentials, speed of thigh muscle contraction and relaxation, and self-reported sport and recreation-related function improve to a greater degree for those receiving biofeedback compared to those who do not (Oravitan & Avram, 2013). This suggests that biofeedback may be particularly effective for targeting neuromuscular control after injury.

Akkaya and colleagues (2011) randomized 45 patients into three groups (n = 15) following arthroscopic partial meniscectomy (Akkaya, Ardic, Ozgen, Akkaya, Sahin, & Kilic, 2011). All three groups received the same home exercise program. In addition, group two was prescribed a quadriceps EMG biofeedback protocol to be carried out five days per week for two weeks, and group three was prescribed a quadriceps electrical stimulation program to be completed five days per week for two weeks. After two weeks of the intervention, the biofeedback group reported using a walking aid for a significantly shorter time, and had better functional outcomes (as measured by the Lysholm Knee Scoring Scale), compared to the control group. Maximum and average quadriceps contractions also favored the biofeedback group compared to both other conditions.

Similarly, Kirnap et al. (2005) randomized 20 patients to a control rehabilitation program and 20 patients to a rehabilitation program that included EMG biofeedback following arthroscopic meniscectomy. The biofeedback protocol began on the third postoperative day and was applied five days per week for two weeks. These authors found that the biofeedback group demonstrated better Lysholm Knee Scale scores and average contraction values than the controls at two- and six-week time points after surgery. Range of motion, particularly knee flexion, also favored the biofeedback group.

For those undergoing ACL surgery, EMG biofeedback has been related to significantly improved range of motion and quadriceps function during the first six weeks of rehabilitation, but there is limited evidence to support its effect on swelling or pain (Christanell, Hoser, Huber, Fink, Luomajoki, 2012; Draper, 1990; Draper & Ballard, 1991). There has also been some investigation of biofeedback for osteoarthritis (OA) patients. One study found that there was no additive effect of EMG biofeedback with strength training for knee OA patients after 3 weeks of intervention (Yilmaz, Senocak, Sahin, Baydar, Gulbahar, Bircan, et al., 2010). A single case study of a patient following total knee arthroplasty, however, suggested that biofeedback might be useful for improving knee biomechanics in this population (McClelland, Zeni, Haley, & Snyder-Mackler, 2012). Given the consistent evidence supporting the use of real-time kinematic, kinetic, and temporospatial biofeedback for short-term improvements in gait (Tate & Milner, 2010), it is reasonable to suggest that this type of intervention may impart some benefit to OA patients, although there is limited information regarding its potential long-term effects. More research will be necessary in this population to determine the value added by biofeedback in rehabilitation settings.

Brain and Spinal Injuries

Biofeedback has long been applied in the area of neurological rehabilitation. Particularly for those with severe brain injury, reacquiring basic voluntary movements like breath control and fine motor skills are paramount in the early stages of recovery. Visual biofeedback has demonstrated efficacy for helping these patients regulate heart rate variability (HRV) (Kim, Zemon, Cavallo, Rath, McCraty, & Foley, 2013), and real-time gesture recognition feedback has been used to promote short-term improvements in fine motor control (Yungher & Craelius, 2012).

Thornton and Carmody (2009) reported the effects of quantitative EEG (QEEG) biofeedback (e.g., brain wave measurements) on auditory and reading memory after traumatic brain injury (TBI). These authors reported significant memory improvements (effect sizes ranging from 1.75 to 1.85) in their sample of 15 adult TBI patients, although they did not provide details about injury severity, time since injury, or level of memory impairment at baseline in their sample.

With growing awareness of sport related concussion in recent years, researchers have begun to search for active rehabilitation techniques to use for concussed athletes. One of the hallmark symptoms of post-concussion syndrome is impaired autonomic function, characterized by increased heart rate and decreased HRV. Although there is a paucity of evidence in this area, it has been hypothesized that HRV biofeedback could be a promising treatment in this patient group (Lagos, Bottiglieri, Vaschillo, & Vaschillo, 2012). To date, however, biofeedback has not been widely considered as a therapeutic option for these athletes.

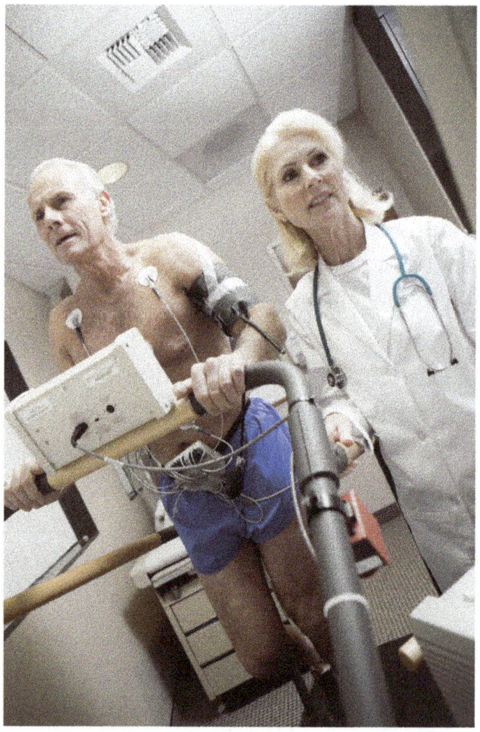

Image © Monkey Business Images, 2014. Used under license from Shutterstock, Inc..

The role of EMG biofeedback in the rehabilitation of other spine-related injuries has been investigated. There is some evidence to support its use for normalizing flexion-relaxation in chronic low back pain patients (Neblett, Mayer, Brede, & Gatchel, 2010), and it has been shown to increase voluntary EMG responses in individuals with spinal cord injury (De Biase, Politti, Palomari, Barros-Filho, & De Camargo, 2011). One study examined EMG biofeedback as a potential therapy modality for long-term pain following whiplash injury, but reported that it had no significant effect (Ehrenborg & Archenholtz, 2010).

Injury Prevention

A limited amount of research has investigated the potential role of biofeedback in injury prevention. Given that specific biofeedback strategies have been shown to positively improve sport and exercise technique, it stands to reason that similar approaches could be used to alter high-risk motor patterns or behaviors to prevent potential acute or chronic injury. To this end, one study demonstrated that augmented feedback, consisting of a self-modeling video of a high-risk motion pattern along with verbal correction, resulted in significant improvements in high-risk vertical drop jump performance (Myer, Stroube, DiCesare, Brent, Ford, Heidt Jr, et al., 2013). Of note, this technique was robust enough to elicit change when feedback was provided during one task (performing a tuck jump), then transferred to another similar task (vertical drop jump). Although this study did not use biofeedback explicitly, it provides proof of concept that such techniques could be successfully applied in this context.

Conversely, Edvardsson, Ivarsson, and Johnson (2012) found that cognitive-behavioral biofeedback had limited injury prevention benefit. They used a biofeedback instrument to measure HRV and GSR using finger sensors, providing graphical curves in response to cognitive-behavioral stress management sessions. They found no significant difference in coping skills, anxiety, life event stress, or injury between intervention group participants and controls over a nine-week period of the Swedish elite football high school season.

Clearly, much additional research is needed to determine the potential benefit of including biofeedback as a component of injury prevention interventions. It is plausible that various techniques could be used to target modifiable injury risk factors, but it is not yet evident which approach would be most successful, nor what the appropriate timing or dose of biofeedback might be.

New Technologies

The most common biofeedback technique used in rehabilitation is EMG, but with the advent of new technologies, researchers and clinicians are adapting a number of additional strategies for treating patients. For example, it has been shown that real-time vibrotactile biofeedback can be provided to injured individuals during balance tasks to improve their performance (Alahakone & Senanayake, 2010). Similarly, the Nintendo Wii™ balance pad, which includes a force plate, has been used in conjunction with interactive training games to promote balance and proprioceptive awareness for patients with neurological injury (Gil-Gomez, Llorens, Alcaniz, & Colomer, 2011). This approach has been met with positive reviews from patients and therapists (Lange, Flynn, Chang, Ahmed, Geng, Utsav, et al., 2010), and demonstrates the practical application of mobile technologies that allow biofeedback to be used in both clinical and home settings.

Advancements in biotechnology have also led to the development of wearable sensors that can be embedded in clothing. Garments that include force and impact sensors, accelerometers, heart and respiration rate sensors, temperature gauges, and more are providing an opportunity for athletes and coaches to receive real-time biofeedback during sport activities. While these technologies are only just beginning to appear in training settings, they have the potential to be integrated into rehabilitation programs, particularly for athletes who are transitioning back into sport, or for those in remote locations without immediate access to rehabilitation facilities.

Some General Recommendations

When implementing a biofeedback intervention, it is important to remember that not all patients will respond the same way. Like any psychological skill, it takes practice to interpret biofeedback information and coordinate it with physical actions. Additional recommendations include:

- Some patients will have preferences for visual or auditory signals when receiving biofeedback information. When there is no option to tailor the signal, patients may need additional guidance from their therapist while first learning the prescribed technique.
- It is important that patients do not become reliant on the biofeedback equipment. A weaning period toward the end of treatment can help the individual monitor his or her awareness of ongoing biological processes (e.g., heart rate) and the ability to initiate corresponding behaviors to regulate those processes.

CHAPTER SUMMARY

Biofeedback has long been considered a valuable part of injury rehabilitation, and is increasingly being used in sport and exercise. In sport, in addition to enhancing athletic performance, biofeedback training can reduce performance anxiety, increase muscle strength, reduce pain and fatigue, increase flexibility, and regulate heart rate. One of the primary goals for the use of biofeedback in exercise is to train participants to self-regulate. With respect to injury rehabilitation, there is substantial evidence that biofeedback has added benefit when included in rehabilitation programs following knee surgery and neurological injury. A number of new technologies are making biofeedback less expensive and more portable, which increases its viability in many settings (e.g., research, fitness facilities, clinical practice). Given these advancements, it is likely that biofeedback will become even more widely used. Coaches will employ it to improve their athletes' performances. Exercisers will use biofeedback to train at the appropriate intensities, and in injury rehabilitation it is likely to be prescribed for a number of injury types, and may become a standard intervention approach in therapy.

REVIEW QUESTIONS

1. What are some common biofeedback devices?
2. What are the five steps in the Wingate five-step approach to biofeedback training?
3. Describe the potential benefits of biofeedback training for cardiac rehabilitation patients.
4. How does the use of light-weight and portable commercially-available biofeedback instruments potentially limit the ultimate goals of biofeedback training?
5. What are some of the benefits associated with EMG biofeedback following knee surgery?
6. What types of biofeedback have been used in injury prevention studies, and what new research questions have been raised as a result of these studies?

SUGGESTED READINGS

Akkaya, N., Ardic, F., Ozgen, M., Akkaya, S., Sahin, F., & Kilic, A. (2011). Efficacy of electromyographic biofeedback and electrical stimulation following arthroscopic partial meniscectomy: a randomized controlled trial. *Clinical Rehabilitation, 26*(3), 224–236.

Beauchamp, M. K., Harvey, R. H., & Beauchamp, P. H. (2012). An Integrated Biofeedback and Psychological Skills Training Program for Canada's Olympic Short-Track Speedskating Team, *Journal of Clinical Sport Psychology, 6*, 67–84.

Christanell, F., Hoser, C., Huber, R., Fink, C., & Luomajoki, H. (2012). The influence of electromyographic biofeedback therapy on knee extension following anterior cruciate ligament reconstruction: a randomized controlled trial. *Sport Medicine, Arthroscopy, Rehabilitation, Therapy & Technology, 4*, 41–50.

Dunbar, C. C. & Kalinski, M. I. (2004). Using RPE to regulate exercise intensity during a 20-week training program for postmenopausal women: A pilot study. *Perceptual and Motor Skills, 99*, 688–690.

Giggins, O. M., Persson, U. M., & Caulfield, B. (2013). Biofeedback in rehabilitation. *Journal of Neuro-Engineering and Rehabilitation, 10*, 60–70.

McManus, A. M., Masters, R. S. W., Laukkanen, R. M. T., Yu, C. C. W., Sit, C. H. P., & Ling, F. C. M. (2008). Using heart-rate feedback to increase physical activity in children. *Preventive Medicine, 47*, 402–408.

Petruzzello, S. J., Landers, D. M., & Salazar, W. (1991). Biofeedback and sport/exercise performance: Applications and Limitations. *Behavior Therapy, 22*, 379–392.

REFERENCES

Akkaya, N., Ardic, F., Ozgen, M., Akkaya, S., Sahin, F., & Kilic, A. (2011). Efficacy of electromyographic biofeedback and electrical stimulation following arthroscopic partial meniscectomy: a randomized controlled trial. *Clinical Rehabilitation, 26*(3), 224–236.

Alahakone, A. U., & Senanayake, A. (2010). A real-time interactive biofeedback system for sports training and rehabilitation. *Proceedings of the Institution of Mechanical Engineers, Part P: Journal of Sports Engineering and Technology.* 181–190.

Association for Applied Psychophysiology and Biofeedback (2008). http://www.aapb.org/i4a/pages/index.cfm?pageid=1

Bar-Eli, M., & Blumenstein, B. (2004). Performance enhancement in swimming: the effect of mental training with biofeedback. *Journal of Medicine and Science in Sport, 7*, 454–464.

Bar-Eli, M., Dreshman, R., Blumenstein, B., & Weinstein, Y. (2002). The effect of mental training with biofeedback on the performance of young swimmers. *Applied Psychology: An International Review, 51*, 567–581.

Beauchamp, M. K., Harvey, R. H., & Beauchamp, P. H. (2012). An Integrated Biofeedback and Psychological Skills Training Program for Canada's Olympic Short-Track Speedskating Team, *Journal of Clinical Sport Psychology, 6*, 67–84.

Blumenstein, B. (2002). Biofeedback applications in sport and exercise: Research findings. In B. Blumenstein, M. Bar-Eli, & G. Tenenbaum (Eds.), *Brain and body in sport and exercise: Biofeedback applications in performance enhancement* (pp. 37–54). Chichester, UK: Wiley.

Blumenstein, B., Bar-Eli, M., & Tenenbaum, G. (1997). A five step approach to mental training incorporating biofeedback. *The Sport Psychologist, 11*, 440–453.

Blumenstein, B., & Weinstein, Y. (2011). Biofeedback training: Enhancing athletic performance. *Biofeedback, 39*, 101–104.

Boucher, T., Wang, S., Trudelle-Jackson, E., & Olson, S. (2009). Effectiveness of surface electromyographic biofeedback-triggered neuromuscular electrical stimulation on knee rehabilitation. *North American Journal of Sports Physical Therapy, 4*(3), 100–109.

Caird, S., McKenzie, A., & Sleivert, G. (1999). Biofeedback and relaxation techniques improve running economy in sub-elite long distance runners. *Medicine and Science in Sports and Exercise, 31*, 717–722.

Christanell, F., Hoser, C., Huber, R., Fink, C., & Luomajoki, H. (2012). The influence of electromyographic biofeedback therapy on knee extension following anterior cruciate ligament reconstruction: a randomized controlled trial. *Sport Medicine, Arthroscopy, Rehabilitation, Therapy & Technology, 4*, 41–50.

Collins, D. (1995). Psychophysiology and sport performance. In S. J. H. Biddle (Ed.), *European perspectives on exercise and sport psychology* (pp. 154–178). Leeds, UK: Human Kinetics.

Crews, D. J. (1991). The influence of attentive states on golf putting as indicated by cardiac and electrocortical activity. *Medicine and Science in Sports and Exercise, 25*, 116–126.

Daniels, F. S., & Landers, D. M. (1981). Biofeedback and shooting performance: A test of disregulation and systems theory. *Journal of Sport Psychology, 4*, 271–282.

De Biase, M. E. M., Politti, F., Palomari, E. T., Barros-Filho, T. E. P., & De Camargo, O. P. (2011). Increased EMG response following electromyographic biofeedback treatment of rectus femoris muscle after spinal cord injury. *Physiotherapy, 97*, 175–179.

Draper, V. (1990). Electromyographic biofeedback and recovery of quadriceps femoris muscle function following anterior cruciate ligament reconstruction. *Physical Therapy, 70*(1), 11–17.

Draper, V., & Ballard, L. (1991). Electrical stimulation versus electromyographic biofeedback in the recovery of quadriceps femoris muscle function following anterior cruciate ligament surgery. *Physical Therapy, 71*, 455–464.

Dunbar, C. C. & Kalinski, M. I. (2004). Using RPE to regulate exercise intensity during a 20-week training program for postmenopausal women: A pilot study. *Perceptual and Motor Skills, 99*, 688–690.

Dursun N., Dursun E., & Kiliç Z. (2001). Electromyographic biofeedback-controlled exercise versus conservative care for patellofemoral pain syndrome. *Archives of Physical Medicine and Rehabilitation, 82*, 1692–1695.

Edmonds, W. A., Tenenbaum, G., Mann, D. T. Y., Johnson, M., & Kamata, A. (2008). The effect of biofeedback training on affective regulation and simulated car-racing performance: A multiple case study analysis. *Journal of Sports Sciences, 26*, 761–773.

Edvardsson, A., Ivarsson, A., & Johnson, U. (2012). Is a cognitive-behavioural biofeedback intervention useful to reduce injury risk in junior football players? *Journal of Sports Science and Medicine, 11,* 331–338.

Ehrenborg, C., & Archenholts, B. (2010). Is surface EMG biofeedback an effective training method for persons with neck and shoulder complaints after whiplash-associated disorders concerning activities of daily living and pain—a randomized controlled trial. *Clinical Rehabilitation, 24,* 715–726.

Fredrikson, M. & Engel, B. T. (1985). Learned control of heart rate during exercise in patients with borderline hypertension. *European Journal of Applied Physiology, 54,* 315–320.

Giggins, O. M., Persson, U. M., & Caulfield, B. (2013). Biofeedback in rehabilitation. *Journal of NeuroEngineering and Rehabilitation, 10,* 60–70.

Gil-Gomez, J. A., Llorens, R., Alcaniz, M., & Colomer, C. (2011). Effectiveness of a Wii balance board-based system (eBaViR) for balance rehabilitation: a pilot randomized clinical trial in patients with acquired brain injury. *Journal of NeuroEngineering and Rehabilitation, 8,* 30–39.

Goldstein, D. S., Ross, R. S., & Brady, J. V. (1977). Biofeedback heart rate training during exercise. *Biofeedback and Self-Regulation, 2(2),* 107–125.

Kim, S., Zemon, V., Cavallo, M. M., Rath, J. F., McCraty, R., & Foley, F. W. (2013). Heart rate variability biofeedback, executive functioning and chronic brain injury. *Brain Injury, 27*(2), 209–222.

Kirnap, M., Calis, M., Turgut, A., Halici, M., & Tuncel, M. (2005).The efficacy of EMG-biofeedback training on quadriceps muscle strength after arthroscopic meniscectomy. *New Zealand Medical Journal, 118,* 1224.

Krebs, D. E. (1981). Clinical electromyographic feedback following meniscectomy: a multiple regression experimental analysis. *Physical Therapy, 61,* 1017–1021.

Lagos, L., Bottiglieri, T., Vaschillo, B. & Vaschillo, E. (2012). Heart rate variability biofeedback for post-concussion syndrome: implications for treatment. *Biofeedback, 40*(4), 150–153.

Lange, B. S., Flynn, S. M., Chang, C. Y., Ahmed, A., Geng, Y., Utsav, K., et al. (2010). Development of an interactive rehabilitation game using the Nintendo WiiFit Balance Board for people with neurological injury. *Proceedings of the 8th International Conference Disability, Virtual Reality & Associated Technologies.*

Levitt, R., Deisinger, J. A., Wall, J. R., Ford, L., & Cassisi, J. E. (1995). EMG feedback-assisted postoperative rehabilitation of minor arthroscopic knee surgeries. *Journal of Sports Medicine and Physical Fitness, 35*(3), 218–223.

Lucca, J. A. & Recchiuti, S. J. (1983). Effect of electromyographic biofeedback on an isometric strengthening program. *Physical Therapy, 63,* 200–203.

McClelland, J., Zeni Jr, J., Haley, R. M., & Snyder-Mackler, L. (2012). Functional and biomechanical outcomes after using biofeedback for retraining symmetrical movement patterns after total knee arthroplasty: a case report. *Journal of Orthopaedic & Sports Physical Therapy, 42,* 135–144.

McManus, A. M., Masters, R. S. W., Laukkanen, R. M. T., Yu, C. C. W., Sit, C. H. P., & Ling, F. C. M. (2008). Using heart-rate feedback to increase physical activity in children. *Preventive Medicine, 47,* 402–408.

Moleiro, M. A., & Cid, F. V. (2001). Effects of biofeedback training on voluntary heart rate control during dynamic exercise. *Applied Psychophysiology and Biofeedback, 26,* 279–292.

Myer, G. D., Stroube, B. W., DiCesare, C. A., Brent, J. L., Ford, K. R., Heidt Jr, R. S., & Hewett, T. E. (2013). Augmented feedback supports skill transfer and reduces high-risk injury landing mechanics: A double-blind, randomized controlled laboratory study. *American Journal of Sports Medicine, 41,* 669–677.

Neblett, R., Mayer, T. G., Brede, E., & Gatchel, R. J. (2010). Correcting abnormal flexion-relaxation in chronic lumbar pain: Responsiveness to a new biofeedback training protocol. *Clinical Journal of Pain, 26,* 403–409.

Neblett, R., & Perez, Y. (2010). Surface electromyography biofeedback training to address muscle inhibition as an adjunct to postoperative knee rehabilitation. *Biofeedback, 38*(2), 56–63.

Ng G., Zang A., & Li, C. (2006). Biofeedback exercise improved the EMG activity ration of the medial and lateral vasti muscles in subjects with patellofemoral pain syndrome. *Journal of Electromyography & Kinesiology, 18,* 128–133.

Oravitan, M., & Avram, C. (2013). The effectiveness of electromyographic biofeedback as part of a meniscal repair rehabilitation programme. *Journal of Sports Science and Medicine, 12,* 526–532.

Perski, A., & Engel, B. T. (1980). The role of behavioral conditioning in the cardiovascular adjustment to exercise. *Biofeedback and Self-Regulation, 5(1),* 91–104.

Petruzzello, S. J., Landers, D. M., & Salazar, W. (1991). Biofeedback and sport/exercise performance: Applications and Limitations. *Behavior Therapy, 22,* 379–392.

Ren, W. D. (1995). A study of EMG biofeedback for improving archery postural consistency. In F. H. Fu & M. L. Ng (Eds.), *Sport psychology: Perspectives and practices toward the 21st century* (pp. 261–265). Hong Kong: Hong Kong Baptist University.

Silkman, C., & McKeon, J. (2010). The effectiveness of electromyographic biofeedback supplementation during knee rehabilitation after injury. *Journal of Sport Rehabilitation, 19,* 343–351.

Sprenger, C. K., Carlson, K., & Wessman, C. (1979). Application of electromyographic biofeedback following medial meniscectomy: a clinical report. *Physical Therapy, 59,* 167–169.

Tate, J. J., & Milner, C. E. (2010). Real-time kinematic, temporospatial, and kinetic biofeedback during gait retraining in patients: a systematic review. *Physical Therapy, 90,* 1123–1134.

Thornton, K. E., & Carmody, D. P. (2009). Traumatic brain injury rehabilitation: QEEG biofeedback treatment protocols. *Applied Psychophysiology and Biofeedback, 34,* 59–68.

van der Vlist, B., Bartneck, C., & Maueler, S. (2011). moBeat: Using interactive music to guide and motivate users during aerobic exercise. *Applied Psychophysiology Biofeedback, 36,* 135–145.

Wilk, K., Macrina, L. C., Cain, E. L., Dugas, J. R., & Andrews, J. R. (2012). Recent advances in the rehabilitation of anterior cruciate ligament injuries. *Journal of Orthopaedic & Sports Physical Therapy, 42,* 153–171.

Yilmaz, O. O., Senocak, O., Sahin, E., Baydar, M., Gulbahar, S., Bircan, C., et al. (2010). Efficacy of EMG-biofeedback in knee osteoarthritis. *Rheumatology International, 30,* 887–892.

Yip S., & Ng, G. (2006). Biofeedback supplementation to physiotherapy exercise programme for rehabilitation of patellofemoral pain syndrome: a randomized controlled pilot study. *Clinical Rehabilitation, 20,* 1050–1057.

Yungher, D., & Craelius, W. (2012). Improving fine motor function after brain injury using gesture recognition feedback. Disability and Rehabilitation: *Assistive Technology,* 1–5.

Zaichkowsky, L. D., & Fuchs, C. Z. (1988). Biofeedback applications in exercise and athletic performance. In K. B. Pandolf (Ed.), *Exercise and sports sciences reviews* (pp. 381–421). New York: Macmillan.

Chapter 9

Coping with Self-Presentational Concerns

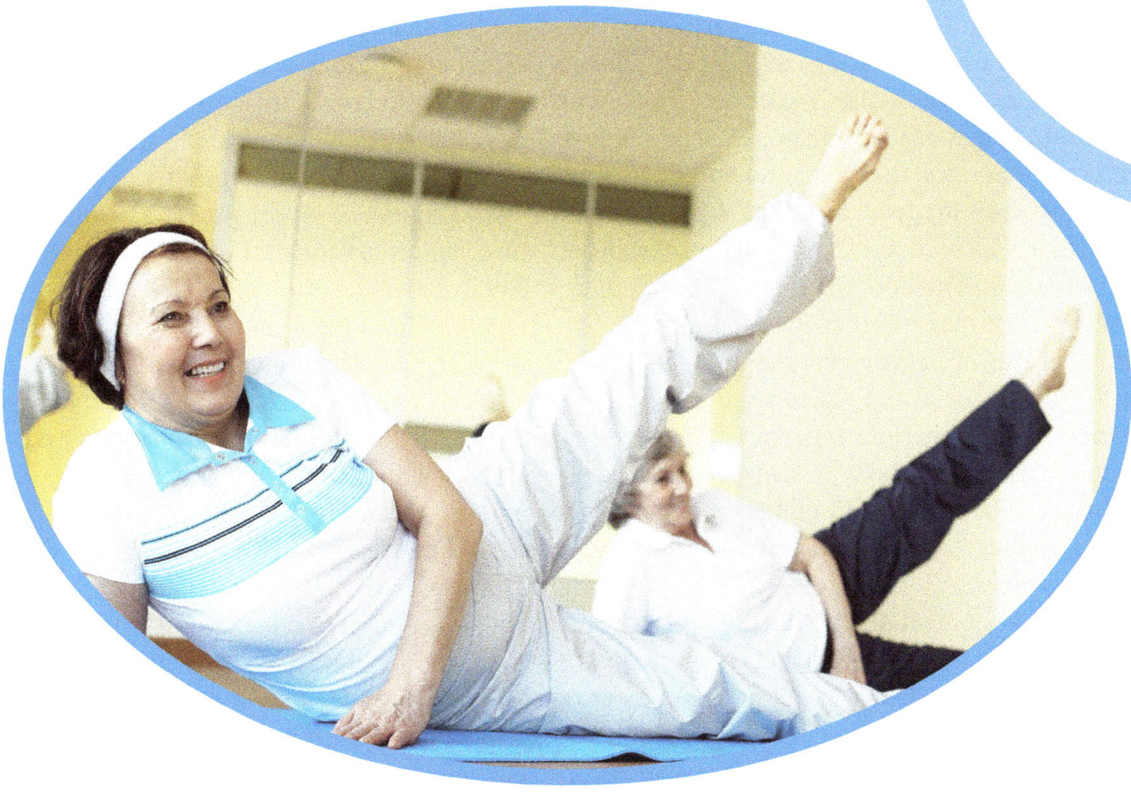

Image © Pressmaster, 2014. Used under license from Shutterstock, Inc.

Introduction

The thoughts that other people have about us may not always be at the forefront of our minds, but we are very frequently aware of how we are perceived by others. The way that our actions are viewed by others can have distinct implications for numerous aspects of our lives, from everyday activities to important events. In fact, the way that we present ourselves to other people is an underlying feature of all interpersonal behavior (Leary & Kowalski, 1990). The term ***self-presentation*** is used to describe people's efforts to regulate or maintain power over how others may perceive them. Sometimes this is referred to as impression management (Leary & Kowalski, 1990).

Leary and Kowalski (1990) proposed that there were two underlying components of self-presentation that we use in trying to control the impressions that other people form of us: impression motivation and impression construction. ***Impression motivation*** refers to the degree to which a person is motivated to present themselves in a certain way, and ***impression construction*** represents the methods that people employ to create the impressions that they strive to convey. For example, a person may be motivated to control how their appearance is perceived when surrounded by attractive others (impression motivation), and may strive to convey the impression that they are also attractive by dressing a particular way (impression construction). In their model, Leary and Kowalski explained that both impression motivation and impression construction are dependent upon specific situational and personal factors. Impression motivation is influenced by variables that include: (a) the value that a person holds over the desired goal, (b) the relevance of the impression to this goal, and (c) the discrepancy between the person's desired and current image (Martin Ginis & Leary, 2004). On the other hand, impression construction is dependent upon dispositional factors, such as the person's desired and undesired identity images, and their self-concept, as well as variables such as: (a) their current or potential social image, (b) limitations of the role, and (c) values of the audience (Martin Ginis & Leary, 2004). A limitation of the self-presentation literature is that researchers often do not identify which component has been assessed, nor do they distinguish between the two constructs. Nonetheless, the two-component model provides a solid framework that may be used in the examination of self-presentational concerns (Martin Ginis & Leary, 2004).

In any social situation, when people doubt their ability to create the impression that they are trying to convey, they may experience social anxiety (Leary, 1992). Researchers have demonstrated that a heightened fear of negative evaluation is associated with increased social anxiety (Leary, 1983). One specific type of social anxiety, termed social physique anxiety (SPA), refers to a person's anxiety over how their body or physique is perceived by others (Hart, Leary, & Rejeski, 1989). SPA has received considerable attention as a self-presentational variable, especially within the sport and exercise literature (refer to the 2004 special issue of the *Journal of Applied Sport Psychology* for a review; Prapavessis, 2004). Some researchers have suggested SPA is the "most widely studied aspect of self-presentation in exercise psychology research" (Gammage, Hall, & Martin Ginis, 2004, p. 1639).

In the development of a measure of SPA, the Social Physique Anxiety Scale (SPAS; Hart et al., 1989), relationships between this construct and participants' sex, height, weight, and feelings toward their bodies were demonstrated. Significant correlations were found between the SPAS and general measures of self-presentational concerns, as well as SPAS and assessments representative of weight and overall physical attractiveness. These relationships provided construct validation for the scale. Specifically, Hart et al. found that women who rated their SPA highest were heavier, had a higher percentage of body fat, and were taller than those who reported lower levels of SPA.

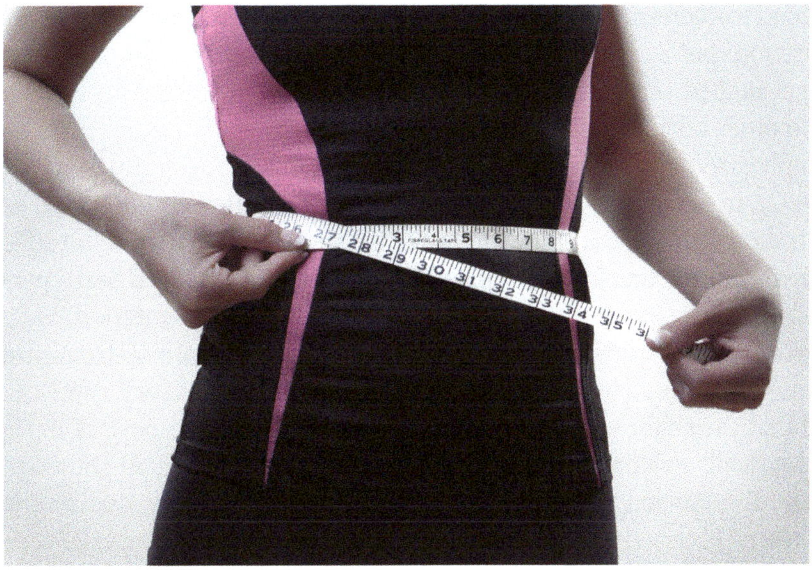

Further support for the validity of the original SPAS has been demonstrated through its employment in various studies in sport and exercise, including the examination of relationships between SPA and exercise setting preferences (Crawford & Eklund, 1994; Eklund & Crawford, 1994; Spink, 1992), motivation to exercise and exercise behavior (Frederick & Morrison, 1996; Lantz, Hardy, & Ainsworth, 1997), and self-efficacy (McAuley, Bane, & Mihalko, 1995). The original version of the SPAS, however, had only a single-factor structure which was, at one time, questioned by researchers (Eklund, Mack, & Hart, 1996). In their attempt to provide support for a unidimensional scale, Martin and her colleagues revised the SPAS to include only nine items (Martin, Rejeski, Leary, McAuley, & Bane, 1997). Since then, this nine-item version of the questionnaire has been used extensively in research investigating self-presentation in exercise (e.g., Gammage, Martin Ginis, & Hall, 2004; Katula, McAuley, Mihalko, & Bane, 1998; Kruisselbrink, Dodge, Swanburg, & MacLeod, 2004). The results of these studies have provided additional support for its improved validity and reliability compared to that of the original 12-item scale (Katula et al., 1998).

One prominent result that was uncovered in the development of the SPAS was that female participants scored higher than males (Hart et al., 1989). A number of other studies have since supported this finding (Frederick & Morrison, 1996; Haase, Prapavessis, & Owens, 2002; Kruisselbrink et al., 2004; Lantz et al., 1997). That women score higher on SPA has been explained by differences between males and females on body image and body dissatisfaction (Miller, Linke, & Linke, 1980; Silberstein, Striegel-Moore, Timko, & Rodin, 1988). The immense value that society places on the physical appearance of women has also contributed to differences in body image between men and women (Melbye, Tenenbaum, & Eklund, 2008). Western culture defines the ideal female body type as ultrathin, toned, and attractive (Melbye et al., 2008). Women typically strive to achieve this often unattainable ideal body, and consequently suffer body dissatisfaction (Silberstein et al., 1988). On the other hand, men may strive to achieve a body that is either thinner or more muscular, depending on their values and original body type (Martin Ginis, Prapavessis, & Haase, 2008). Women have also been found to be more critical of their bodies, and tend to overestimate their size and shape (Hart et al., 1989). Taken together, these findings support the notion that women are more prone to experience anxiety when they believe that their physique is being evaluated. This likely elicits greater impetus for women to manage the impressions that they convey to other people.

It has been emphasized that self-presentation may exist in any social situation, including sport and exercise (Leary, 1992). In his review, Leary proposed that the activities an individual selects, the motivation to take part in these activities, and the quality of the performance may all be affected by the degree of self-presentational concern that is experienced. Leary also acknowledged that a person's choice of the setting where activity takes place may be influenced by their self-presentation. Further, he suggested that environments that act to mitigate concerns over potential evaluations from other people may be sought by those who are attuned to how other people perceive them (Leary, 1992). For example, some women explained that they choose not to exercise in public settings because of the apprehension they feel about being physically evaluated (Bain, Wilson, & Chaikind, 1989). At the extreme, some people may be completely discouraged from participating in physical activity due to their excessive self-presentational concerns (Leary, 1992). For instance, young women who experienced great concern for how they would be perceived by their peers expressed that they would rather avoid participation in mandatory swimming classes and suffer punishment for their choice than participate in a situation that presented the potential for negative peer evaluation (James, 2000).

Conceived initially as a stable personality trait by Hart and colleagues (1989), SPA has also been shown to fluctuate with the demands of the situation (e.g., Gammage, Hall, & Martin Ginis, 2004; Gammage, Martin Ginis, et al., 2004; Kruisselbrink et al., 2004; Martin Ginis et al., 2008). The examination of situational or state-levels of SPA has highlighted a number of environmental factors that may act to heighten women's awareness of how her body is perceived by others in the exercise setting. For example, women have indicated increased SPA in response to exercise settings that include the presence of men (Kruisselbrink et al., 2004), revealing or physique-salient clothing (Martin Ginis et al., 2008), and mirrors and windows (Gammage, Martin Ginis, et al., 2004). As was proposed by Leary (1992), the relationship between these environmental features and a person's self-presentational concerns may possess the potential to deter some people from participating in exercise altogether. Researchers have provided evidence of some of the negative outcomes (i.e., non-adherence, non-participation, lack of enjoyment or satisfaction) that may result from exercising in environments that are full of evaluative potential, especially for those high in SPA (e.g., Gammage, Hall, et al., 2004; Lantz et al., 1997). How self-presentational variables influence adherence to exercise programs is of particular importance because of the public health issue surrounding the current low physical activity participation rates (Hausenblas, Brewer, & Van Raalte, 2004).

With respect to the characteristics of the environment that have been associated with self-presentational concerns, researchers have considered two general categories, the social environment and the physical environment. The social environment includes characteristics of the other people who are present in the environment, how they relate socially, and function as a whole. Hausenblas and colleagues (2004) have referred to the social environment as the "nature of the audience" (p. 10). In group dynamics research, the presence of others has been shown to both alleviate and heighten social anxiety (see Carron, Burke, & Prapavessis, 2004, for a review). A good example of this is apparent in a study conducted by Jackson and Latanté (1981). These researchers found that as the size of the audience increased, the social anxiety of their participants increased in response to imagined scenarios of themselves performing the national anthem. However, when other people were performing alongside the participants, their social anxiety was reduced. The participants experienced further reductions in anxiety as the number of people performing with them increased.

The physical environment is made up of features of the location as a whole, as well as specific elements that may be found within the environment. Characteristics of the physical exercise environment have been shown to influence a person's self-presentation. With respect to exercise, for example, women who are highly anxious tend to choose environments where there is little potential for physical evaluation, preferring to exercise alone in private, rather than public settings (Spink, 1992). Public exercise settings are avoided by obese women, primarily because of their apprehension over their physical evaluation (Bain et al., 1989). Focht and Hausenblas (2004) demonstrated how women's perceptions of evaluative threat were influenced by exercising in a standard exercise facility (i.e., in a university fitness centre with the presence of other exercisers and mirrors) compared to a private laboratory condition (i.e., without mirrors or other exercisers). Their sample included women who reported high levels of SPA. They found that female exercisers reported significantly higher ratings of perceived evaluative threat and state anxiety in the fitness facility compared to the laboratory condition. These researchers concluded that "self-presentational aspects of the exercise environment can negatively impact the psychological responses to exercise" (p. 366). Their findings lend support to a previous study (Focht & Hausenblas, 2003) that demonstrated associations between state anxiety and SPA for inactive women who exercised in a typical exercise facility.

In the following sections we will examine self-presentational concerns in sport, exercise, and injury rehabilitation and interventions that have investigated how people can cope with these concerns. In doing so, both the social and physical characteristics of the environment will be considered.

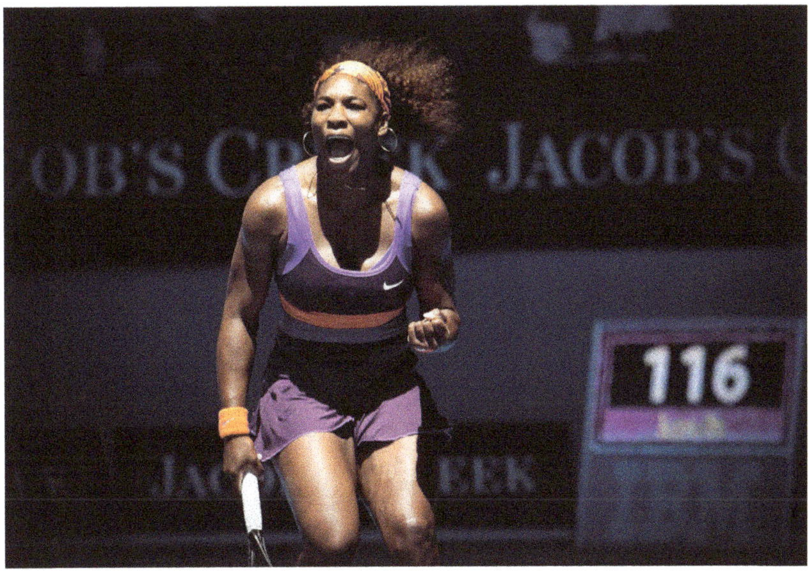

Self-Presentation in Sport

Self-presentation in sport has been examined from four primary perspectives: self-handicapping, stereotype cognitions, SPA, and competitive anxiety. We will consider each of these in turn.

Self-Handicapping

Athletes often make statements prior to a competition such as "I haven't been able to practice much lately so I hope I don't embarrass myself" or "I haven't been feeling well and it affected my training." Such statements may represent an attempt at self-presentation by self-handicapping. A distinction is often made between self-reported and behavior forms of self-handicapping. Self-reported handicaps are verbal claims that temporary states (e.g., illness, bad mood) and trait-like qualities (e.g., obesity, competitive anxiety) might interfere with performance. Behavioral handicaps are deliberate, observable acts that could interfere with performance such as withholding effort, actively assisting opponents, and choosing to perform under sub-optimal conditions.

Individuals differ in the tendency to use self-handicapping strategies and these tendencies are often assessed with the Self-Handicapping Scale (SHS; Jones & Rhodewalt, 1982). The SHS measures people's tendencies to focus on and employ potential handicaps such as mental and physical state, unfavorable circumstances, lack of effort and procrastination before evaluative performances. It appears to be psychometrically sound and has been used in a number of sport related studies.

When self-handicapping is used as an impression management strategy by athletes, it can sometimes provide benefits in this regard; however, there is also the possibility of negative consequences. These will occur if the handicap gives the impression that you are either not very good or not in control. Prapavessis, Grove, and Eklund (2004) have proposed a model that outlines the factors influencing the self-presentational consequences of self-handicapping strategies (see Figure 9-1).

Descriptive information about the types of handicaps that are likely to be claimed by athletes has been obtained from using an open-ended, "impediments approach" to examining self-handicapping in sport. In these studies, athletes are asked to list any events that had disrupted their preparation for competition during the past week. A list of the common impediments was compiled by Prapavessis et al. (2004) and is presented in Table 9–1. The frequency of citation for various categories fits very well with the model shown in Figure 9–1. More specifically, the most frequently-cited impediments such as school commitments and injury/illness tend to be situational, uncontrollable, and/or socially desirable. Also, the least frequently-cited impediments like personal problems and sport-based conflicts seem to be more dispositional, controllable, and/or socially undesirable.

Studies have examined the relationship between achievement goals and self-handicapping. For example, Thill and Curry (2000) manipulated achievement goals during the learning of a golf task and assessed the use of self-handicapping strategies among participants. Sixteen male and 16 female recreational golfers participated in the study. All golfers participated in four conditions over the course of the study. Two of these conditions were particularly relevant to self-handicapping. In the task involvement condition, the golfers practiced with different clubs, and emphasis was placed on skill acquisition and style. In the relative social comparison condition, golfers played a one-on-one competition against an opponent. The competition component was emphasized by placing the results on a large board for public display.

FIGURE 9–1 Factors Influencing the Self-presentational Consequences of Self-handicapping Strategies

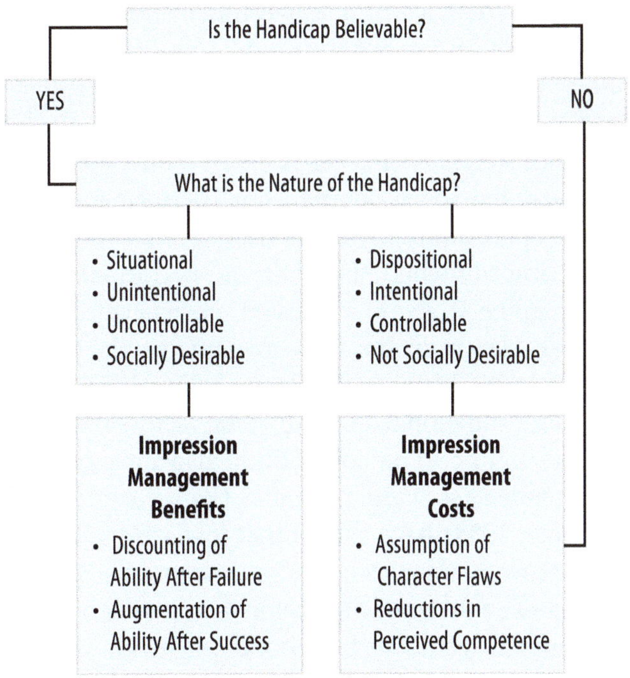

Proposed by Prapavessis et al. (2004)

TABLE 9–1 Percentages for the Types of Impediments Cited by Athletes Prior to Competition

General Nature of the Impediment Cited	Proportion of Citations [1]
School activities, commitments, or obligations	30.5
Physical state, injury, or illness	20.5
Sport-related problems or disruptions	14.8
Commitments or problems related to family/friends	13.8
Work obligations or travel commitments	11.7
Personal problems and/or life stress	4.9
Conflicts with teammates or coaches	3.7

Note. [1]Values are weighted by sample size and based on data from 668 participants in studies conducted by Carron, Prapavessis, and Grove (1994), Hausenblas and Carron (1996), Ryska, Yin, and Cooley (1998), and Prapavessis and Grove (1998).

The researchers found that a learning environment emphasizing competition and other-referenced standards of performance led to an increase in the reported frequency of self-handicapping. In contrast, a learning environment emphasizing self-referenced standards led to a decrease in the reported frequency of self-handicapping. The latter learning environment poses a lack of threat to the self and accordingly, self-handicapping strategies are not required.

In another study (Coudevylle & Famose, 2005) also couched in achievement motivation theory, basketball players performed an evaluated basketball drill in a private condition that emphasized personal accomplishments and improvements (mastery climate), or a public condition that emphasized competition and performance-related social comparisons (performance climate). Before performing the drill, players were given the opportunity to take as many practice shots as they desired and to indicate any possible performance impediments. Players in the performance climate took fewer practice shots (a behavioral self-handicapping strategy) and listed more performance impediments (a claimed self-handicapping strategy) than players in the mastery climate. The effects were influenced by sex; compared to women, men were more likely to employ behavioral (i.e., fewer practice shots) but not claim self-handicaps. Clearly, both situational and individual factors moderate self-handicapping.

The desire to practice before an important competition also appears to be related to individual differences in self-handicapping tendencies. Various studies (Bailis, 2001; Deppe & Harackiewicz, 1996; Rhodewalt, Saltzman, & Wittmer, 1984) have shown that low self-handicappers feel more competent and enjoy the competition more when they spend more time practicing prior to competition. In contrast, high self-handicappers decrease their practice before competing but actually feel more competent and enjoy their involvement more. It seems the behavioral self-handicapping strategy of reduced practice may be beneficial for athletes with high self-handicapping tendencies because it offers them and their audience a viable alternative to personal ability as an explanation for a poor performance and thereby provides them some "breathing room."

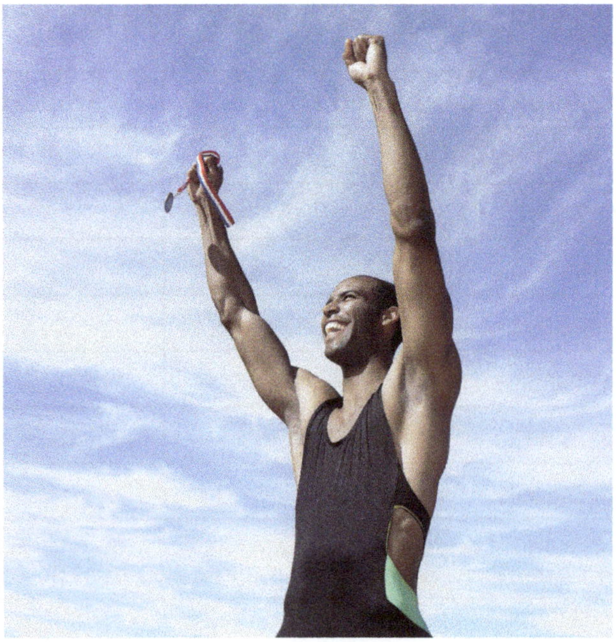

Stereotype Cognitions

Sometimes people make stereotypical inferences about athletes who participate in certain sports. For example, when people were asked to give their impressions of tennis, golf, snow skiing, bowling, and motocross racing athletes, impressions of bowlers were least positive. Specifically, they found bowlers less active and daring compared to skiers and racers (Sadalla, Linder, & Jenkins, 1988).

Athletes have been found to employ self-presentation strategies to manage their identity in an effort to maintain or improve their situation. Halbert (1997) interviewed 12 women professional boxers and determined that women boxers face widespread discrimination at the gyms and in competitions (e.g., trainers and managers often fail to assist them with their training; they receive verbal sexual harassment). They are also victims of numerous stereotype labels (e.g., husky, butch, ugly, and lesbian). These women used strategies such as wearing feminine uniforms and emphasizing feminine appearance (e.g., long hair and make-up) in public places outside the ring. They also concealed information (e.g., hide lesbianism and bisexuality) and avoided potentially harmful situations (e.g., do not associate with stereotyped people).

Social Physique Anxiety

It has been suggested that physique-salient sport athletes (e.g., diving, figure skating) may experience greater SPA than non self-presentational sport athletes (volleyball, badminton) due to the heightened focus on physical appearance. In contrast, it has been argued that athletes who participate in sports that emphasize the physique do so because they are confident about making a favorable physical impression; they are not worried about their physique. Research, however, generally has not supported either argument. Crocker, Snyder, Kowalski, and Hoar (2000) and Haase and Prapavessis (2001) found no differences in SPA for athletes competing in sports in which body aesthetics may be included in subjective scoring (e.g., diving, gymnastics) and those in sports that are objectively evaluated (e.g., basketball, rowing). Although more research is needed, there seems to be little need to develop interventions to help athletes cope with SPA.

Competitive Anxiety

Leary (1992) maintains that competitive anxiety is a sport-specific class of social anxiety. That is, the feelings of tension and apprehension often associated with participating in sport are really context-specific social anxieties stemming from doubts about one's ability to achieve self-presentational goals in the competitive environment. Competition is fraught with self-presentational risks. Athletes risk conveying a variety of negative images of themselves (e.g., lack of skill, poor fitness, inability to handle pressure) to a number of evaluative others such as spectators, coaches, teammates, and opponents. Research (e.g., Hudson & Williams, 2001; Wilson & Eklund, 1998) supports the view that competitive anxiety can reasonably be conceptualized as substantially a social anxiety experience. It is evident, however, that a few issues are not self-presentational in nature (e.g., anxiety associated with injury fears).

This overall approach is consistent with previous findings by Smith, Smoll, and Cumming (2007) who investigated the effects of a motivational climate intervention for coaches on young athletes' sport performance anxiety. The study involved 37 coaches (33 males and 4 females) who coached basketball in community-based programs in a city in the western United States. Twenty of these coaches participated in a 75-minute coach-development workshop. During this workshop coaches were encouraged to increase four specific behaviors: positive reinforcement, mistake-contingent encouragement, corrective instruction given in a positive and encouraging fashion, and sound technical instruction. Coaches were urged to encourage athletes to learn from mistakes. They also were encouraged to emphasize that success means giving maximum effort and becoming the best one can be, rather than winning or outperforming others. This overall approach is consistent with a mastery motivational climate, was designed to increase positive coach-athlete interactions, enhance team solidarity and mutual supportiveness, reduce fear of failure, and create a more enjoyable learning environment that increases intrinsic motivation for the activity. The other 17 coaches served as the control group and did not participate in the workshop.

The athletes in this study were 216 basketball players (117 boys and 99 girls) between the ages of 10 and 14 years. The athletes completed the Sport Anxiety Scale-2 (Smith, Smoll, Cumming, & Grossbard, 2006) during team practice sessions on two separate occasions. The first session occurred in the week preceding the administration of the coach-development workshop (intervention) and early in the preseason practice period. The second administration occurred at a team practice approximately 12 weeks later during the final week of the competitive season. Smith et al. (2007) found that relative to athletes who played for the coaches in the control group, those who played for the coaches in the intervention group exhibited decreases in anxiety from preseason to late season. Control group athletes reported increases in anxiety over the season. The intervention had equally positive effects on boys' and girls' teams.

Some General Recommendations

It is possible to make recommendations for conducting interventions for three of the four perspectives from which self-presentation in sport has been examined.

- An intervention emphasizing self-referenced standards will likely lead to a decrease in the reported frequency of self-handicapping.
- Interventions generally are not required to help athletes cope with SPA.
- Interventions aimed at developing a mastery motivational climate can be effective in reducing competitive anxiety.

Self-Presentation in Exercise

Self-presentational processes play an important role in the regulation of exercise behavior and in its associated cognitive and affective outcomes (Leary, 1992). There are numerous ways in which self-presentational concerns can influence behavior. For example, researchers have shown that self-presentational concerns are represented in some of the most commonly-reported reasons for exercising and that they also can influence which exercise activities we select, how often and how intensely we exercise, and where (i.e., under what environmental circumstances) we exercise. In the two decades since Leary (1992) described the prominent role that self-presentational processes can play in regulating our exercise behavior, the body of research in this area has expanded greatly. In this section of the chapter we present and discuss the multitude of ways in which self-presentational concerns can influence behavior in the exercise domain and suggest how the research that has been conducted in this area to date can inform the development and delivery of exercise-promotion interventions.

Some Important Concepts

Before we proceed to a discussion of the role of self-presentation in exercise, it is important to define some related constructs. Although these constructs are conceptually different from self-presentation, research examining these constructs has informed our understanding of self-presentation in exercise.

Body image. Body image is a multi-dimensional construct that reflects the way we see, think, feel, and act toward our own bodies. Our perceptions about our own bodies as they actually exist as well as how we would ideally like them to exist contribute to the way in which we present ourselves. Physical appearance is only one aspect of ourselves which we present to the world; however, our physical appearance does have a strong influence on the way that we are perceived by others (Dion, Berscheid, & Walster, 1972). Physical appearance is particularly salient in the physical activity domain, thus, body image plays an important role in this context.

The way in which we perceive our bodies can range from being healthy and positive to unhealthy and negative. A healthy body image is characterized by positive thoughts, feelings, and actions toward our bodies whereas an unhealthy body image is characterized by negative thoughts, feelings, and actions. Perceiving our bodies in a negative way is called body image disturbance and is often driven by unrealistic aspirations for thinness or muscularity.

Social anxiety and social physique anxiety. As described in the opening of this chapter, social anxiety occurs when people are uncertain or anxious about their ability to create the impression that they wish to convey (Leary, 1992). When this uncertainty or anxiety occurs with respect to the way in which people wish to present themselves physically, it is called SPA. Research in the area of self-presentation in exercise has focused, to a great extent, on causes and consequences of SPA.

Self-presentational efficacy. Just as people can feel unsure about their ability to self-present as desired, they also can feel confident in their abilities. Self-presentational efficacy refers to the degree to which people are confident that they can create the impressions of themselves that they wish to convey.

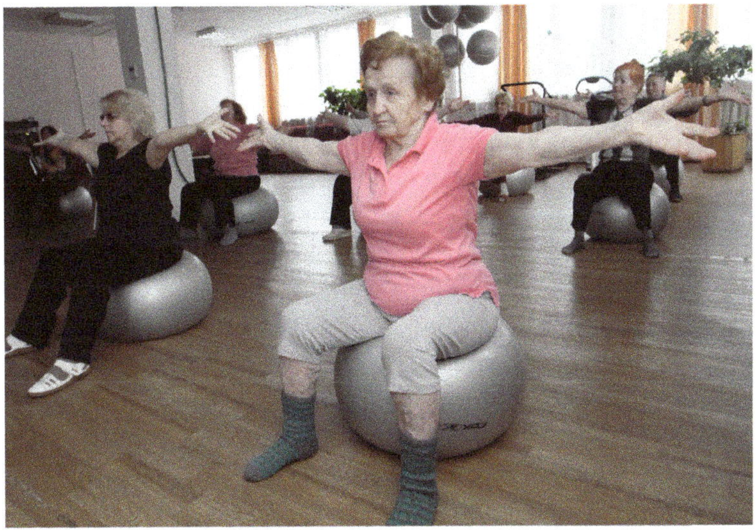

Image © De Visu, 2014. Used under license from Shutterstock, Inc.

Self-Presentational Concerns and Reasons for Exercising

Although there are many different reasons for exercising, such as staying healthy, having fun, or chasing and achieving goals (Ryan & Deci, 2007), there are at least two reasons for exercising that directly reflect self-presentational processes: creating and maintaining an ideal physical appearance and achieving a desirable social identity (Leary, 1992). Physical appearance motives are often cited as the most compelling reason to be physically active. Whether it is to remain thin and toned to match a typical female body ideal or to gain muscle mass to match a more typical male body ideal, both women and men endorse physical appearance as a primary motivator for engaging in exercise. Indeed, some researchers have shown a positive relationship between self-presentational concern and physical activity, suggesting that concern about one's physical appearance can be an incentive for engaging in physical activity (e.g., Lichtenberger, Martin Ginis, MacKenzie, & McCartney, 2003). One indicator that exercisers find appearance-related motives may be the high frequency with which regular exercisers report using appearance-related mental imagery that involves being toned, losing weight, or achieving a body ideal (Cumming, 2008; Cumming & Stanley, 2009; Gammage, Hall, & Rodgers, 2000; Giacobbi, Hausenblas, & Penfield, 2005; Hall, Rodgers, Wilson, & Norman, 2010; Hausenblas, Hall, Rodgers, & Munroe, 1999; Munroe-Chandler, Kim, & Gammage, 2004; Stanley, Cumming, Standage, & Duda, 2012; Thogersen-Ntoumani, Cumming, Ntoumanis, & Nikitaras, 2012; Wilson, Rodgers, Hall, & Gammage, 2003).

In contrast to evidence suggesting that self-presentational processes can be motivating, some researchers have demonstrated that self-presentational concern can be a disincentive for physical activity (e.g., Culos-Reed, Brawley, Martin, & Leary, 2002; Frederick & Ryan, 1993; McAuley et al., 1995). The reason for these mixed findings is unclear; however, one factor that may determine whether someone finds self-presentational reasons facilitative or debilitative is the personal importance that they attach to the self-presentational reason for exercising. In turn, the degree of importance placed on a self-presentational reason for exercising may be influenced by other individual-level factors such as an individual's self-presentational efficacy (Sinden, Martin Ginis, & Angove, 2003) or age (Treasure, Lox, & Lawton, 1998). Thus, one important area for future research involves uncovering the conditions under which self-presentational processes are motivating and de-motivating.

Achieving a desirable social identity is a second self-presentation related reason for which Leary (1992) suggested individuals may engage in physical activity. In general, physical activity is valued in our society and active individuals are perceived more favourably than inactive individuals. Evidence of this phenomenon is presented by Martin, Sinden, and Fleming (2000). In this study, 627 men and women read a description of a young man or woman who was described as an exerciser, non-exerciser, or control, then rated the young man or woman on 8 physical appearance and 12 personality characteristics. The results showed that across the 20 characteristics, the ratings of the non-exercisers were significantly less favorable than the ratings of the exercisers or controls. These findings were replicated by Mack (2003) and then extended by Martin Ginis, Latimer, and Jung (2003) to demonstrate that this positive exerciser bias could be generalized across different levels of exercise. Specifically, Martin Ginis et al. (2003) showed that individuals described as "exercisers," "active living participants," or "excessive exercisers" were rated more positively than "non-exercisers" and controls in terms of physical appearance. For personality traits, "exercisers" and "active living participants" were rated higher than the other groups. Overall, these findings show that by being an active person, one might gain praise, attention, respect, or other social rewards. Thus, self-presenting as an exerciser could have important benefits to individuals who value this type of social identity.

As we have seen, self-presentational motives facilitate exercise among some people (Frederick & Morrison, 1996; Krane, Stiles-Shipley, Waldron, & Michalenok, 2001; Russell, 2002; Yeung & Hemsley, 1997), but self-presentational concerns are debilitating for others (e.g., Finkenberg, DiNucci, McCune, Chenette, & McCoy, 1998; Hausenblas & Fallon, 2002; Hausenblas, Symons Downs, Fleming, & Connaughton, 2002; Lantz et al., 1997; Motl & Conroy, 2000; Ransdell, Wells, Manore, Swan, & Corbin, 1998; Treasure et al., 1998). Thus, the challenge for interventionists is to determine for which individuals, or under which conditions, self-presentational motives can lead to increased exercise motivation and behavior and for which individuals and under which conditions self-presentational issues detract from motivation and behavior. Then, interventions can be tailored to either capitalize on or inhibit these motives.

Self-Presentational Concerns and Choice of Activity

The type of physical activity in which someone engages could be influenced, at least in part, by self-presentational concerns. Although there are many factors that influence the type of activity that someone chooses, such as the enjoyment they derive from participating, or the resources they have available, our selection of physical activities may also be used for impression management. From the sports context we know that people who engage in one sport are perceived differently than people who participate in another. As discussed in the section on self-presentation in sport, subjective evaluations of athletes from five different sports (i.e., tennis, golf, snow skiing, bowling, and motocross racing) showed that bowlers are generally considered to be the least active and daring, as well as the least sensual and attractive (Sadalla et al., 1988). In contrast, skiers are perceived as being the most active and daring (Sadalla et al.). Although this study was conducted in a sports context, it is reasonable to assume that different exercise activities also are associated with differential stereotypes. For example, someone who engages in water aerobics may be perceived as being relatively delicate whereas someone who participates in

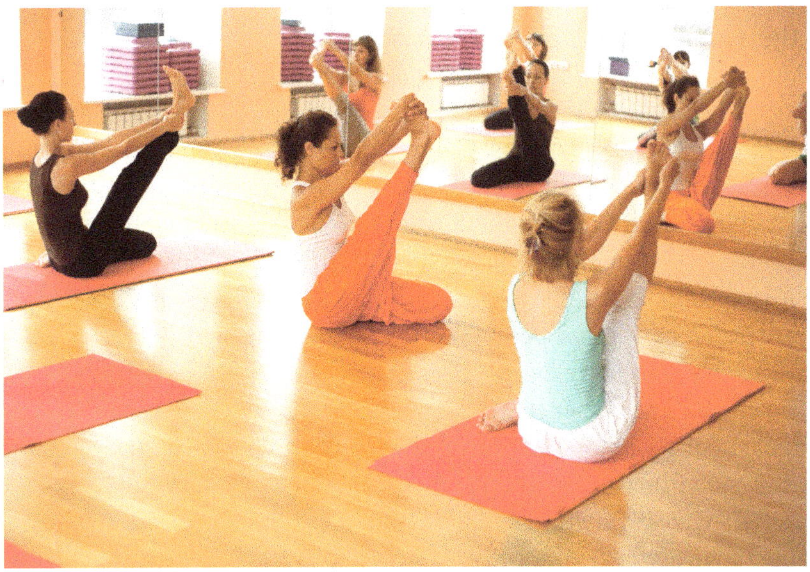

CrossFit may be perceived as being relatively tough. The implications of these associations are that individuals may select or forego certain physical activities because of the associated stereotypes. This may be particularly prevalent for activities that connote a gender stereotype (Jackson & Marsh, 1986). For example, whereas swimming laps may not be associated with particularly strong male or female characteristics, taking aerobics or dance classes may be perceived as relatively feminine and lifting weights may be perceived as relatively masculine. Women and men who wish to self-present in a manner aligned with gender stereotypes may choose their exercise activities accordingly.

Self-Presentational Concerns and Preferences for Exercise Contexts

Self-presentational concerns can have an impact on the physical and social contexts in which people choose to exercise, and even on whether they chose to exercise at all.

Influence of the physical context. Researchers have found that the physical characteristics of an exercise environment can influence the thoughts, feelings, and behaviors of individuals in those environments. The presence of mirrors in the exercise environment is one such characteristic (e.g., Katula et al., 1998). When Martin Ginis, Jung, and Gauvin (2003) randomly assigned 58 sedentary women to exercise in front of either a mirrored or a non-mirrored wall, they found that women in the mirrored condition felt worse after exercising than women in the non-mirrored condition. Interestingly, these effects were not moderated by the women's body image concern, suggesting that exercising in mirrored environments may have negative consequences for sedentary women. In another study that employed a similar design among female university students, however, Lamarche, Gammage, and Strong (2009) found that exercising in front of a mirror led to increased self-presentational efficacy and decreased state social anxiety. These mixed findings suggest that the degree to which environmental characteristics that increase the salience of physical appearance are motivating or de-motivating may depend on characteristics of the individual exercisers. Interventionists are advised to consider the characteristics and preferences of individual exercisers when determining the physical location for exercise interventions.

Influence of the social context. Self-presentational concerns are substantially influenced by our social context. SPA, for example, is characterized by individuals' reservations to present themselves physically in front of others. In turn, these social reservations can dramatically impact our exercise preferences and behaviors, as well as the psychosocial outcomes of exercising. From the behavioral perspective, decades of research in this area have confirmed that self-presentational concerns lead people to avoid exercising in public settings (e.g., Bain et al., 1989; James, 2000; Spink, 1992). Researchers have shown that among individuals high in SPA, negative feeling states can arise from exercising in public whereas more positive feeling states arise from exercising privately (Focht & Hausenblas, 2006).

Beyond the mere presence of other people, certain characteristics of other people in the social context influence the way that people respond to the social context. Gender is one such characteristic: researchers have shown that the presence of members of the opposite sex can lead to apprehension in an exercise setting, particularly among women (Eklund & Crawford, 1994; Yin, 2001). The physicality of others in an exercise environment is another factor that can be influential. For example, when men who were non-exercisers were exposed to images of muscular male models, they reported greater body-focused negative affect than after they viewed control images (Halliwell, Dittmar, & Orsborn, 2007). The implications of this study suggest that in a real-world setting, men who are non-exercisers may experience body-focused negative affect if they exercise in a gym full of really muscular men.

The presence of other people in an exercise environment is not always de-motivating. For example, in the study conducted by Halliwell et al. (2007), when the same images of muscular male models were shown to men who went to the gym regularly, the men actually reported less negative body-focused affect. Although it was not assessed, it is likely that these men who worked out at the gym regularly had higher levels of self-presentational efficacy which allowed them to view a physical social comparison as motivating rather than de-motivating.

Although people often wish to impression manage in the presence of their peers, researchers also have found that the presence of friends can help to buffer the social anxiety associated with self-presentation. When asked to rate the anxiety they would feel in a situation that provokes SPA, male and female university students reported that, compared to facing this situation alone, they would experience less anxiety if they were in the company of their best friend, and even less anxiety still if they were in the company of a group of friends (Carron & Prapavessis, 1997). Although this study was not conducted within an exercise setting, it has implications for the exercise domain. If exercising in public is perceived as a SPA-arousing situation, exercising with a buddy or in a group of close friends may be a way to reduce the anxiety and experience exercising more positively.

Given the strong relationship between SPA and preferences for the physical and social contexts in which exercise takes place, self-presentational concerns should be taken into account when designing and implementing physical activity promotion interventions. For example, using a women-only section of the gym may be one way to relieve some anxiety among individuals who are high in SPA. Encouraging new exercisers to wear comfortable, loose-fitting clothing and to exercise in private spaces without imposing windows or mirrors could be an advantage for this population as well. If it is not possible to eliminate the presence of others, such as in an aerobics class, select a location within the exercise space that limits the potential for social evaluation (e.g., the back of the room), select exercise activities with other exercisers at the same level (e.g., a beginner level aerobics class), or invite a friend along for the workout.

Self-Presentational Concerns Influence the Effort Exerted During Exercise

We tend to exercise more intensely in the presence of others. Most people who have run on the treadmill at a gym can remember a time when the presence of someone else running on a nearby treadmill motivated them to run faster than they might have otherwise. In a classic test of this idea, Worringham and Messick (1983) observed solitary joggers as they ran along a running path past a female confederate who either watched them or faced in the opposite direction. When the confederate was watching, participants ran significantly faster than when she was not. These findings highlight our inherent tendency to self-present as capable exercisers.

There are at least two important implications tied to our desire to self-present in this way. The first is that our desire to be perceived as physically capable may lead us to engage in self-handicapping. Unfortunately, researchers have shown that engaging in self-handicapping leads to reduced interest in and withdrawal from physical activity (Ommundsen, 2001) and may negatively impact self-perceptions such as self-esteem, task self-efficacy, and self-presentational efficacy (Martin & Brawley, 2002).

Engaging in excessive, harmful, or unsafe behavior is a second implication of our inherent desire to self-present as highly capable exercisers in the presence of others. For example, in a study conducted by Martin and Leary (2001) 28% of university-aged men surveyed reported lifting excessive weights at the gym in order to achieve self-presentational ideals (e.g., to appear tougher). In addition, Buckley, Yesalis, Friedle, Anderson, Streit, and Wright (1988) reported that among teenage boys in the United States who use steroids, self-presentational motives were the second most cited reason for steroid use, after improving athletic performance. Although lifting excessive weights is less common among women (Martin & Leary, 2001), women may be inclined to engage in excessive or harmful amounts of other types of exercise to achieve self-presentational ideals (Eklund & Crawford, 1994; Hausenblas & Martin, 2000).

Measurement of Self-Presentational Processes in Exercise

Over the past three decades, research on the influence of self-presentational processes in exercise has flourished. During this time, multiple self-report measures have been established and validated to assess various aspects of self-presentation.

The Self-Presentation in Exercise Scale (SPES; Conroy, Motl, & Hall, 2000) was established based on Leary and Kowalski's (1990) two-factor model of self-presentational tendencies. Initial work to validate this measure showed preliminary evidence of its convergent and discriminant validity with other theoretically salient measures. Subsequent attempts to confirm the factor structure of the SPES, however, were unsuccessful, leading a new group of researchers to suggest a reconstitution of the SPES into an 8-item questionnaire that retained the two factors. Attempts to cross-validate this revised SPES in two samples again provided only partial support for the validity of the questionnaire (Gammage, Hall, Prapavessis, et al., 2004). Although the development and testing of this questionnaire conducted to date marks an important step forward for self-presentation research, more work is required before this questionnaire captures a completely accurate representation of self-presentational processes in exercise.

A second questionnaire that is applied frequently in the examination of self-presentational processes in exercise is SPAS (Hart et al., 1989), which was discussed in the introduction to this chapter. Although this scale appears to be reliable, researchers should remain mindful that SPA represents only one component of self-presentation (albeit a component that is particularly relevant in the exercise domain).

Using Exercise to Reduce Self-Presentational Concern

A substantial body of correlational research has demonstrated that self-presentational efficacy is positively related and SPA is negatively related to exercise behavior (e.g., Gammage, Hall, & Martin Ginnis, 2004; Martin Ginis, Lindwall, & Prapavessis, 2007). The majority of the studies examining this link, however, have either not involved any real participation in exercise (e.g., Culos-Reed et al., 2002; Gammage, Hall, & Martin Ginnis, 2004; Strong, Martin Ginis, Mack, & Wilson, 2006; Woodgate, Martin Ginis, & Sinden, 2003), or have examined these relationships following only a single exercise bout (e.g. Lamarche et al., 2009; Lamarche & Gammage, 2010). In an initial longitudinal test examining the impact of a structured 12-week cardiovascular exercise program on self-presentational variables, Pearson, Hall, and Gammage (2013) showed that among participants who adhered to the program, SPA significantly decreased and self-presentational efficacy expectations significantly increased over time. These findings indicate that exercise may be an effective intervention tool for increasing self-presentational beliefs over time. More research is needed to replicate these findings.

Some General Recommendations

- As we have seen throughout this section, the degree to which self-presentational factors are motivating or de-motivating in an exercise context depends on individual-level factors. Thus, we advise interventionists to consider the individual with whom they are working to determine if it is more appropriate to highlight self-presentational factors to capitalize on its motivating potential or to protect against self-presentational concerns reduce or eliminate their de-motivating influence. As a general rule, sedentary individuals who are beginning an exercise program, individuals who do not exercise regularly, or individuals who may be particularly vulnerable to SPA should be protected against self-presentational pressure. For these people, all efforts should be made to enhance self-presentational efficacy and limit the situations that may arouse social anxiety. In contrast, individuals who exercise regularly may benefit from circumstances that trigger self-presentational processes.
- To reduce self-presentational concerns, consider the physical and social characteristics of an exercise environment. Exercising in private places without windows or mirrors can help to make exercisers feel less self-presentational pressure. Utilizing single-gender facilities (i.e., women only gyms), exercising among people at a similar level of ability, and exercising in the presence of friends are all factors that can enhance the social context of exercise and reduce self-presentational burden.

Self-Presentation in Injury Rehabilitation

Impression management can pose significant challenges to athletes and exercisers who are recuperating from injury. Because the physical and psychological effects of injury are often incongruent with desired projections of strength, skill, and independence, impression motivation in this setting is often fueled by a discrepancy between the individual's desired and current image (Leary & Kowalski, 1990). Elite-level athletes in particular may feel the pressure of evaluation by peers, coaches, spectators, and others, resulting in negative behaviors such as playing while injured or returning to sport before making a complete recovery (Tenenbaum & Eklund, 2007).

Aspects of the environment can trigger social anxiety, which results from being unsure of one's ability to portray a desired impression. For athletes, visual indications of their injury (e.g., crutches, casts, slings) can project unwanted images of weakness or fragility that may cause distress. SPA may also become a concern if injuries result in visible changes to the athlete's appearance, such as scarring or missing teeth. Although not all injured athletes experience these self-presentational concerns (in fact, some sport cultures look upon scars as a "badge of honor"), women are generally more prone to SPA than men (Frederick & Morrison, 1996; Haase et al., 2002; Hart et al., 1989; Kruisselbrink et al., 2004; Lantz et al., 1997).

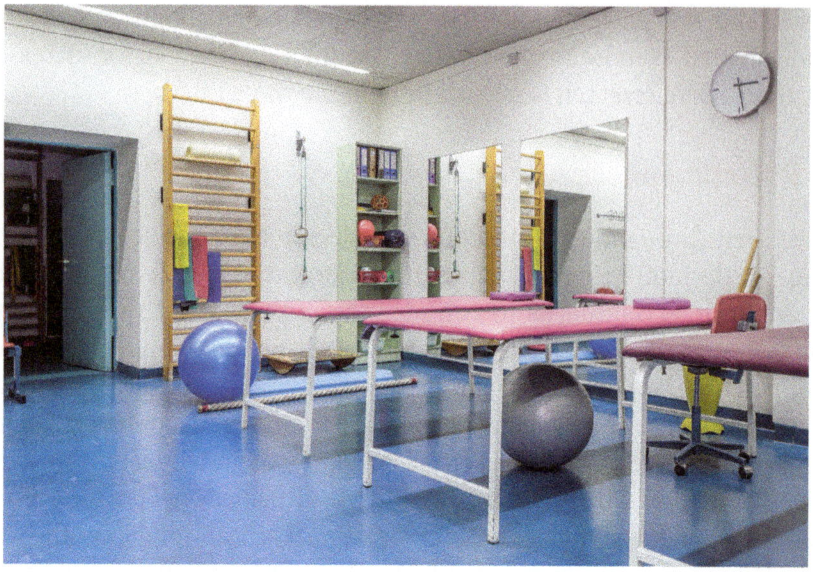

Interestingly, it has been demonstrated that changes in objective and subjective measures of fitness or physical function are potential mediators of exercise training on SPA (Martin Ginis, Eng, Arbour, Phillips, & Hartman, 2005; McAuley et al., 1995; McAuley, Marquez, Jerome, Blissmer, & Katual, 2002). This suggests that rehabilitation exercises may positively affect SPA if the athlete can experience incremental improvements during the treatment program. However, there has been limited research into determining whether findings from the exercise domain are generalizable to rehabilitation settings.

Driediger (2012) conducted two cross-sectional studies to determine whether the same self-presentational concerns exist in injury rehabilitation as in exercise settings. In the first study, 54 male and 135 female undergraduate students were recruited to investigate the relationship between dispositional SPA and ratings of self-presentation variables, along with preferences for characteristics of the social and physical injury rehabilitation environment. The results indicated that, in rehabilitation settings, a positive, significant relationship does exist between SPA and a number of self-presentation variables, including descriptors of physique and negative affect. As in the exercise literature, women reported significantly higher SPA than men, and preferred environments that reduced the potential for evaluation (e.g., private treatment spaces, ability to wear baggy clothing). In the second study, the results were replicated with a sample of 62 women who were actually initiating physiotherapy treatment. This study also found significant correlations between SPA and self-presentational concerns that were consistent with the exercise literature.

Self-Presentation and the Environment

Social physique anxiety. As we have seen, SPA is a salient issue for those participating in sport, exercise, and injury rehabilitation. It has been shown to fluctuate based on situational characteristics such as the social and physical environment (e.g., Gammage, Hall, Prapavessis et al., 2004; Gammage, Martin Ginis et al., 2004; Kruisselbrink et al., 2004; Martin Ginis et al., 2008). For those undergoing therapy, the features of the rehabilitation setting may increase self-presentational concerns, particularly if the individual demonstrates high SPA (Driediger, 2012). It has also been hypothesized that the type of injury that the patient is receiving treatment for might also increase these worries, but this has not been empirically supported (Driediger, 2012).

Importantly, the consequences of SPA and related impression construction in the rehabilitation setting can be especially detrimental. Impression management may lead individuals to decrease their adherence to, or effort during, their rehabilitation program, which can ultimately prevent a full recovery from the injury. Driediger (2012) conducted two rounds of qualitative interviews with a sample of 10 women (aged 18–64 years) who were undergoing physiotherapy treatment for a variety of injuries. These women were high in SPA (mean score = 36.4/60, standard deviation = 7.8 on the SPAS) and reported feeling anxiety about others' impressions of their physical appearance. Participants were notably concerned that their inability to perform physiotherapy exercises as well as expected would result in negative perceptions, and they expressed discomfort at the idea of having to wear physique-salient clothing. They were also worried that others would attribute their injury to their body type (e.g., those with knee problems feared that others would assume this was because they were overweight). These types of concerns clearly have implications for the patient's willingness to attend physiotherapy sessions, which would compromise the quality of their care.

An interesting, but under-researched area in rehabilitation is the effect of injury severity on SPA. It has been suggested that people with physical disabilities may be particularly prone to SPA due to self-consciousness regarding their limited functional ability (Prapavessis, Grove, et al., 2004). Although this question has not been addressed in general rehabilitation populations, it is possible that those with debilitating, disfiguring, or long-term injuries may exhibit greater tendencies to impression manage than those with less severe injuries.

Social environment. The majority of attention to the social environment has focused on gender differences in exercise and clinical settings. These studies have been primarily interested in understanding the experiences of females working out or undergoing rehabilitation in either mixed-gender or female-only situations. Although there have been relatively few investigations into this issue, findings have consistently indicated that most women have greater self-presentational concerns in the presence of men (Driediger, 2012; Kruisselbrink et al., 2004). During rehabilitation, however, women have also expressed concerns about receiving treatment in the company of other women. Driediger (2012) found that the women in her study held a definite preference for being around other female patients, but they indicated that they would be most comfortable if those patients were their age or older because they perceived less judgment from women their own age. They also felt that the presence of young, fit women in the clinic would actually prevent them from continuing with their rehabilitation program.

Despite clear preferences to be treated alongside other female patients, one study (Driediger, 2012) found that women did not express a preference for their therapist to be female. It was speculated that other therapist characteristics, such as knowledge and empathy, were more important to these individuals when they were receiving treatment, but this hypothesis requires further investigation.

The number of people present in treatment clinics has also been shown to trigger self-presentational concerns. Women have indicated preferences for having few people present during their appointments because of an increased awareness of being evaluated in large groups (Driediger, 2012). Yet, people generally prefer not to be the only patient present because of the focused attention they would receive from clinic staff (Driediger, 2012). Additionally, injury type can influence impression management concerns.

In her qualitative study, Driediger (2012) reported that participants experienced a heightened fear of negative evaluation when their injury was not obvious. Many of the women stated that they would feel most comfortable in a clinic that focused only on their type of injury.

Taking a different perspective, one international study found that patients' self-presentational styles influenced the type of support and attention they received from their physiotherapists (Ford & Gordon, 1997). The therapists indicated that they preferred athletes who were self-reliant and open, instead of unaffected, withdrawn, or negative. If therapists become less supportive because of the way a patient is presenting himself or herself, this is likely to affect that patient's adherence to the treatment program. Moreover, considering the reciprocal nature of the therapist-patient relationship, it is important to address the influence of the patient's impression management on treatment quality in order to ensure that health outcomes are optimized.

Physical environment. With regard to the physical environment, the concerns and preferences expressed by patients in the injury rehabilitation literature are similar to those found in the exercise domain (for a review, see Hausenblas et al., 2004). Performing exercises in front of a mirror can elicit negative feeling states (Martin Ginis, Jung, et al., 2003), and patients have reported avoiding areas of the clinic that have mirrors because it heightens their body awareness (Driediger, 2012). Treatment facilities may also have windows that allow people from outside the room to see in. These have the potential to increase the threat of evaluation (e.g., Focht & Hausenblas, 2003; Focht & Hausenblas, 2004; Gammage, Martin Ginis et al., 2004; Katula et al., 1998). Whereas exercisers can choose to avoid settings with windows or other anxiety-causing features, patients may not have a choice in the location of the clinic where they are treated. As such, the design of the clinic space itself may inadvertently dictate the type of clientele it attracts, or may influence rehabilitation program adherence.

Open-concept clinics are often favored by therapists because they allow flexibility in the types of treatment that they can offer, but these spaces are associated with the most potential for evaluation due to the lack of privacy they afford. Patients may be willing to tolerate receiving treatment here, depending upon the number of people present or what they are required to do, but high-SPA individuals would likely experience heightened anxiety in doing so (Driediger, 2012). These patients are typically more comfortable being treated in either curtained areas or private rooms that reduce or eliminate the risk of evaluation (Driediger, 2012). Of note, clinicians should be aware that patients might not explicitly communicate their discomfort with the treatment setting. Driediger (2012) found that women perceived that others would criticize them if they asked for additional privacy, so it is recommended that therapists give patients that choice up front if it is available.

Self-Presentation Interventions

Physiotherapy patients have reported using protective self-presentational strategies when faced with situations that they perceive to be evaluative. These include psychological techniques such as self-talk and thought-blocking, and avoidance behaviors like scheduling appointments during slow hours at the clinic (Driediger, 2012). Practitioners can assist patients who have self-presentation concerns by promoting these types of psychological strategies and facilitating treatments under low-evaluation conditions.

Self-Presentation and Injury Risk

In both athletic and non-athletic situations, many individuals desire to appear attractive, physically fit, brave, and "cool," while avoiding being labeled as unskilled or weak. Such impression motivations can lead to the adoption of a number of risky behaviors, which Martin Ginis and Leary (2004) have categorized as either acts of *commission* or acts of *omission*. For example, to finish running a race despite a broken ankle would be classified as commission (e.g., actively engaging in a particular behavior); failing to wear a helmet while riding a bicycle would be omission (e.g., choosing *not* to engage in a given behavior). In both situations, the individual has opted to forego reasonable precautions in order to construct a specific impression on others.

Athletes and exercisers who are motivated to impression manage in the presence of others (such as coaches, teammates, opponents, or other exercisers) have been observed to perform health-jeopardizing actions. To illustrate, Martin and Leary (2001) investigated the behavior of recreational weight lifters, and participants in their study admitted to lifting more weight than they could do safely in order to impress others. It has also been speculated that self-presentational concerns contribute to a large proportion of accidental injuries occurring as individuals attempt activities that they do not have the ability or experience to succeed in (Leary, Tchividjian, & Kraxberger, 1994; Driediger, 2012). It is easy to imagine a novice runner joining a training group and injuring himself by attempting to keep up to the pace of the other runners, or a young snowboarder being hurt while performing a skill beyond her repertoire in order to "one-up" her friend.

It is important to note that those presenting with high levels of impression-motivation and self-monitoring are more likely than their peers to sacrifice their health and well-being for self-presentational reasons (Martin Ginis & Leary, 2004). Adolescents are particularly prone to risky behavior while trying to convey certain impressions, and it has been shown that the desire to avoid seeming overcautious emerges as early as six or seven years old (Leary et al., 1994).

Although there is evidence that men are typically more motivated to appear brave or reckless than women (Leary et al., 1994), SPA can be associated with risk behaviors in female populations. Eating disorders, which are an often under-appreciated contributor to injury risk (Beals & Manore, 2002; Nattiv, Loucks, Manore, Sanborn, Sundgot-Borgen, & Warren, 2007), are also an important consideration during injury rehabilitation. In two studies that explored the influence of SPA on eating behaviors in otherwise healthy individuals, significant associations emerged. SPA predicted 21% of the variance in eating-disordered attitudes and behaviors in a combined sample of female athletes and non-athletes (Haase & Prapavessis, 2001), and negative perfectionism and SPA predicted 41% of the variance in disturbed eating attitudes and behaviors in a sample of elite female athletes (Haase et al., 2002).

Those who are unable to be physically active because of a long-term injury may begin to exhibit unhealthy eating behaviors in an attempt to prevent weight gain or other changes to their physical appearance. In rehabilitation clinics that are primarily frequented by high-performance athletes, the potential for negative peer evaluation could be seen as a strong motivator for impression management in this regard. There has been no research to date that explicitly examines the relationship between eating behaviors and SPA in rehabilitation, but it can be hypothesized that such an association exists, especially for sports with weight restrictions (e.g., wrestling, rowing) or that are based upon judged scores (e.g., gymnastics, diving).

How It Is Measured

Recently, three questionnaires were developed by Driediger (2012) to assess self-presentation in injury rehabilitation settings. Although the limited use of these questionnaires to date prevents an assessment of their generalizability to clinical application, they are promising instruments for future study.

Self-Presentation in Injury Rehabilitation Questionnaire (SPIRQ). This is a 32-item questionnaire designed to assess self-presentational concerns in physiotherapy settings. Its development was guided by two established measures of self-presentation in sport and exercise: the Self-Presentation in Sport Questionnaire (Wilson & Eklund, 1998), and the Self-Presentation in Exercise Questionnaire (Conroy et al., 2000), with emphasis on general self-presentational concerns that include, but are not limited to, physical appearance (McGowan, Prapavessis, & Wesch, 2008; Gammage, Hall, Prapavessis et al., 2004). When responding to the questionnaire items, participants are asked to imagine that they are undergoing rehabilitation for a specified injury. Treatment vignettes are presented, including photos and descriptions of the treatment facility and information about the people who are present in the clinic. Respondents rate how the other people in the clinic would perceive them by scoring each item on a scale ranging from 1 (not at all true) to 5 (completely true).

Injury Rehabilitation Social Environment Preferences Questionnaire. This 14-item questionnaire evaluates individual preferences for the social environment within a physiotherapy clinic. The items address the characteristics of other people present in the clinic, such as sex, physique, physical ability, level of interaction, and the perceived need to impress these people. There are also items that focus on the clothing that patients may be required to wear. Respondents rate their preference for each item on a 5-point scale ranging from 1 (not preferred) to 5 (completely prefer).

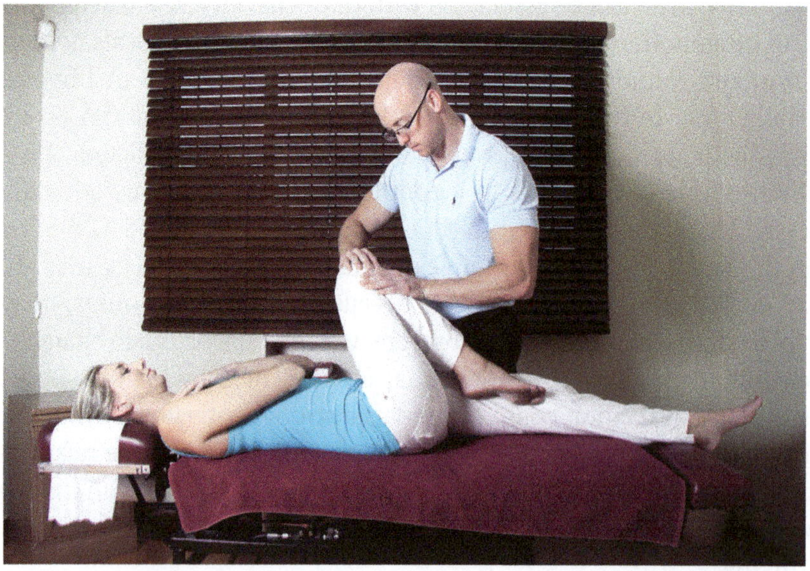

Injury Rehabilitation Treatment Environment Preferences Questionnaire. This brief, 3-item questionnaire assesses preferences for specific treatment settings. Items depict the characteristics of different locations within a typical physiotherapy clinic that have varying degrees of potential evaluation by others, alongside a written description and photograph. Respondents initially read over the written descriptions for each item without providing a rating. They are then instructed to observe the photographs and rate each treatment setting on a 5-point scale ranging from 1 (not preferred) to 5 (completely prefer).

Some General Recommendations

Some recommendations can be forwarded regarding coping with self-presentational concerns in injury rehabilitation.

- Physical self-presentation confidence (PSPC) can be enhanced through exercise training interventions (Lox, McAuley, & Tucker, 1995), and greater PSPC has been related to greater persistence and endurance (Tenenbaum, Lidor, Lavyan, Morrow, Tonnel, & Gershgoren, 2005). Emphasizing positive physical changes associated with rehabilitation exercises may increase patients' PSPC, and in turn promote greater effort and adherence to rehabilitation programs.
- Individuals undergoing rehabilitation may engage in self-handicapping (e.g., impair their own performance intentionally because they are worried about failing). These individuals can then internalize credit for succeeding against obstacles when they achieve desired outcomes, or externalize failure when they do not succeed. This is most likely to occur when performance is important, or will be compared with others. Practitioners should be alert for signs of both behavioral handicaps (e.g., the individual actually creates obstacles to performance) and claimed handicaps (e.g., the individual states that an obstacle exists) (Prapavessis et al., 2004).
- Athletes returning to sport may worry about appearing unfit, unskilled, or not as good as they were before the injury. Elite athletes in particular might express concerns about not meeting performance expectations, letting down their teammates and coaches, and not being able to uphold their reputation as an athlete. These issues can impact the athlete's quality of experience in re-entering competition, and could be associated with performance decrements or self-handicapping (Podlog, Dimmock, & Miller, 2011).

CHAPTER SUMMARY

In the domains of sport, exercise, and injury rehabilitation, researchers have shown that self-presentational concerns have a substantial influence on our thoughts, feelings, and actions. In certain cases, the desire to self-present as a capable athlete or exerciser can be motivating and can help to enhance effort and persistence. In other cases, self-presentational concerns can be debilitating and can influence people to avoid practicing, exercising, or engaging in rehabilitation activities. Much of the research on self-presentational processes in the domains of sport, exercise, and injury rehabilitation has been guided by Leary and Kowalski's (1990) model of self-presentation that outlines two components of our self-presentational desires; impression motivation and impression construction. Impression motivation represents the way in which people wish to self-present whereas impression construction represents the actions they take to present in that way.

Two phenomena that arise due to self-presentational concerns across the domains of sport, exercise, and injury rehabilitation are SPA and self-handicapping. SPA represents the uncertainty or anxiety occurs when people are faced around presenting themselves physically in social contexts. Whereas SPA can be critically-debilitating factor in the domains of exercise and injury rehabilitation, it appears not to be of paramount concern in sport. Self-handicapping, however, affects behavioral processes in all three contexts. Self-handicapping refers to highlighting actual or claimed impediments to performance to protect one's self-esteem against the potential of failure in the future. Importantly, self-handicapping can lead athletes to practice less, exercisers to avoid workouts, and patients to discontinue rehabilitation exercises.

Self-presentational processes can be heavily influenced by environmental factors, both physical and social. Physical characteristics of a space, such as an abundance of mirrors, windows to public spaces, and open-concept designs can increase the salience of self-presentational concerns and, in turn, influence motivation and behavior. Social characteristics such as the presence of observers (e.g., audiences in the context of sport or other patients in rehabilitation settings) or the presence of other participants (e.g., teammates or exercise buddies) also can influence our impression motivation and impression construction.

REVIEW QUESTIONS

1. In this chapter we discussed two reasons for exercising that directly reflect self-presentational processes. Describe these two reasons.
2. In what ways can the social context influence a person's self-presentational beliefs? In what ways might the social context influence behavior?
3. Discuss the potential dangers associated with the desire to self-present as a capable exerciser.
4. Explain the relationship between patient self-presentation and treatment quality in clinical settings.
5. How can the social and physical environment influence rehabilitation program adherence?
6. Identify some of the gaps in the research literature that should be addressed to improve our understanding of self-presentation in rehabilitation.

SUGGESTED READINGS

Hausenblas, H. A., Brewer, B. W., & Van Raalte, J. L. (2004). Self-presentation and exercise. *Journal of Applied Sport Psychology, 16(1),* 3–18.

Leary, M. R. (1992). Self-presentational processes in exercise and sport. *Journal of Sport & Exercise Psychology, 14,* 339–351.

Martin Ginis, K. A., & Leary, M. R. (2004). Self-presentational processes in health-damaging behavior. *Journal of Applied Sport Psychology, 16,* 59–74.

Podlog, L, Dimmock, J, & Miller, J. (2011). A review of return to sport concerns following injury rehabilitation: Practitioner strategies for enhancing recovery outcomes. *Physical Therapy in Sport, 12,* 36–42.

REFERENCES

Bailis, D. S. (2001). Benefits of self-handicapping in sport: A field study of university athletes. *Canadian Journal of Behavioral Sciences, 33*, 213–223.

Bain, L. L., Wilson, T., & Chaikind, E. (1989). Participant perceptions of exercise programs for overweight women. *Research Quarterly for Exercise and Sport, 60*, 134–143.

Beals, K. A., & Manore, M. M. (2002). Disorders of the female athlete triad among collegiate athletes. *International Journal of Sport Nutrition and Exercise Metabolism, 12*(3), 281–293.

Buckley, W. A., Yesalis, C. E., Friedle, C. E., Anderson, W., Streit, A., & Wright, J. (1988). Estimated prevalence of anabolic steroid use among male high school seniors. *Journal of the American Medical Association, 260*, 3341–3445.

Carron, A. V., Burke, S. M., & Prapavessis, H. (2004). Self-presentation and group influence. *Journal of Applied Sport Psychology, 16*, 41–58.

Carron, A., & Prapavessis, H. (1997). Self-presentation and group influence. *Small Group Research, 28*, 500–516.

Carron, A. V., Prapavessis, H., & Grove, J. R. (1994). Group effects and self-handicapping. *Journal of Sport & Exercise Psychology, 16*, 246–257.

Conroy, D. E., Motl, R. W., & Hall, E. G. (2000). Progress toward construct validation of the self-presentation in exercise questionnaire (SPEQ). *Journal of Sport & Exercise Psychology, 22*, 21–38.

Coudevylle, G., & Famose, J. P. (2005). Le climat motivationnel comme determinant principal des declarations et des comportements d' auto-handicap en basketball [Motivational climate as a principal determinant of self-handicapping claims and behaviors in basketball]. *Actes dh Congrès, Société Française de Psychologie du Sport, Congrès International*, 80–81.

Crawford, S., & Eklund, R. C. (1994). Social physique anxiety, reasons for exercise, and attitudes toward exercise settings. *Journal of Sport & Exercise Psychology, 16*, 70–82.

Crocker, P. R. E., Snyder, J., Kowalski, K., & Hoar, S. (2000). Don't let me be fat or physically incompetent! The relationship between physical self-concept and social physique anxiety in Canadian high performance female adolescent athletes. *Avante, 6*, 1–8.

Culos-Reed, S. N., Brawley, L. R., Martin, K. A., & Leary, M. R. (2002). Self-presentation concerns and health behaviors among cosmetic surgery patients. *Journal of Applied Social Psychology, 32*(3), 560–569.

Cumming, J. (2008). Investigating the relationship between exercise imagery, leisure-time exercise behavior, and self-efficacy. *Journal of Applied Sport Psychology, 20*, 184–198.

Cumming, J., & Stanley, D. M. (2009). Are images of exercising related to feeling states? *Journal of Imagery Research in Sport and Physical Activity, 4*, 1–20.

Deppe, R. K., & Harackiewicz, J. M. (1996). Self-handicapping and intrinsic motivation: Buffering intrinsic motivation from the threat of failure. *Journal of Personality & Social Psychology, 70*, 868–876.

Dion, K., Berscheid, E., Walster, E. (1972). What is beautiful is good. *Journal of Personality and Social Psychology, 24*(3), 285–290.

Driediger, M. (2012). *Self-presentation and social physique anxiety in injury rehabilitation settings.* (Doctoral dissertation). Retrieved from University of Western Ontario—Electronic Thesis and Dissertation Repository. (Paper 525)

Eklund, R. C., & Crawford, S. (1994). Active women, social physique anxiety, and exercise. *Journal of Sport & Exercise Psychology, 16,* 431–448.

Eklund, R. C., Mack, D., & Hart, E. (1996). Factorial validity of the social physique anxiety scale for females. *Journal of Sport & Exercise Psychology, 18,* 281–295.

Finkenberg, M. E., DiNucci, J. M., McCune, S. L., Chenette, T., & McCoy, P. (1998). Commitment of physical activity and anxiety about physique among college women. *Perceptual and Motor Skills, 87,* 1393–1394.

Focht, B. C., & Hausenblas, H. A. (2003). State anxiety responses to acute exercise in women with high social physique anxiety. *Journal of Sport & Exercise Psychology, 25,* 123–144.

Focht, B. C., & Hausenblas, H. A. (2004). Perceived evaluative threat and state anxiety during exercise in women with social physique anxiety. *Journal of Applied Sport Psychology, 16,* 361–368.

Focht, B. C., & Hausenblas, H. A. (2006). Exercising in public and private environments: Effects on feeling states in women with social physique anxiety. *Journal of Applied Biobehavioral Research, 11,* 147–165.

Ford, I. W., & Gordon, S. (1997). Perspectives of sport physiotherapists on the frequency and significance of psychological factors in professional practice: Implications for curriculum design in professional training. *Australian Journal of Science and Medicine in Sport, 29,* 34–40.

Frederick, C. M., & Morrison, C. S. (1996). Social physique anxiety: Personality constructs, motivations, exercise attitudes, and behavior. *Perceptual and Motor Skills, 82,* 963–972.

Frederick, C. M., & Ryan, R. M. (1993). Differences in motivation for sport and exercise and their relations with participation and mental health. *Journal of Sport Behavior, 16,* 124–146.

Gammage, K. L., Hall, C. R., & Martin Ginis, K. A. (2004). Self-presentation in exercise contexts: Differences between high and low frequency exercisers. *Journal of Applied Social Psychology, 34,* 1638–1651.

Gammage, K. L., Hall, C. R., Prapavessis, H., Maddison, R., Haase, A., & Martin, K. A. (2004). Re-examination of the factor structure and composition of the self-presentation in exercise questionnaire (SPEQ). *Journal of Applied Sport Psychology, 16,* 82–91.

Gammage, K. L., Hall, C. R., & Rodgers, W. M. (2000). More about exercise imagery. *The Sport Psychologist, 34,* 348–359.

Gammage, K. L., Martin Ginis, K. A., & Hall, C. R. (2004). Self-presentational efficacy: Its influence on social anxiety in an exercise context. *Journal of Sport & Exercise Psychology, 26,* 179–190.

Giacobbi, P. R. Jr., Hausenblas, H. A., & Penfield, R. D. (2005). Further refinements in the measurement of exercise imagery: The Exercise Imagery Inventory. *Measurement in Physical Education and Exercise Science, 9,* 251–266.

Haase, A. M., Prapavessis, H. (2001). Social physique anxiety and eating attitudes in female athletic and non-athletic groups. *Journal of Science and Medicine in Sport, 4*(4), 396–405.

Haase, A. M., Prapavessis, H., & Owens, R. G. (2002). Perfectionism, social physique anxiety, and disordered eating: A comparison of male and female elite athletes. *Psychology of Sport and Exercise, 3*, 209–222.

Halbert, C. (1997). Tough enough and woman enough: Stereotypes, discrimination, and impression management among women professional boxers. *Journal of Sport and Social Issues, 21*, 17–36.

Hall, C. R., Rodgers, W. M., Wilson, P. M., & Norman, P. (2010). Imagery use and self-determined motivations in a community sample of exercisers and non-exercisers. *Journal of Applied Social Psychology, 40*, 135–152.

Halliwell, E., Dittmar, H., & Orsborn, A. (2007). The effects of exposure to muscular male models among men: Exploring the moderating role of gym use and exercise motivation. *Body Image, 4(3)*, 278–287.

Hart, E. A., Leary, M. R., & Rejeski, W. J. (1989). The measurement of social physique anxiety. *Journal of Sport & Exercise Psychology, 11*, 94–104.

Hausenblas, H. A., Brewer, B. W., & Van Raalte, J. L. (2004). Self-presentation and exercise. *Journal of Applied Sport Psychology, 16*, 3–18. doi: 10.1080/10413200490260026

Hausenblas, H., & Carron, A. V. (1996). Group cohesion and self-handicapping in female and male athletes. *Journal of Sport & Exercise Psychology, 18*, 132–143.

Hausenblas, H. A., & Fallon, E. A. (2002). Relationship between body image, exercise behavior, and exercise dependence symptoms. *International Journal of Eating Disorders, 32*, 179–185.

Hausenblas, H. A., Hall, C. R., Rodgers, W. M., & Munroe, K. J. (1999). Exercise imagery: Its nature and measurement. *Journal of Applied Sport Psychology, 11*, 171–180.

Hausenblas, H. A., & Martin, K. A. (2000). Bodies on display: Predictors of social physique anxiety in female aerobic instructors. *Women in Sport and Physical Activity Journal, 9*, 1–14.

Hausenblas, H. A., Symons Downs, D., Fleming, D., & Connaughton, D. P. (2002). Body image in middle school children. *The Journal of Eating and Weight Disorders 7*, 244–248.

Hudson, J., & Wilson, M. (2001). Associations between self-presentation and competitive A-trait: A preliminary investigation. *Social Behavior and Personality, 29*, 1–10.

Jackson, J. M., & Latané, B. (1981). All alone in front of all of those people: Stage fright as a function of the number and type of co-performers and audience. *Journal of Personality and Social Psychology, 40*, 73–85.

Jackson, S. A., & Marsh, H. W. (1986). Athletic or antisocial? The female sport experience. *Journal of Sport Psychology, 8*, 198–211.

James, K. (2000). "You can feel them looking at you": The experiences of adolescent girls at swimming pools. *Journal of Leisure Research, 32*, 262–280.

Jones, E. E., & Rhodewalt, F. (1982). *The Self-Handicapping Scale.* (Available from F. Rhodewalt, Department of Psychology, University of Utah)

Katula, J. A., McAuley, E., Mihalko, S. L., & Bane, S. M. (1998). Mirror, mirror on the wall ... exercise environment influences on self-efficacy. *Journal of Social Behavior and Personality, 13*, 319–332.

Krane, V., Stiles-Shipley, J. A., Waldron, J., & Michalenok, J. (2001). Relationships among body satisfaction, social physique anxiety, and eating behaviors in female athletes and exercisers. *Journal of Sport Behavior, 24*, 1–18.

Kruisselbrink, L. D., Dodge, A. M., Swanburg, S. L., & MacLeod, A. L. (2004). Influence of same-sex and mixed-sex exercise settings on the social physique anxiety and exercise intentions of males and females. *Journal of Sport & Exercise Psychology, 26*, 616–622.

Lamarche, L., & Gammage, K. L. (2010). The effects of leader gender on self-presentational concerns in exercise. *Psychology and Health, 25*, 769–781.

Lamarche, L., Gammage, K. L., & Strong, H. A. (2009). The effect of mirrored environments on self-presentational efficacy and social anxiety in women in a step aerobics class. *Psychology of Sport and Exercise, 10(1)*, 67–71.

Lantz, C. D., Hardy, C. J., & Ainsworth, B. E. (1997). Social physique anxiety and perceived exercise behavior. *Journal of Sport Behavior, 20*, 83–93.

Leary, M. R. (1983). A brief version of the fear of negative evaluation scale. *Personality and Social Psychology Bulletin, 9*, 371–375.

Leary, M. R. (1992). Self-presentational processes in exercise and sport. *Journal of Sport & Exercise Psychology, 14*, 339–351.

Leary, M. R., & Kowalski, R. M. (1990). Impression management: A literature review and two-component model. *Psychological Bulletin, 107*, 34–47.

Leary, M. R., Tchividjian, L. R., & Kraxberger, B. E. (1994). Self-presentation can be hazardous to your health: Impression management and health risk. *Health Psychology, 13*(6), 461–470.

Lichtenberger, C. M., Martin Ginis, K. A. M., MacKenzie, C. L., & McCartney, N. (2003). Body image and depressive symptoms as correlates of self-reported versus clinician-reported physiologic function. *Journal of Cardiopulmonary Rehabilitation and Prevention, 23(1)*, 53–59.

Lox, C. L., McAuley, E., & Tucker, R. S. (1995). Exercise as an intervention for enhancing subjective well-being in an HIV-1 population. *Journal of Sport & Exercise Psychology, 17*(4), 345–362.

Mack, D. E., Strong, H. A., Kowalski, K. C., & Crocker, P. R. E. (2007). Does friendship matter? An examination of social physique anxiety in adolescence. *Journal of Applied Social Psychology, 37*(6), 1248–1264.

Mack, M. G. (2003). Does exercise status influence the impressions formed by college students? *College Student Journal, 37(4)*, 483–489.

Martin, K. A., & Brawley, L. R. (2002). Self-handicapping in physical achievement settings: The contributions of self-esteem and self-efficacy. *Self and Identity, 1*(4), 337–351.

Martin, K. A., & Leary, M. R. (2001). Self-presentational determinants of health risk behaviour among college freshmen. *Psychology and Health, 16*, 17–27.

Martin, K. A., Rejeski, W. J., Leary, M. R., McAuley, E., & Bane, S. (1997). Is the Social Physique Anxiety Scale really multidimensional? Conceptual and statistical arguments for a unidimensional model. *Journal of Sport & Exercise Psychology, 19*, 359–367.

Martin, K. A., Sinden, A. R., & Fleming, J. C. (2000). Inactivity may be hazardous to your image: The effects of exercise participation on impression formation. *Journal of Sport & Exercise Psychology, 22*(4), 283–291.

Martin Ginis, K. A., Eng, J. J., Arbour, K. P., Phillips, S. M., & Hartman, J. W. (2005). Mind over muscle? Sex differences in the relationship between body image change and subjective and objective physical changes over a 12-week strength-training program. *Body Image, 2*, 363–372.

Martin Ginis, K. A., Jung, M. E., & Gauvin, L. (2003). To see or not to see: Effects of exercising in mirrored environments on sedentary women's feeling states and self-efficacy. *Health Psychology, 22*, 354–361.

Martin Ginis, K. A., Latimer, A. E., & Jung, M. E. (2003). No pain no gain? Examining the generalizability of the exerciser stereotype to moderately active and excessively active targets, *Social Behavior and Personality, 31*(3), 283–290.

Martin Ginis, K. A., Leary, M. R. (2004). Self-presentational processes in health-damaging behavior. *Journal of Applied Sport Psychology, 16*, 59–74.

Martin Ginis, K. A., Lindwall, M., & Prapavessis, H. (2007). Who cares what other people think? Self-presentation in sport and exercise. In G. Tenenbaum, & R. Eklund (Eds.), *Handbook of sport psychology* (3rd ed., pp. 136–157). New York: Wiley.

Martin Ginis, K. A., Prapavessis, H., & Haase, A. M. (2008). The effects of physique-salient and physique non-salient exercise videos on women's body image, self-presentational concerns, and exercise motivation. *Body Image, 5*, 164–172. doi: 10.1016/j.bodyim.2007.11.005

McAuley, E., Bane, S. M., & Mihalko, S. L. (1995). Exercise in middle-aged adults: Self-efficacy and self-presentational outcomes. *Preventive Medicine, 24*, 319–328.

McAuley, E., Marquez, D. X., Jerome, G. J., Blissmer, B., & Katual, J. (2002). Physical activity and physique anxiety in older adults: Fitness and efficacy influences. *Aging and Mental Health, 6*, 222–230.

McGowan, E., Prapavessis, H., & Wesch, N. (2008). Self-presentational concerns and competitive anxiety. *Journal of Sport & Exercise Psychology, 30*, 383–400.

Melbye, L., Tenenbaum, G., & Eklund, R. (2008). Self-objectification and exercise behaviors: The mediating role of social physique anxiety. *Journal of Applied Biobehavioral Research, 12*, 196–220.

Miller, T. M., Linke, J. G., & Linke, R. A. (1980). Survey on body image, physical attractiveness, and depression. *Journal of Consulting and Clinical Psychology, 77*, 561–566.

Motl, R. W., & Conroy, D. E. (2000). Validity and factorial invariance of the Social Physique Anxiety Scale. *Medicine and Science in Sports and Exercise, 32*, 1007–1017.

Munroe-Chandler, K. J., Kim, A. J., & Gammage, K. L. (2004). Using imagery to predict weightlifting dependency in men. *International Journal of Men's Health, 3*, 129–139.

Nattiv, A., Loucks, A. B., Manore, M. M., Sanborn, C. F., Sundgot-Borgen, J., & Warren, M. P. (2007). American College of Sports Medicine position stand. The female athlete triad. *Medicine and Science in Sports and Exercise, 39*(10), 1867–1882.

Ommundsen, Y. (2001). Self-handicapping strategies in physical education classes: The influence of implicit theories of the nature of ability and achievement goal orientation. *Psychology of Sport and Exercise, 2*, 139–156.

Pearson, E. S., Hall, C. R., & Gammage, K. L. (2013). Self-presentation in exercise: Changes over a 12-week cardiovascular programme for overweight and obese sedentary females. *European journal of Sport Science, 13*(4), 407–413.

Podlog, L, Dimmock, J, & Miller, J. (2011). A review of return to sport concerns following injury rehabilitation: Practitioner strategies for enhancing recovery outcomes. *Physical Therapy in Sport, 12,* 36–42.

Prapavessis, H. (2004). Introduction to self-presentation in exercise and sport. *Journal of Applied Sport Psychology, 16,* 1–2.

Prapavessis, H., & Grove, J. R. (1998). Self-handicapping and self-esteem. *Journal of Applied Sport Psychology, 10,* 175–184.

Prapavessis, H., Grove, J. R., & Eklund, R. C. (2004). Self-presentational issues in competition and sport. *Journal of Applied Sport Psychology, 16,* 19–40.

Ransdell, L. B., Wells, C. L., Manore, M. M., Swan, P. D., & Corbin, C. B. (1998). Social physique anxiety in postmenopausal women. *Journal of Women & Aging, 10,* 19–39.

Rhodewalt, F., Saltzman, A. T., & Wittmer, J. (1984). Self-handicapping among competitive athletes: The role of practice in self-esteem protection. *Basic & Applied Social Psychology, 5,* 197–209.

Russell, W. D. (2002). Comparison of self-esteem, body satisfaction, and social physique anxiety across males of different exercise frequency and racial background. *Journal of Sport Behavior, 25,* 74–90.

Ryan, R. M., & Deci, E. L. (2007). Active human nature: Self-determination theory and the promotion and maintenance of sport, exercise, and health. In M. S. Hagger & N. L. D. Chatzisarantis (Eds.), *Intrinsic motivation and self-determination in exercise and sport* (pp. 1–19). Champaign, IL: Human Kinetics.

Ryska, T. A., Yin, Z., & Cooley, D. (1998). Effects of trait and situational self-handicapping on competitive anxiety among athletes. *Current Psychology: Developmental, Learning, Personality, Social, 17,* 48–56.

Sadalla, E. K., Linder, D. E., & Jenkins, B. A. (1988). Sport preference: A self-presentational analysis. *Journal of Sport and Exercise Psychology, 10,* 214–222.

Silberstein, L. R., Striegel-Moore, R. H., Timko, C., & Rodin, J. (1988). Behavioral and psychological implications of body dissatisfaction: Do men and women differ? *Sex Roles, 19,* 219–232.

Sinden, A. R., Martin Ginis, K. A., & Angove, J. (2003). Older Women's Reactions to Revealing and Non-revealing Exercise Attire. *Journal of Aging & Physical Activity, 11*(4).

Smith, R. E., Smoll, F. L., & Cumming, S. P. (2007). Effects of a motivational climate intervention for coaches on young athletes' sport performance anxiety. *Journal of Sport & Exercise Psychology, 29,* 39–59.

Smith, R. E., Smoll, F. L., Cumming, S. P., & Grossbard, J. R. (2006). Measurement of multidimensional sport performance anxiety in children and adults: The Sport Anxiety Scale-2. *Journal of Sport & Exercise Psychology, 28,* 479–501.

Spink, K. S. (1992). Relation of anxiety about social physique to location of participation in physical activity. *Perceptual and Motor Skills, 74,* 1075–1078.

Stanley, D. M., Cumming, J., Standage, M., & Duda, J. L. (2012). Images of exercising: Exploring the links between exercise imagery use, autonomous and controlled motivation to exercise, and exercise intention and behavior. *Psychology of Sport and Exercise, 13*, 133–141.

Strong, H. A., Martin Ginis, K. A., Mack, D. E., & Wilson, P. M. (2006). Examining self-presentational exercise motives and social physique anxiety in men and women. *Journal of Applied Biobehavioral Research, 11*, 209–225.

Tenenbaum, G., & Eklund, R. C. (2007). *Handbook of sport psychology* (3rd ed.). Hoboken, NJ: John Wiley & Sons.

Tenenbaum, G., Lidor, R., Lavyan, N., Morrow, K., Tonnel, S., & Gershgoren, A. (2005). Dispositional and task-specific social-cognitive determinants of physical effort perseverance. *Journal of Psychology, 139*, 139–157.

Thill, E. E., & Cury, F. (2000). Learning to play golf under different goal conditions: their effects on irrelevant thoughts and on subsequent control strategies. *European Journal of Social Psychology, 30*, 101–122.

Thogersen-Ntoumani, C., Cumming, J., Ntoumanis, N., & Nikitaras, N. (2012). Exercise imagery and its correlates in older adults. *Psychology of Sport and Exercise, 13*, 19–25.

Treasure, D. C., Lox, C. L., & Lawton, B. R. (1998). Determinants of physical activity in a sedentary, obese female population. *Journal of Sport and Exercise Psychology, 20*, 218–224.

Wilson, P., & Eklund, R. C. (1998). The relationship between competitive anxiety and self-presentational concerns. *Journal of Sport & Exercise Psychology, 20*, 81–97.

Wilson, P. M., Rodgers, W. M., Hall, C. R., & Gammage, K. L. (2003). Do autonomous exercise regulations underpin different types of exercise imagery. *Journal of Applied Sport Psychology, 15*, 294–306.

Woodgate, J., Martin Ginis, K. A., & Sinden, A. R. (2003). Physical activity and social physique anxiety in older women: The moderating effects of self-presentation efficacy. *Journal of Applied Biobehavioral Research, 8*, 116–127.

Worringham, C. J., & Messick, D. M. (1983). Social facilitation of running: An unobtrusive study. *Journal of Social Psychology, 121*, 23–29.

Yeung, R. R., & Hemsley, D. R. (1997). Personality, exercise and psychological well-being: Static relationships in the community. *Personality and Individual Differences, 22*, 47–53.

Yin, Z. (2001). Setting for exercise and concerns about body appearance of women who exercise. *Perceptual and Motor Skills, 93*, 851–855.

Chapter 10

Coping with Emotions in Sport

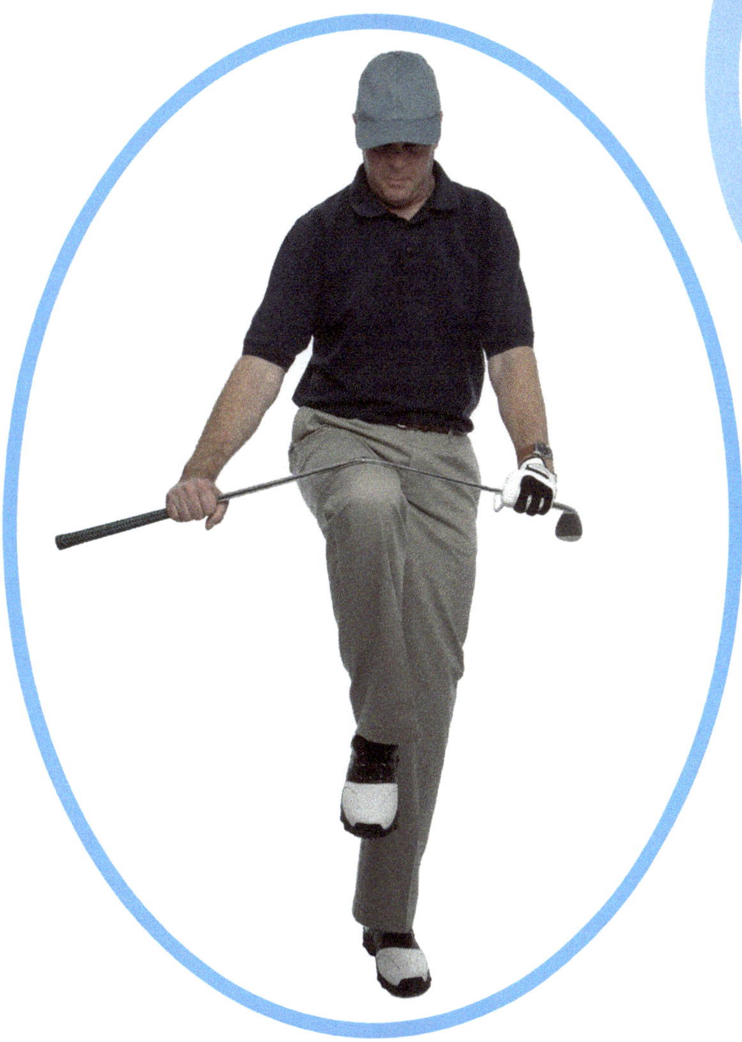

Introduction

If athletes do not believe that they have the resources to deal with the demands encountered in the competition environment, then they will probably experience negative emotions, such as anxiety and anger, and possibly suffer from negative behavior such as physical tension. Intuitively, we all know what it is like to experience an emotion toward something or somebody, but psychologists have had a difficult time actually defining what is emotion. Arriving at a list of necessary and sufficient conditions for something to be called an emotion has been very problematic. What separates an emotion from non-emotion, such as anger from non-anger, is probably a matter of degree (Gross, 2007).

Much of the research considering emotions in sport has employed Lazarus' (2000) cognitive-motivational-relational (CMR) theory of emotions. This research has investigated the stressors encountered by performers, the appraisals and the emotional response associated with appraisals, and subsequent coping responses to stressors. There are a wide variety of stressors encountered by athletes from poor practice performance and weak teammates, to late travel arrangements and an unfavorable competition format. It has been found that unexpected stressors were appraised as more threatening than those that were expected during performance (Dugdale, Eklund, & Gordon, 2002). Appraisals of events are suggested to comprise primary and secondary appraisals. Primary appraisals refer to whether an event or situation is personally relevant to the athlete. If an athlete appraises an event as having no relevance, no emotions will arise. Secondary appraisals are concerned with an athlete's perceived coping options. If an athlete feels he or she cannot manage the demands of the situation, this will certainly influence the specific emotions experienced. Uphill and Jones (2007), interviewing international athletes from a range of sports, provided some support for the association of appraisals with a variety of emotions, including anger, anxiety, guilt, happiness, pride, relief, sadness, and shame. Moreover, CMR suggests the experience of emotions need not be detrimental. For example, the emotion of anxiety might benefit performance through an increase in mobilized energy and/or concentration on the task at hand. We chose this example since it is anxiety that has received by far the most research attention in sport (Woodman, Davis, Hardy, Callow, Glasscock, & Yuill-Proctor, 2009).

Coping strategies can be classified into one of two categories (Lazarus, 2000). Problem-focused coping entails taking action to change some aspect of the person–environment relationship, either by altering an aspect of the environment itself or by changing one's situation within it. For example, a figure skater in training could decide to work on an easier jump to cope with her disappointment of continually not being able to land the more difficult jump she has been attempting. Emotion-focused coping, on the other hand, influences only what is in the mind of an athlete. Specifically, strategies to cope with a particular event may involve either a re-direction of attention or a re-interpretation (re-appraisal) of the person–environment relationship. A squash player, for example, who gets an unfavorable call from a referee on a critical point may reduce his anger by re-focusing attention to task-relevant cues. Athletes use numerous coping strategies (Giacobbi, Foore, & Weinberg, 2004; Holt & Hogg, 2002), with higher level athletes employing more coping strategies than lower skilled athletes (Nicholls, Polman, Levy, Taylor, & Cobley, 2007). The specific coping strategies employed by athletes are considered later in this chapter.

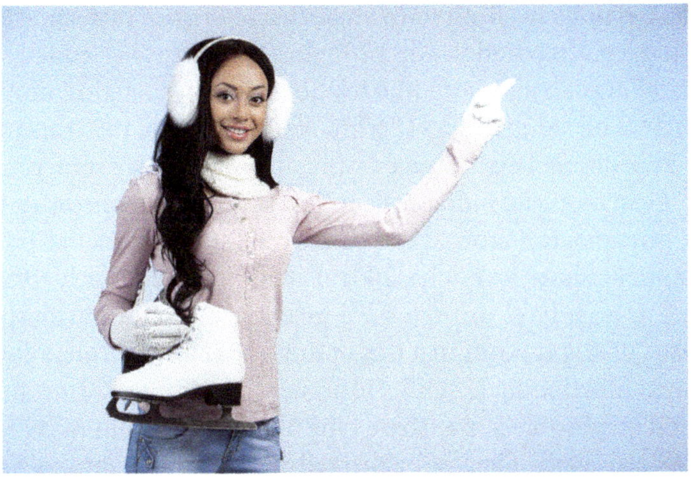

Emotions are sometimes conceptualized as pre-performance and post-performance emotions (Woodman et al., 2009). Although anxiety can be readily conceptualized as a pre-performance emotion, other negative emotions are more readily thought of as post-performance emotions. For example, an athlete may feel angry at having performed below potential, ashamed of a particularly poor performance in front of the home crowd, or guilty of letting the coach down with a poor performance. Many positive emotions are best thought of as post-performance emotions. For example, an athlete may feel happy to have won, relieved at having achieved a performance goal, or proud to have made the finals of a major competition.

Consequences of Emotions

Consequences of emotions can be considered in both the short-term (e.g., behavioral response) and long-term (e.g., health outcomes), and at the intrapersonal and interpersonal levels (Uphill, McCarthy, & Jones, 2009). We will discuss the short-term consequences of emotions in sport, primarily because there is minimal research on the long-term consequences. Our focus will also be at the intrapersonal level since this is the level most interventions have examined. This is not to indicate that research on interpersonal aspects of emotion is less important. For example, a coach who is visibly anxious before an important game may then communicate this anxiety to his players. There has not, however, been intervention research directed at this issue.

The consequences of emotions for individual athletes can be categorized as physiological, cognitive, and motivational (Uphill et al., 2009).

Physiological Consequences

Of the physiological consequences, arousal has been considered the most often. It is likely that the arousal accompanying some emotions may be of sufficient intensity to affect sport performance (Uphill et al., 2009). A simple relationship, however, between the physiological arousal accompanying emotions and athletes' performance is unlikely. Both individual characteristics (for some athletes the intensity of the arousal accompanying a given emotion will be higher than for other athletes) and the nature of the task the athlete is undertaking can influence this relationship. Physiological arousal has been positively associated with performance on aerobic tasks (Parfitt, Hardy, & Pates, 1995) and strength tasks (Perkins, Wilson, & Kerr, 2001). In addition, heightened emotional intensity may sometimes be beneficial to performance, especially if it can motivate individuals to invest greater resources to the current task (Lazarus, 2000). In contrast, physiological arousal can be harmful to performance on tasks that require fine motor control (Noteboom, Fleshner, & Enoka, 2001; Parfitt, Jones, & Hardy, 1990).

Finding the optimal arousal level to perform a given task should obviously benefit sport performance. Yuri Hanin (1980; 2000) proposes that this optimal level for an athlete can be represented by the individual zone of optimal functioning (IZOF). He argues that by monitoring an athlete over a number of competitions, it should be possible to use some type of intervention to make sure the athlete is in his or her IZOF. Research by Movahedi, Sheikh, Bagherzadeh, Hemayattalab, and Ashayeri (2007) suggests that this optimal arousal level may be associated with the level at which the athlete practices. Male physical education students were randomly assigned to a high-arousal (n = 19) or low-arousal group (n = 18). To manipulate participants' level of arousal, the authors used motivational techniques. They used heart rate and the Sport Competition Anxiety Test (Martens, 1977) to measure the level of arousal that participants achieved. At the determined and given arousal state, the two groups performed basketball free throws for 18 sessions. Both groups performed a retention test at the two arousal levels immediately after the last exercise session, in the posttest, and after 10 days. It was found that both groups learned the task similarly and achieved their peak performance at their experienced arousal level. When tested at an arousal level that differed from the one that they experienced throughout practice sessions, participants' performance deteriorated. Performance of the task seemed to have been integrated with the arousal level of the participants during the learning of the task, suggesting a practice-specificity-based explanation for achieving peak performance.

Cognitive Consequences

Emotions may lead to changes in a range of cognitive functions that could influence sport performance. The emotion considered the most in sport is undoubtedly anxiety. Studies have demonstrated that competitive anxiety affects the amount of information that is processed. An increase in competitive anxiety is associated with the narrowing of attentional focus (Janelle, Singer, & Williams, 1999). The consequences of this can be positive or negative. Performance may be improved if unimportant distracting cues are blocked out. In contrast, an athlete's performance may be diminished if important task-relevant cues are missed.

Competitive anxiety also affects the type of information that is processed. Highly anxious athletes attend to threatening task-irrelevant information to a greater extent than low anxious athletes. Moran, Byrne, and McGlade (2002) presented eight expert female gymnasts with three digital slides of a model performing a skill, the 'back flip' on the beam, that is known to cause anxiety. The slides differed in the amount of anxiety that they elicited in the viewer; this was accomplished by varying the height of the beam and the presence or absence of safety mats. The gymnasts were asked to imagine themselves in the position of the depicted model and to describe the anxiety that they felt. Their eye movements were recorded as they viewed the slides. The results revealed that anxiety was associated with an increase in the number of fixations to peripheral areas. Moreover, the more threatening slides elicited significantly more fixations than the less feared images. The implications of these types of findings are that attention that is selectively focused on task-irrelevant cues when an athlete is anxious can be detrimental for performance.

Elevated levels of competitive anxiety can also influence the type of cognitive processing that occurs during performance. With increased anxiety there can be a shift from automatic processing to more conscious, controlled processing (Liao & Masters, 2002). Heightened conscious control of a previously automated skill seems to disrupt the coordinated fluidity of that skill. Mullen and Tattersall (2005) had participants complete 60 golf putts. They completed 3 blocks of 10 putts in single task, task-relevant shadowing, and task-irrelevant tone-counting conditions. Each set of 3 × 10 putts was completed in low and high anxiety conditions. They found that performance was impaired in the high anxiety shadowing and tone-counting conditions, supporting the conscious processing hypothesis as an explanation of the anxiety/performance relationship.

Motivational Consequences

It has been proposed that emotions may also influence athletes' motivation (Hanin, 2000) but research examining the influence of emotions on motivation is scarce. In fact, Uphill and colleagues (2009) note that the processes by which emotions may influence motivation are unclear. It might be expected that negative emotions would undermine motivation but this need not be the case. For example, anxiety may contribute to enhanced cognitive effort in some circumstances (Smith, Bellamy, Collins, & Newell, 2001). Positive emotions would typically be expected to support motivation and this seems to be true for sport enjoyment. Scanlan and her colleagues have identified enjoyment as a key predictor of sport commitment and a primary reason for initiating and maintaining involvement in youth and elite sport (Carpenter & Scanlan, 1998; Scanlan, Russell, Beals, & Scanlan, 2003).

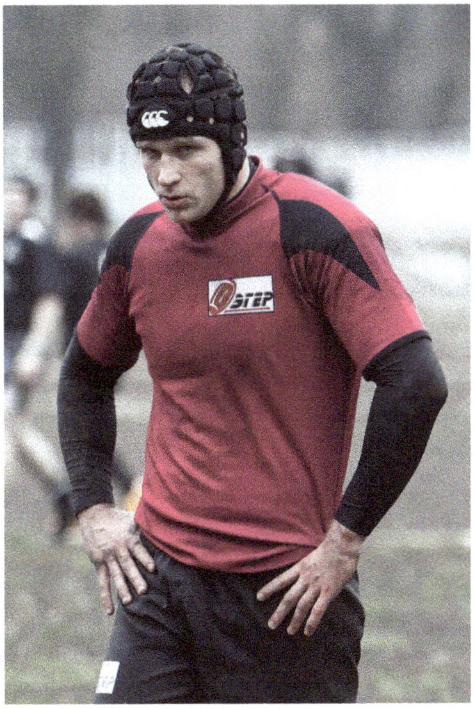

Image © Alexander Ishchenko, 2014. Used under license from Shutterstock, Inc.

Coping Strategies in Sport

The ways in which athletes can cope with emotions are almost limitless (Richards & Gross, 2000). Nicholls, Jones, Polman, and Borkoles (2009) examined acute sport related stressors, coping, and emotion among professional rugby union players during training and matches. Five professional rugby union players maintained diaries for 31 days in which stressors, coping strategies, an evaluation of coping effectiveness, and an evaluation of emotional intensity were recorded. Stressors were more frequently reported in training compared with matches. The various coping strategies employed and the frequency with which they were used is given in Table 10-1. Increased concentration was the most frequently cited coping strategy on training days, whereas blocking was the most frequently cited coping strategy on

TABLE 10–1 Coping Strategies and Frequencies Reported by Rugby Players

Coping Strategy	Frequency of Use
Increased concentration	50
Blocking	41
Increased effort	33
Focused on own role	31
Visualization	15
Played through injury	10
Thought stopping	10
Carried on playing	9
Acceptance	6
Used strapping	5
Adhered to routine	5
Rationalization	4
Warmed up	3
Stopped playing	3
Practiced	3
Positive self talk	2
Nothing	2
Re-directed anger toward opponent	1
Relaxed	1
Behavioral avoidance	1

Nicholls et al. (2009)

match days. Coping effectiveness was significantly higher during training compared with matches. Also, as would be expected, higher levels of emotional intensity were significantly associated with lower levels of coping effectiveness.

In another study, Filaire, Maso, Sagnol, Ferrand, and Lac (2001) had judo competitors complete a measure of coping strategies just prior to a major competition. The competitors were classified as winners or losers depending on the number of fights they won. It was shown that winners used more positive reappraisal (i.e., reinterpreting a stimulus in ways that change its emotional 'punch'), whereas losers employed more avoidance-oriented coping, self-blame, and sought more social support.

Amiot and colleagues conducted a study to determine whether the affective states of athletes would change from pre-competition to post-competition as a result of their use of coping strategies (Amiot, Gaudreau, & Blanchard, 2004). The use of task-oriented coping during competition produced increased positive affect, while disengagement-oriented coping was associated with increased negative affect. These results were supported by Gaudreau and Antl (2008) when they examined coping and life satisfaction. Athletes employing task-oriented coping during a competition were more satisfied about their life following the competition.

Given all the various coping strategies athletes can employ to handle their emotions, Gross and Thompson (2007) group the various strategies into five categories: situation selection, situation modification, attention deployment, cognitive change, and response modulation. Situation selection is the process of actively choosing to place oneself in a certain situation or context, rather than others. By selecting some situations as opposed to others, one may be able make it more or less likely that a desirable emotional state is attained. For example, a squash player may choose to play in a lower competitive category (e.g., B instead of A) to minimize the anxiety associated with playing against very strong opponents. Situation modification involves attempting to modify external aspects of the environment or the people therein. A runner may choose to change her running group because she enjoys herself more in the company of the other group.

Attention deployment refers to how an individual directs their attention within a given situation to influence their emotions. For example, the strategy of focusing on the thoughts and feelings associated with anger may be desirable in some circumstances (e.g., in contact sports such as football and hockey). Alternatively, one can use distraction to focus on non-emotional aspects of the situation. Athletes will often focus their attention just prior to competing on the upcoming task so they are less anxious and more confident.

Cognitive change entails changing the meaning or significance of an event or situation. How one appraises a situation is thought to alter the quality and intensity of the emotional response. Uphill et al. (2009) discuss some of the strategies that practitioners use to assist athletes change cognitions associated with an emotional response. These include: goal setting, reappraisal, imagery, and self-talk. The final category is response modulation. This refers to strategies designed to regulate the physiological, behavioral, cognitive, and experiential aspects of emotion as directly as possible. In sport, regulating the physiological arousal associated with emotion has received the most consideration. Some of the strategies successfully employed to regulate the physiological arousal levels of athletes, and concomitantly influence the experience of emotion, are progressive muscular relaxation, centering, playing up-beat music, and using relaxing or energizing imagery.

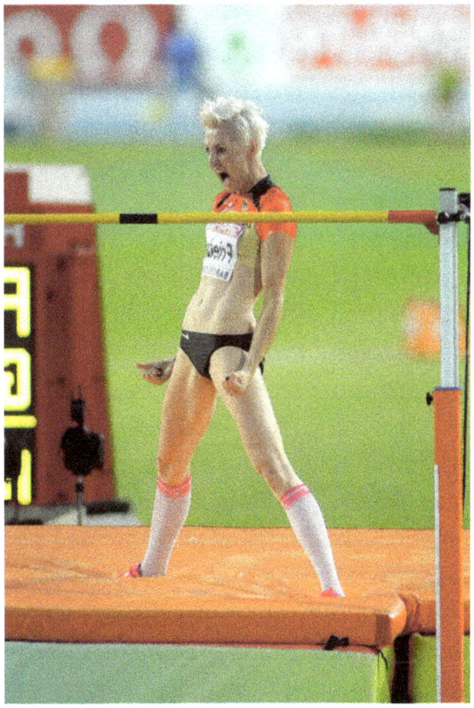

Coping Interventions

To examine the effects of manipulating emotions in assisting athletes to enter their optimal zones of functioning as described by IZOF theory, Robazza, Pellizzari, and Hanin (2004) had eight athletes from two different sports implement an individualized multimodal self-regulation intervention. A multiple baseline single-subject design was employed. Initially, the athletes recalled emotional content and intensities from their previous best and worst performances. This information served as individualized criteria and guidelines for the athletes' self-regulation. Next, the psychological and behavioral preparation procedures currently employed by each athlete were identified to gain information necessary for the development of most effective individualized self-regulation strategies. The identification process took into account preparatory routines and behaviors associated with goal setting, imagery, focusing, self-talk, arousal regulation, and emotion control.

Following a baseline phase during which each athlete monitored his pre-competition emotions, the mental skills intervention was implemented. The athletes were provided with psychological skills training during 10 individual, once-per-week meetings, each meeting lasting two hours. Athletes were informed that the mental training procedures would be beneficial in improving self-regulation skills, with the purpose of reaching a pre-performance state as near as possible their own optimal states. The intervention comprised several phases and evolved at different rates within and across sessions depending on the athlete's progress. The goal of the first phase was to improve individual awareness of content and intensity of pre-performance emotions and bodily symptoms, and their facilitating-inhibiting functional effects. The goal of the second phase was to enable the athletes to achieve optimal conditions by applying their effective self-regulation strategies and dismissing ineffective habits. In the final phase, suggestions were provided to the athletes to improve, refine, and expand their self-regulation strategies. The athletes were encouraged to achieve an optimal content and intensity of emotions and physiological symptoms by consistently applying self-regulation prior to practice and competition.

It was demonstrated that the intervention was effective in adjusting the patterns of both emotions and symptoms as intended. Five of the six athletes modified their pre-competition states toward patterns related to best performance in the expected direction after intervention (four of them also got more distant from worst performance), and their performance improved. While the overall findings certainly supported the intervention, Robazza and colleagues cautioned that getting athletes into the optimal zone pre-event does not guarantee that the athletes will stay in the zone until the task is completed.

In a more recent study, Mosewich, Crocker, Kowalski, and DeLongis (2013) investigated the influence of a self-compassion intervention on negative cognitive states and self-compassion in varsity women athletes. Self-compassion entails giving oneself care and compassion during difficult times. Self-compassion may play an important role in emotion regulation, providing a strategy to deal with negative cognitions and emotions associated with failure and negative events. At the same time, it may present an opportunity to learn from the experience and promote a more positive state of mind. The athletes were randomly assigned to either a self-compassion intervention or an attention control group. Participants in both groups listened to a psychoeducation presentation, participated in an applied example writing task, and received a book of writing modules to complete over the next seven days. The content covered, however, differed between the two groups. One week following the completion of the writing modules, athletes completed a questionnaire. A final follow-up questionnaire was completed one month later. The questionnaires assessed self-compassion, state rumination, state self-criticism, and concern over mistakes.

The self-compassion intervention began with a 10-minute presentation that consisted of an overview of basic stress and coping ideas in sport and information on self-compassion. Next, the athletes participated in an applied example of self-compassionate writing. They were instructed to "Think about a negative event in sport that occurred over the past week that was personally demanding." They were asked to provide a description of the event, including what happened leading up to the event, who was at the event, what happened, and any thoughts and actions that happened during the event. After completing this task, athletes responded to three prompts designed to promote thinking about the event in a self-compassionate manner. The athletes then were given a module booklet to use for their writing tasks over the next week. The booklet contained five exercises to be completed over the course of the next seven days, and each module was some variation of the example applied task. For the attention control participants the focus was on general writing and the topics chosen were not expected to have any influence on the study variables. The content consisted of where and how writing is often used in sport (e.g., training diaries, journaling).

The self-compassion intervention was successful, resulting in higher levels of self-compassion, and lower levels of state self-criticism, state rumination, and concern over mistakes, compared with an attention control group. This research provides support for the utility of a self-compassion intervention in sport and speaks to the importance of helping athletes to develop a wide array of coping strategies.

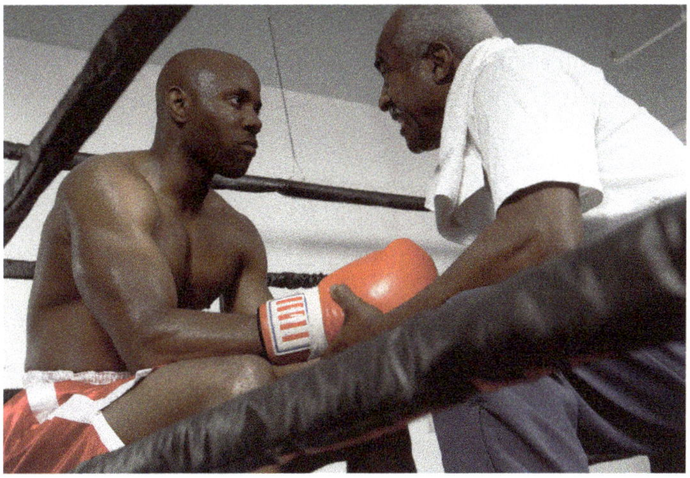

Measuring Emotions and Coping Strategies

There have been instruments developed to measure both emotions and coping strategies in sport. In 2005, Jones, Lane, Bray, Uphill, and Catlin developed the Sport Emotion Questionnaire (SEQ) as a sport-specific measure of pre-competitive emotion. It assesses anger, anxiety, dejection, excitement, and happiness with 22 items. The SEQ shows good evidence of validity and reliability. The SEQ is unique in that it is specifically designed to measure emotion rather than mood or affect. Furthermore, the SEQ allows athletes to report on a broader range of emotional states than other measures typically used to examine emotion in sport, such as the Positive and Negative Affect Schedule (PANAS: Watson, Clark, & Tellegen, 1988) or the Profile of Mood States (POMS: McNair, Lorr, & Droppleman, 1971). Although the SEQ measures five emotions, this is obviously not an exhaustive list and emotions such as guilt, shame, relief, and pride may also be experienced, which the SEQ fails to assess.

For the assessment of coping strategies employed by athletes in competitive sport settings, Gaudreau and Blondin (2002) developed the Coping Strategies in Sport Competition Inventory. The questionnaire consists of 39 items assessing 10 coping strategies: thought control, mental imagery, relaxation, energy expenditure, logical analysis, seeking support, venting of unpleasant emotion, mental distraction, disengagement/resignation, and social withdrawal. There is support for both the validity and reliability of the instrument. This inventory is an improvement over earlier instruments employed to measure coping in sport because it is sport-specific and can be used with both individual and team sport athletes.

CHAPTER SUMMARY

Individuals experience an array of different emotions in sport settings and how athletes cope with these emotions can influence their sport performance, as well as cognitive, motivational, and physiological aspects of their performance. Athletes employ problem-focused coping and emotion-focused coping strategies. They use numerous coping strategies, with higher level athletes employing more coping strategies than lower skilled athletes. Gross and Thompson (2007) group the various strategies into five general categories: situation selection, situation modification, attention deployment, cognitive change, and response modulation. Coping interventions conducted in sport have proven to be effective in regulating emotions and show the importance of helping athletes to develop a wide array of coping strategies.

REVIEW QUESTIONS

1. What is the difference between problem-focused coping strategies and emotion-focused coping strategies?
2. Briefly discuss the three consequences of emotions.
3. Given all the various coping strategies athletes can employ, Gross and Thompson (2007) grouped the various strategies into five categories. What are these five categories?
4. In their study investigating the influence of a self-compassion intervention on negative cognitive states and self-compassion in varsity women athletes, what did Mosewich et al. (2013) find?

SUGGESTED READINGS

Lazarus, R. S. (2000). How emotions influence performance in competitive sports. *The Sport Psychologist, 14*, 229–252.

Uphill, M. A., McCarthy, J. P., & Jones, M. V. (2009). Getting a grip on emotion regulation in sport: Conceptual foundations and practical application. In S. D. Mellalieu & S. Hanton (Eds.), *Advances in applied sport psychology: A review* (pp. 162–194). NY: Routledge.

REFERENCES

Amiot, C. E., Gaudreau, P., & Blanchard, C. M. (2004). Self-determination, coping and goal attainment in sport. *Journal of Sport & Exercise Psychology, 26*, 386–411.

Carpenter, P. J., & Scanlan, T. K. (1998). Changes over time in the determinance of sport commitment. *Pediatric Exercise Science, 10*, 356–365.

Dugdale, J. R., Eklund, R. C., & Gordon, S. (2002). Expected and unexpected stressors in major international competition: appraisal, coping, and performance. *The Sport Psychologist, 16*, 20–33.

Filaire, E., Maso, F., Sagnol, M., Ferrand, C., & Lac, G. (2001). Anxiety, hormonal responses, and coping during a judo competition. *Aggressive Behavior, 27*, 55–63.

Gaudreau, P., & Antl, S. (2008). Athletes' broad dimensions of dispositional perfectionism: Examining changes in life satisfaction and the mediating role of sport-related motivation and coping. *Journal of Sport & Exercise Psychology, 30*, 356–382.

Gaudreau, P., & Blondin, J. P. (2002). Development of a questionnaire for the assessment of coping strategies employed by athletes in competitive sport settings. *Psychology of Sport and Exercise, 3*, 1–34.

Giacobbi Jr., P. R., Foore, B., & Weinberg, R. S. (2004). The sources of stress and coping responses of skilled and moderately skilled golfers. *Journal of Applied Sport Psychology, 16*, 166–182.

Gross, J. J. (2007). *Handbook of emotion regulation*. London: Guilford Press.

Gross, J. J., & Thompson, R. A. (2007). Emotion regulation: conceptual foundations. In J. J. Gross (Ed.), *Handbook of emotion regulation* (pp. 3–24). London: Guilford Press.

Hanin, Y. L. (1980). A cognitive model of anxiety in sports. In W. Straub (Ed.), *Sport psychology: An analysis of athlete behavior* (pp. 236–249). Ithaca, NY: Movement.

Hanin, Y. L. (2000). Successful and poor performance and emotions. In Y. L. Hanin (Ed.), *Emotions in sport* (pp. 157–187). Champaign, IL: Human Kinetics.

Holt, N. L., & Hogg, J. M. (2002). Perception of stress and coping during preparations for the 1999 women's soccer world cup finals. *The Sport Psychologist, 16*, 251–271.

Janelle, C. M., Singer, R. N., & Williams, A. M. (1999). External distraction and attentional narrowing: visual search evidence. *Journal of Sport & Exercise Psychology, 21*, 70–91.

Jones, M. V., Lane, A. M., Bray, S. R., Uphill, M., & Catlin, J. (2005). Development and validation of the Sport Emotion Questionnaire. *Journal of Sport & Exercise Psychology, 27*, 407–431.

Lazarus, R. S. (2000). How emotions influence performance in competitive sports. *The Sport Psychologist, 14*, 229–252.

Liao, C., & Masters, R. S. W. (2002). Self-focused attention and performance failure under psychological stress. *Journal of Sport & Exercise Psychology, 24*, 289–305.

Martens, R. (1977). *Sport Competition Anxiety Test*. Champaign, IL: Human Kinetics.

McNair, D. M., Lorr, M., & Droppleman, L. F. (1971). *Profile of Mood State manual*. San Diego, CA: Educational and Industrial Testing Service.

Moran, A., Byrne, A., & McGlade, N. (2002). The effects of anxiety and strategic planning on visual search behaviour. *Journal of Sports Sciences, 20*, 225–236.

Mosewich, A. D., Crocker, P. R. E., Kowalski, K. C., & DeLongis, A. (2013). Applying self-compassion in sport: An intervention with women athletes. *Journal of Sport & Exercise Psychology, 35*, 514–524.

Movahedi, A., Sheikh, M., Bagherzadeh, F., Hemayattalab, R., & Ashayeri, H. (2007). A practice-specificity-based model of arousal for achieving peak performance. *Journal of Motor Behavior, 39*, 457–462.

Mullen, R., & Tattersall, A. (2005). The effects of anxiety on motor performance: A test of the conscious processing hypothesis. *Journal of Sport & Exercise Psychology, 27*, 212–225.

Nicholls, A. R., Jones, C. R., Polman, R. C. J., & Borkoles, E. (2009). Acute sport-related stressors, coping, and emotion among professional rugby union players during training and matches. *Scandinavian Journal of Medicine and Science in Sports, 19*, 113–120.

Nicholls, A. R., Polman, R. C. J., Levy, A. R., Taylor, J., & Cobley, S. (2007). Stressors, coping, and coping effectiveness: gender, type of sport, and skill differences. *Journal of Sports Sciences, 25*, 1521–1530.

Noteboom, J. T., Fleshner, M., & Enoka, R. M. (2001). Activation of the arousal response can impair performance on a simple motor task. *Journal of Applied Physiology, 91*, 821–831.

Parfitt, C. G., Jones, J. G., & Hardy, L. (1990). Multidimensional anxiety and performance. In J. G. Jones & L. Hardy (Eds.), *Stress and performance in sport* (pp. 43–80). Chichester, England: Wiley.

Parfitt, G., Hardy, L., & Pates, J. (1995). Somatic anxiety and physiological arousal: Their effects upon a high anaerobic, low memory demand task. *International Journal of Sport Psychology, 26*, 196–213.

Perkins, D., Wilson, G. V., & Kerr, J. H. (2001). The effects of elevated arousal and mood on maximal strength performance in athletes. *Journal of Applied Sport Psychology, 13*, 239–259.

Richards, J. M., & Gross, J. J. (2000). Emotion regulation and memory: the cognitive costs of keeping one's cool. *Journal of Personality and Social Psychology, 79*, 410–424.

Robazza, C., Pellizzari, M., & Hanin, Y. (2004). Emotion self-regulation and athletic performance: An application of the IZOF model. *Psychology of Sport and Exercise, 5*, 379–404.

Scanlan, T. K., Russell, D. G., Beals, K. P., & Scanlan, L. A. (2003). Project on elite athlete commitment (PEAK): II. A direct test and expansion of the sport commitment model with elite amateur sportsmen. *Journal of Sport & Exercise Psychology, 25*, 377–401.

Smith, N. C., Bellamy, M., Collins, D. J., & Newell, D. (2001). A test of processing efficiency theory in a team sport context. *Journal of Sports Sciences, 19*, 321–332.

Uphill, M. A., & Jones, M. V. (2007). The antecedents of emotions in elite athletes. *Research Quarterly for Sport and Exercise, 78*, 79–89.

Uphill, M. A., McCarthy, J. P., & Jones, M. V. (2009). Getting a grip on emotion regulation in sport: Conceptual foundations and practical application. In S. D. Mellalieu & S. Hanton (Eds.), *Advances in applied sport psychology: A review* (pp. 162–194). NY: Routledge.

Watson, D., Clark, L. A., & Tellegen, A. (1988). Development and validation of brief measures of positive and negative affects. The PANAS scales. *Journal of Personality and Social Psychology, 54*, 1063–1070.

Woodman, T., Davis, P. A., Hardy, L., Callow, N., Glasscock, I., & Yuill-Proctor, J. (2009). Emotions and sport performance: An exploration of happiness, hope, and anger. *Journal of Sport & Exercise Psychology, 31*, 169–188.

Chapter 11

Group Interventions in Exercise

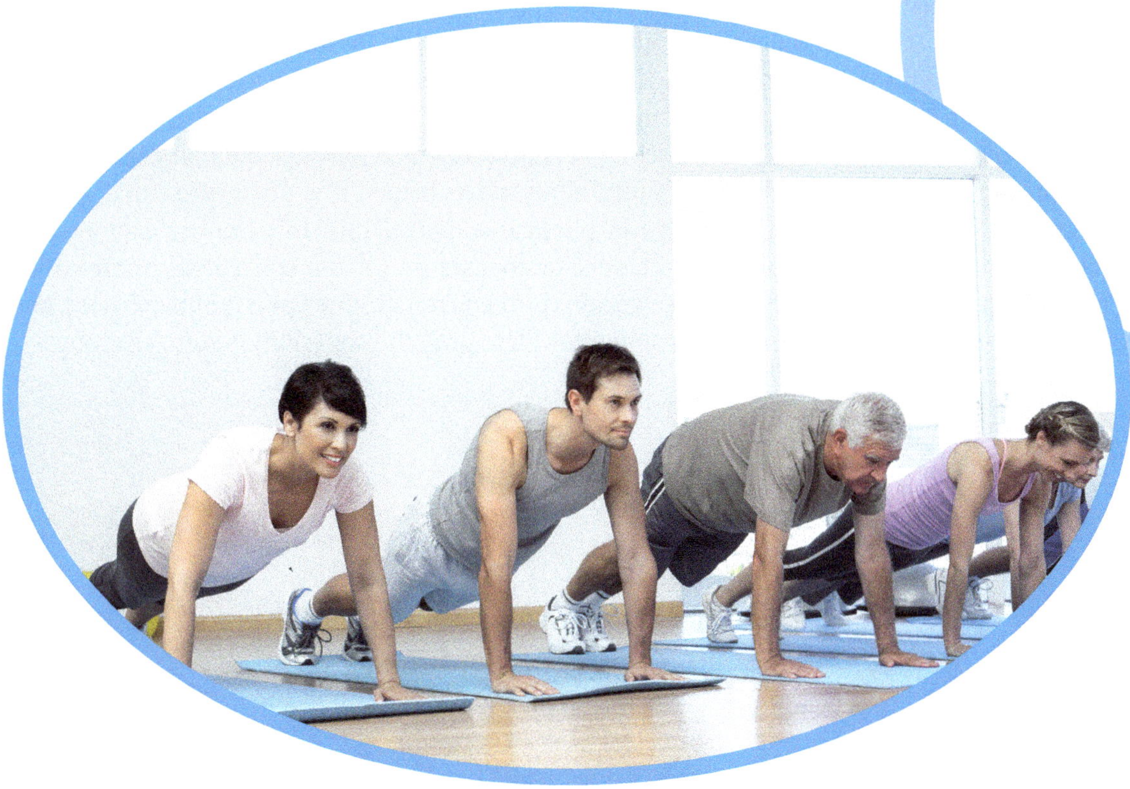

Introduction

Throughout this book we have discussed multiple approaches to stimulating involvement in and maintenance of physical activity. The intervention strategies discussed thus far have primarily focused on individual-level approaches. For example, mental imagery, self-talk, and biofeedback are all inherently personal and impact on individual-level factors that can affect performance. Although individual-level interventions can be applied in group settings, each individual within the group must adopt the intervention approach. Other strategies discussed in this book, such as modeling and self-presentation, are more social in nature. These types of interventions impact the motivation, cognitions, and behaviors of individuals; however, enacting them typically involves interpersonal processes. One final type of intervention that influences psychological and behavioral outcomes in exercise is group-based interventions.

In sports, group dynamics are thought to play an important role in performance. For example, the 2011–2012 regular season of the National Hockey League marked an average performance by the Los Angeles Kings. Accumulating 95 points over the course of the regular season, they finished eighth in the Western Conference, just barely qualifying for a playoff position. Drawing on what many fans, commentators, and the players themselves described as resilience and team unity, the Kings rallied together during the playoffs, knocked out the top three seeds, and won the Stanley Cup (McGran, 2012). Although the surprising success of the L.A. Kings represents a relatively rare event, it exemplifies what research has shown—cohesive teams perform well.

The influence of groups in the exercise context is no different. Consider the popularity of exercise classes, running groups, and "beer league" intramural sports teams. It is no surprise that group processes can impact our motivation to engage in physical activity. Thus, this chapter explores current research on group processes in exercise with specific focuses on (a) the conceptual frameworks that have been applied to examining the exercise group, (b) the factors influencing group cohesion and the effectiveness of exercise groups, and (c) strategies for increasing the cohesion of exercise groups.

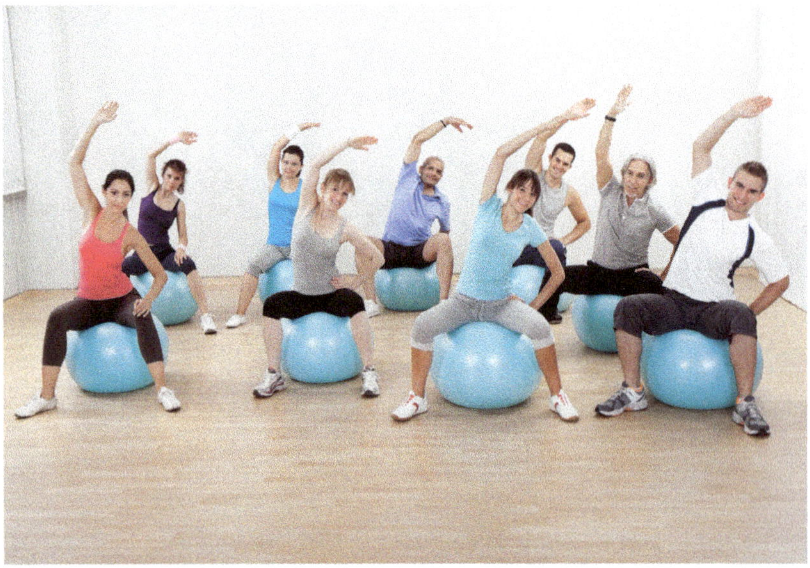

The Advantage of Group Interventions in Exercise

Several reviews and meta-analyses have explored the question of whether group-level interventions are superior to individual level-interventions for impacting outcomes related to exercise participation. The first review, conducted by Dishman and Buckworth, incorporated findings from 127 studies that tested interventions in a variety of settings such as schools, worksites, homes, and health-care settings (Dishman & Buckworth, 1996). The findings from this meta-analysis indicated that interventions delivered in group settings yielded much larger effects than interventions delivered in any other context (e.g., one-on-one interventions, interventions targeting families, etc.). The second review found conflicting evidence. In this study, Atienza reviewed 39 studies and concluded that home-based exercise was superior to group-based exercise for promoting adherence to physical activity (Atienza, 2001). A third review of 38 studies, found no significant differences between home-based, group-based, and education interventions with respect to promoting physical activity over the short-term (Van der Bij, Laurant, & Wensing, 2002).

Across the first three reviews examining the effectiveness of group-level interventions in exercise, drastically different conclusions were drawn. Burke and colleagues suggested that these different findings may have occurred because of the different ways that the group context was operationalized (Burke, Carron, Eys, Ntoumanis, & Estabrooks, 2006). For example, home-based interventions are often operationalized as being individual interventions; however, the degree to which social support is offered in home-based interventions can differ dramatically and may confound the traditional classification of home-based interventions as 'individual.' Likewise, environments which are traditionally classified as group settings can also vary in the degree to which 'the group' is salient. Consider a drop-in aerobics class that has a high variability in class attendees and for which the instructors rotate from week to week. Compare this to a more structured class in which the participants and the instructors stay consistent each week over a 12-week session. In the former example, there is very little from which to establish perceptions of 'groupness' (or group identity) whereas in the latter example, there are a number of characteristics which may help to define the aerobics class as a group. If the instructor in the latter example were to apply group-building strategies (which we will discuss later in the chapter), the group experience may be enhanced even more. Thus, within what is traditionally considered a group setting, there is substantial variability in the salience of 'the group.'

To answer the question of whether group-level interventions are superior to individual level-interventions, Burke and colleagues applied a revised conceptualization of group versus individual which consisted of four different contexts: (a) home-based programs that did not involve contact from researchers or health-care professionals, (b) home-based programs that involved some contact from researchers or health-care professionals, (c) standard exercise classes, and (d) exercise classes in which group-dynamics principles (i.e., team building strategies) were applied. The first of these categories (i.e., home-based programs with no contact) represented truly individual interventions whereas the exercise classes that applied group-dynamics principles represented true groups. The findings of this meta-analysis showed that across five categories of outcomes (i.e., exercise adherence, social interaction, quality of life, physiological effectiveness, and functional effectiveness), exercising in a true group was superior. True groups were higher on all outcome variables when compared to the standard exercise classes and exercising at home with contact (no difference between these two groups). In turn, standard exercise classes and exercising at home with contact were superior to exercising at home without contact.

These findings suggest that group-level interventions are, in fact, superior to individual-level interventions when the degree of social interaction is taken into consideration in classifying interventions as 'group' or 'individual' (Burke et al., 2006).

Why Do Exercise Groups Work?

There are a variety of reasons why exercise groups may lead to more positive exercise-related outcomes such as enjoyment and adherence. First, in exercise groups there is a degree of social support which is not present when exercising alone. In the meta-analysis conducted by Burke and colleagues (discussed in the previous section), exercise outcomes improved as a function of the social contact involved in the intervention (Burke et al., 2006). Outcomes were the weakest for interventions that did not involve any forms of support, were slightly stronger for the two conditions that involved moderate amounts of support (i.e., home-based programs with formal support from a researcher or health care provider or group-based programs with limited social interaction), and were strongest for interventions involving true groups. Indeed, physical activity interventions are most effective when they include social support (Kahn et al., 2002).

A second reason that exercise groups may improve outcomes is through their influence on feeling states. For example, Courneya examined the relationships between perceptions of the group environment and feeling states among 99 women enrolled in a 12-week exercise class at a university fitness center (Courneya, 1995). After 4 weeks in the class, the women completed an assessment of the group environment. Then, during each of the final 8 weeks of the class they completed an assessment of their affect. Scores across the 8 weeks that this measure was administered were combined to create a mean affect score for each participant. The findings from this study showed that perceptions of the group environment were positively correlated with positive affect. Although this study was correlational and causality cannot be inferred, it provides a preliminary indication that individuals who feel a stronger connection to their exercise group may benefit from more positive feelings.

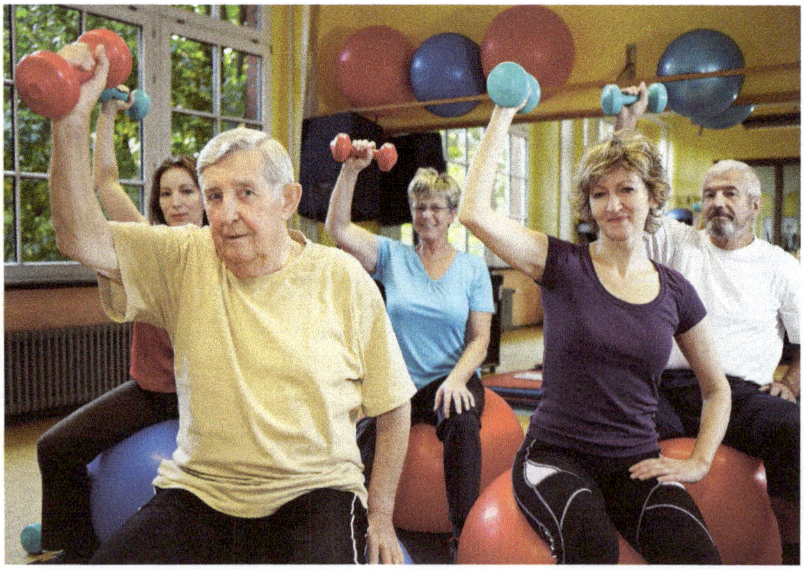

Research applying the theory of planned behavior (Ajzen, 2011) to examining the impact of groups on exercise outcomes has pointed to some additional reasons that group processes may be effective in exercise. For example, Courney and McAuley (1995) recruited 62 women from 11 exercise classes at a university fitness center. The women completed questionnaires assessing their perceptions of the group environment and variables from the theory of planned behavior at baseline and every 4 weeks over the course of the 12-week session. Using path analysis, the researchers showed that attitudes toward exercise, and intentions to exercise, mediated the effect of the group on exercise adherence. Thus, these findings indicate that perceptions of the group experience influence the motivational antecedents of behavior.

The Role of Cohesion in the Success of Exercise Groups

For several decades, group cohesion has been considered one of the most important factors influencing the success of groups. The effects of cohesion in group performance have been demonstrated across many contexts including work groups, the military, sports, and exercise. Group cohesion is defined as "a dynamic process which is reflected in the tendency for a group to stick together and remain united in the pursuit of its instrumental objectives and/or for the satisfaction of member affective needs" (Carron, Brawley, & Widmeyer, 1998, p. 213). This definition highlights four factors which are each critical for the cohesion of groups. First, cohesion is a multidimensional; that is, there are numerous factors that contribute to the cohesion of a group and those factors vary across groups. Second, cohesion is dynamic; the cohesion of a group can change over time. Third, cohesion is instrumental; this means that cohesion in itself is an important reason that a group remains together. Finally, cohesion is affective; as we discussed above, when a group is cohesive, its members experience positive affect.

The literature examining the role of group cohesion in exercise has been based primarily on Carron and colleagues' conceptual model of group cohesion (Carron, Widmeyer, & Brawley, 1985), depicted in Figure 11-1. The model identifies two levels of group cohesion: individual vs. group and task vs. social. The individual level of the model represents individual-level factors that draw a person to the group. For example, an individual may be drawn to the exercise group because he or she personally enjoys the company of the other group members. On the group level, members may be drawn to the group because they feel that the dynamics achieved through supportive interactions are motivating. Both the individual and group levels of cohesion are further bisected by the second level of group cohesion, task vs. social. The task level of cohesion refers to member of the group, both individually and collectively, being drawn to the group because of task-related factors such as achieving group goals. The social level of cohesion refers to members of the group enjoying the interpersonal aspects of group membership such as formulating new friendships. When the two levels of group cohesion are combined, they form four dimensions of group cohesion: attraction to the group—task, attraction to the group—social, group integration—task, and group integration—social.

FIGURE 11–1 Conceptual model of group cohesion

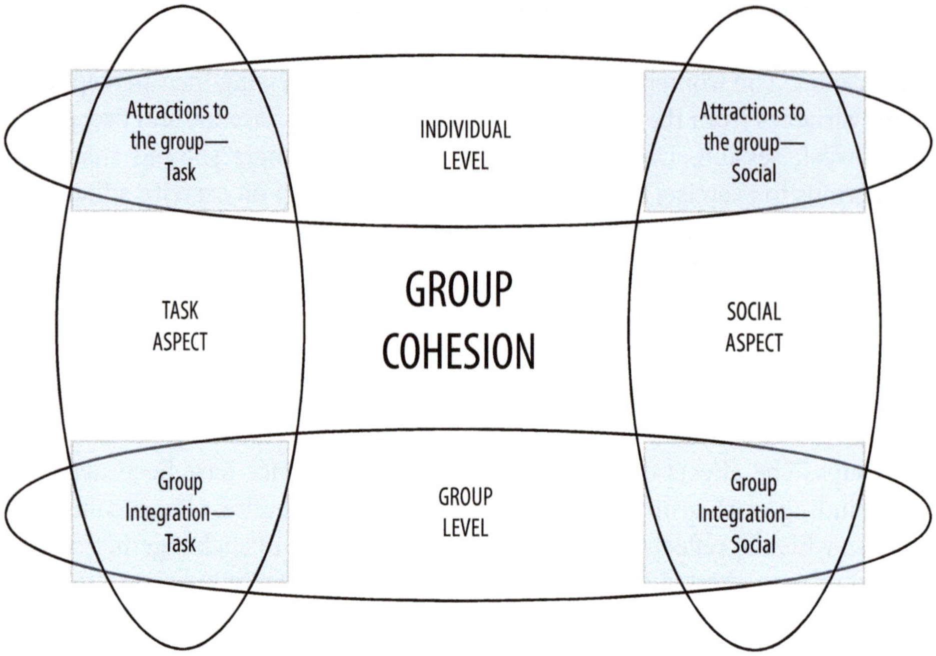

(Carron et al., 1985)

How It Is Measured

In the exercise context, the group environment is typically assessed using the Group Environment Questionnaire (GEQ) (Carron et al., 1985). Although the GEQ was originally developed to assess the group environment in sports teams, it was subsequently revised for an exercise setting (Carron & Spink, 1992). Modification of the GEQ for the exercise context yielded an 18-item questionnaire with four scales representing the four dimensions of group cohesion: attraction to the group—task, attraction to the group—social, group integration—task, and group integration—social. Further modifications to the GEQ were then conducted to create the Physical Activity Group Environment Questionnaire (PAGEQ) which is more appropriate for assessing the physical activity environment among older adults (Estabrooks & Carron, 2000). The PAGEQ includes 21 items also assessing each of the four dimensions of group cohesion.

Factors Influencing Group Cohesion in Exercise

There are four primary factors that influence group cohesion in the exercise domain: personal factors, group factors, leadership factors, and environmental factors (Carron, Shapcott, & Burke, 2007). The research conducted in each of these areas has implications for intervention; thus, we discuss each factor, below.

Personal factors. There are numerous demographic or individual-difference factors that may impact an individual's perceptions of the group experience. From the organizational psychology literature we know that diversity in age, experience, and personality types among group members impact group processes. In the exercise context, research examining the role of personal factors is somewhat limited; however, the research that has been done has focused on the effects of member diversity on cohesion and performance. One of the first studies investigating the role of personal factors on group cohesion in exercise examined the influence of diversity between walking group members in task-related factors and task-unrelated factors on group cohesion and performance (Shapcott, Carron, Burke, Bradshaw, & Estabrooks, 2006). The participants were individuals who were registered for the Walk Kansas community-based physical activity promotion program. Walk Kansas involved participating in small walking groups (with approximately six members per group) for a period of 8 weeks. During the program, participants engaged in group goal setting and a number of other activities aimed at establishing group identity and group cohesion. At the point of program registration, the participants completed questionnaires assessing demographic and psychological variables (including the perceptions of the group environment). Throughout the program, participants reported their levels of physical activity on a weekly basis. The analysis focused on the degree to which diversity on task-related (i.e., self-efficacy, previous physical activity level, and personal goals) and task unrelated factors (i.e., ethnicity and gender) influenced cohesion and performance. With regard to task-related factors, diversity in previous levels of physical activity was negatively related to cohesion and performance—groups with more diversity in previous physical activity levels were less cohesive and did not perform as well as groups whose members were less diverse. With regard to task-unrelated factors, diversity in gender was negatively related to cohesion—groups with more gender diversity were less cohesive. No relationships were observed for the other task-related and task-unrelated factors on cohesion or performance. These findings suggest that exercise groups may benefit from homogeneity with respect to previous experience and gender. The implications that can be drawn from this research suggest that grouping exercisers according to gender and to previous level of experience may be one way to enhance cohesion and performance in the exercise domain. More research is needed to further explore the role of diversity of personal factors in cohesion and performance across different exercise settings.

Leadership factors. Anyone who has attended an aerobics class can attest to the important role an exercise leader has on a variety of outcomes. For example, instructors that are energetic, positive, and encouraging can help the class participants feel motivated and energetic themselves. Indeed, researchers have shown that instructor characteristics and behaviors can influence motivation in an exercise setting (e.g., Edmunds, Ntoumanis, & Duda, 2006). Can leadership behaviors also influence group cohesion? To test this question, Loughead and colleagues recruited 117 older adults from community-based exercise programs to complete questionnaires assessing their perceptions of cohesion in their exercise classes, and their perceptions of the enthusiasm, motivation, and availability of their leaders (Loughead, Colman, & Carron, 2001). The findings showed that perceptions of group cohesion were significantly related to leader characteristics. These findings suggest that the characteristics of an exercise leader may, indeed, influence perceptions of group cohesion among exercise participants.

Environmental factors. Various environmental factors may influence the degree to which exercise groups are cohesive. In the sports domain, group size and level of competition have both been found to influence cohesion (Carron et al., 2007). Because it is less common for exercise groups to compete against one another, level of competition is less relevant in the exercise setting. Group size, however, can vary dramatically from one setting to another and may, in fact, influence cohesion. To test this question,

Carron and Spink conducted a series of four studies (Carron & Spink, 1993). In the first three studies they examined relationships between group size (small groups had fewer than 20 participants and large groups had more than 40 participants) and perceptions of cohesion. Across these three studies their findings were consistent: perceptions of cohesion are stronger among smaller exercise groups. In the fourth study, Carron and Spink implemented team-building interventions in small and large exercise groups. They found the influence of group size on team cohesion disappeared. More specifically, they found that through the team-building intervention they were able to enhance the perceptions of group cohesion among exercisers in larger groups.

Group factors. The group factors that influence cohesion and performance are those related to the specific processes engaged in by the group members, such as goal setting. In Chapter 5 we discussed goal setting as an effective intervention strategy for improving processes and performances in sports teams. Research on group cohesion in the exercise domain has also pointed to group goal setting as an effective intervention strategy in exercise. For example, Burke and colleagues examined the relationship between group goal setting and team performance in the Walk Kansas intervention discussed earlier (Burke, Shapcott, Carron, Bradshaw, & Estabrooks, 2010). An analysis of the relationship between team goal setting and the collective distance walked over the 8-week program (i.e., "performance") showed that groups that collectively set more ambitious goals walked more miles than groups that set less ambitious goals.

There are a variety of other group factors that may influence cohesion and performance in exercise groups. These factors include things like establishing a group identity and group norms, increasing the frequency or quality of within-group interactions and communication, and developing a culture of sacrifice in which members sacrifice their own personal achievement in support of group-wide achievement. To date, few of these strategies have been tested individually; instead, they have been combined into team-building interventions and the effects of these composite interventions have been tested. Below, we discuss common approaches to team building in an exercise setting.

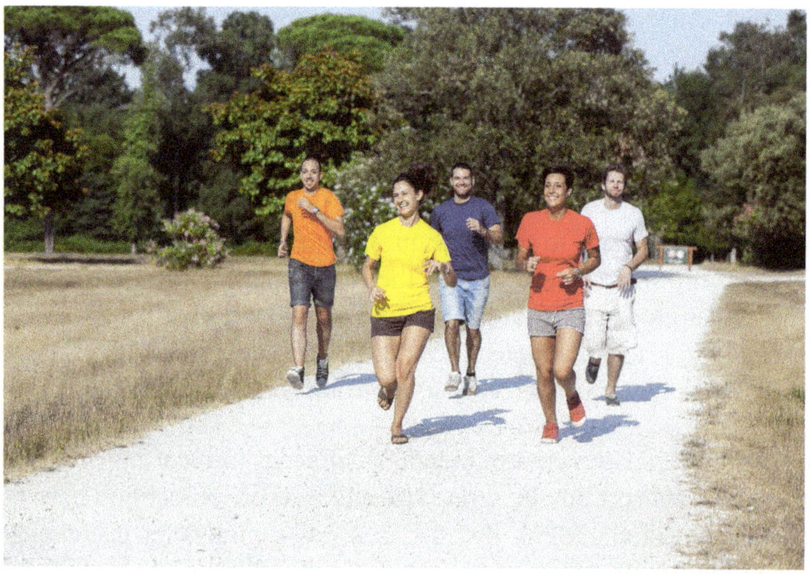

Approaches to Team Building in Exercise Groups

The overall goal of team building is to increase group cohesion in order to improve performance (Carron, Spink, & Prapavessis, 1997). Generally, team-building takes place through either a direct or indirect approach. A direct approach involves a team-building specialist (i.e., an exercise psychologist or some other intervention specialist) working directly with the exercise group to implement the team building activities. In an indirect approach the team-building specialist works with the exercise leader or instructor and trains them to deliver the team-building activities. This approach is considered indirect because the intervention strategies are delivered from the team-building specialist to the exercisers indirectly, through the exercise leader (Carron, Hausenblas, & Eys, 2005). In organization and sport settings both direct and indirect approaches are common. In contrast, team-building interventions in the exercise domain typically involve indirect approaches.

Carron and his colleagues (e.g., Carron & Spink, 1993; Carron & Widmeyer, 1987; Estabrooks & Carron, 1999; Prapavessis, Carron, & Spink, 1996; Spink & Carron, 1993) have developed, adapted, and successfully applied a model of team building to guide the indirect approach. The model involves four stages: (1) the introductory stage, (2) the conceptual stage, (3) the practical stage, and (4) the intervention stage. In the introductory stage the exercise leader is introduced to the general benefits of group cohesion. This stage allows for 'buy-in' from the exercise leaders such that they come to fully endorse the values of the team-building intervention. In the conceptual stage the team-building specialist presents and describes a conceptual model in which the intervention will be grounded. Grounding the intervention in a conceptual model allows for the person administering the intervention to visualize how each of the intervention components will come together to produce a change in the target outcomes (i.e., cohesion and performance). Carron and his colleagues apply a conceptual model of team-building that describes the inputs, throughputs, and outputs associated with team-building interventions (see Figure 11–2; Carron & Spink, 1993). Inputs represent factors that can be targeted by interventions. The model specifies two categories of inputs: group environment and group structure. To

FIGURE 11–2 Conceptual Model of Team Building

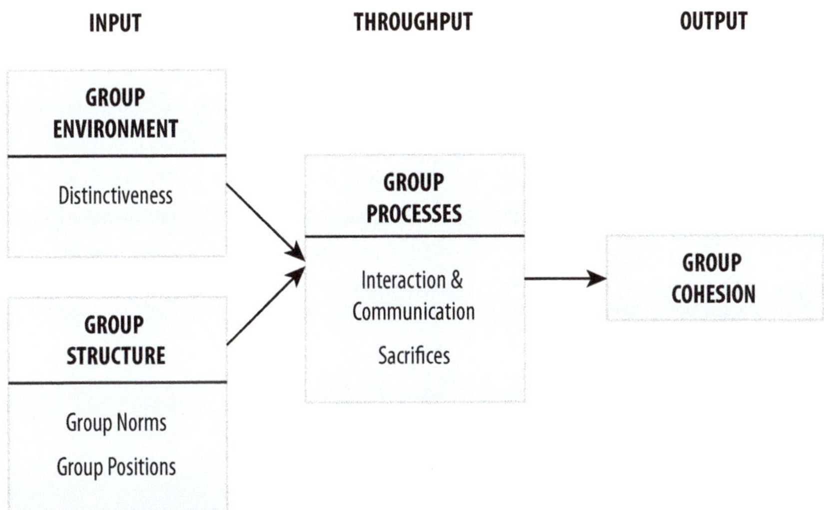

Adapted from Carron and Spink (1993)

influence the group environment, interventions aimed at enhancing the distinctiveness of the group may be most effective. Giving the group a name or providing members with matching t-shirts are two ways distinctiveness of a group may be enhanced. Intervening on the group structure can be done by establishing group norms and/or positions. Establishing positions may be physical (e.g., each exerciser in the class has their own established space in the room) or social (e.g., exercisers may take on distinct roles such as motivator, demonstrator, etc.). According to the model, intervening on these inputs will cause change in the group processes (throughputs). For example, groups with well-established norms may begin to sacrifice personal outcomes for group outcomes. An exerciser may choose to use dumbbells that are slightly too light or slightly too heavy if they perceive that other group members are more in need of a specific weight. Finally, adjustments in these throughputs cause changes in group cohesion (the output).

The practical stage of the team-building model is a chance for the exercise leader to work with the team-building specialist to identify and plan specific team-building activities that can feasibly be integrated into the exercise setting. Although there are many effective team-building strategies, they may not all be feasible within a given exercise context. Thus, this stage allows for planning around which strategies will be most effective and how they will be applied. In Table 11–1 is an overview of team-building strategies frequently employed in exercise. Finally, in the intervention stage the team-building activities are introduced in the group setting and maintained over time. During this stage, monitoring of the team-building activities should occur to ensure they are being implemented effectively and that they are having the expected results. If, through monitoring, it becomes apparent that any of the team-building strategies are ineffective, under-effective, or are not being implemented properly, revisions to the team-building protocol should be made.

Special Considerations for Implementing Team-Building Strategies in Exercise

Group exercise settings are highly variable. In some cases, exercise groups are formed naturally and do not have a formal leader. For example, new mothers who make plans to get together in the mornings and push their strollers around the neighborhood for fitness constitute one type of informal exercise group. In other cases, exercise groups might be highly-structured. An example of this type of group is a 3-month resistance training class in which participants enroll for the entire 3-month session and the group leader remains consistent from week to week. The specific group circumstances and characteristics influence the types of team-building activities that are feasible. In drop-in classes that have different membership each time it may be difficult to establish group norms. In spinning classes where the exercise bicycles are fixed to the floor, it may be difficult to encourage interaction with a variety of other group members during the class. Thus, implementing team-building strategies often requires some creativity, and may not always be an easy task!

TABLE 11–1 Team Building Strategies and their Application in Exercise Settings

Strategy	Examples
Increase distinctiveness of the group	Instructors can use terms that refer to the group as a unit such as "Good morning team! Let's have a great workout today!" The group can create a unique name. Members of the group wear similar apparel. For example, a running group gets matching t-shirts or shoelaces.
Establish group norms	Instructors can establish routines that only apply to one specific group. For example, the instructor may have aerobics group members clap their hands on beat during one specific move. Every time that move comes up, all the group members clap together. Group members establish a routine of helping one another set up their exercise equipment at the beginning of a class session. Group members establish a pattern of cheering each other on between songs in a Zumba class.
Establish group positions	Group members take on distinct roles within the group. One member provides verbal motivation to everyone during tough sets, another helps to set up extra equipment, another is in charge of the music, etc. Group members select physical locations in the exercise space that is theirs every time. In a spinning class, group members always stick to the same bike.
Increase interaction and communication	The group leader includes exercises that involve working in partners such as passing medicine balls back and forth.
Encourage sacrifices	The group agrees to do an extra set of abdominal exercises because they know one member really wants to focus on that area. Members of a hiking group agree to hike trails they've already been on so that other group members can discover them. Walking group members each walk an extra two miles this week to help the group meet its mileage goal.
Set group goals	Work together to identify a goal that everyone can work toward.

Some General Recommendations

- Group-based exercise has an advantage over individual exercise in its ability to stimulate motivation and adherence; but, group-based interventions are most effective when team-building strategies are applied. Therefore, whenever possible, team-building strategies should be incorporated into group exercise settings.
- Consider the circumstances and characteristics of the group and tailor team-building strategies accordingly. Not all strategies will be effective for all groups.
- Although it may be difficult, apply team-building strategies in large groups whenever possible. Carron and Spink (1993) demonstrated that individuals exercising in large groups perceive more group cohesion when team-building strategies are applied. Given the benefits of cohesion on outcomes such as motivation and adherence, team building has important implications in large group settings.
- Allow the group members to contribute to creating and implementing team-building strategies. Among the wide variety of team-building strategies, group goals, group norms, physical and social positions, and sacrificing behaviors, will all be more effective if they are endorsed by the group members. Including exercise participants in establishing these norms and behaviors will help to ensure that they are more fully endorsed by the group.

CHAPTER SUMMARY

Groups can be used to motivate participation in and maintenance of physical activity. The majority of the research examining group-influences in exercise has centered on the construct of group cohesion. Cohesion is characterized by the individual and group level factors that draw people toward the group as well as the task-related and social benefits of group membership. The cohesiveness of a group is influenced by personal, leadership, environmental, and group factors. The influence of a group on an individual's motivation and behavior is particularly strong when the group experience is enhanced with team-building activities. There is a wide variety of team-building activities that can be applied in the exercise setting; however, exercise leaders should be careful to select activities that best align with the resources and characteristics of the exercise group.

REVIEW QUESTIONS

1. Explain what Carron and Spink (1993) mean by "inputs, throughputs, and outputs" in their conceptual model of team building.
2. Discuss the environmental factors that influence cohesion in exercise groups.
3. In your opinion, how might diversity in task-unrelated factors among group members impact on group cohesion?
4. Provide three examples for how interaction and communication might be enhanced in exercise groups.

SUGGESTED READINGS

Carron, A., Shapcott, K., & Burke, S. (2007). Group cohesion in sport and exercise: Past, present and future. In M. R. Beauchamp & M. A. Eys (Eds.), *Group dynamics in exercise and sport psychology: Contemporary themes* (pp. 117–140). Milton Park, Oxon: Routledge.

Carron, A., Spink, K., & Prapavessis, H. (1997). Team building and cohesiveness in the sport and exercise setting: Use of indirect interventions. *Journal of Applied Sport Psychology, 9*(1), 61–72.

REFERENCES

Ajzen, I. (2011). Theory of planned behavior. In P. A. M. Van Lange, A. W. Kruglanski, & E. T. Higgins. *Handbook of Theories of Social Psychology* (pp. 438–459). Thousand Oaks, CA: Sage Publications Ltd.

Atienza, A. A. (2001). Home-based physical activity programs for middle-aged and older adults: summary of empirical research. *Journal of Aging and Physical Activity, 9*, S38–S58.

Burke, S., Carron, A., Eys, M., Ntoumanis, N., & Estabrooks, P. (2006). Group versus individual approach? A meta-analysis of the effectiveness of interventions to promote physical activity. *Sport and Exercise Psychology Review, 2*(1), 19–35.

Burke, S., Shapcott, K., Carron, A., Bradshaw, M., & Estabrooks, P. (2010). Group goal setting and group performance in a physical activity context. *International Journal of Sport and Exercise Psychology, 8*(3), 245–261.

Carron, A., Brawley, L., & Widmeyer, N. (1998). The measurement of cohesiveness in sport groups. In J. Duda (Ed.), *Advances in sport and exercise psychology measurement*, (pp. 213–226). Morgantown, WV: Fitness Information Technology.

Carron, A., Hausenblas, H., & Eys, M. (2005). *Group dynamics in sport*. Morgantown, WV: Fitness Information Technology: Inc.

Carron, A., Shapcott, K., & Burke, S. (2007). Group cohesion in sport and exercise: Past, present and future. In M. R. Beauchamp & M. A. Eys (Eds.), *Group dynamics in exercise and sport psychology: Contemporary themes* (pp. 117–140). Milton Park, Oxon: Routledge.

Carron, A., & Spink, K. (1992). Internal consistency of the Group Environment Questionnaire modified for an exercise setting. *Perceptual and Motor Skills, 74*, 304–306.

Carron, A., & Spink, K. (1993). Team building in an exercise setting. *Sport Psychologist, 7*, 8–18.

Carron, A., Spink, K., & Prapavessis, H. (1997). Team building and cohesiveness in the sport and exercise setting: Use of indirect interventions. *Journal of Applied Sport Psychology, 9*, 61–72.

Carron, A., & Widmeyer, W. (1987). Developing effective groups *Workshop presented for the Faculty of Part-time and Continuing Education*. London, ON, Canada.

Carron, A., Widmeyer, N., & Brawley, L. (1985). The development of an instrument to assess cohesion in sport teams: The Group Environment Questionnaire. *Journal of Sport Psychology, 7*, 244–266.

Courneya, K. (1995). Cohesion correlates with affect in structured exercise classes. *Perceptual and Motor Skills, 81*, 1021–1022.

Courneya, K., & McAuley, E. (1995). Cognitive mediators of the social influence-exercise adherence relationship: A test of the theory of planned behavior. *Journal of Behavioral Medicine, 18*, 499–515.

Dishman, R., & Buckworth, J. (1996). Increasing physical activity: a quantitative synthesis. *Medicine and Science in Sports and Exercise, 28*, 706–719.

Edmunds, J., Ntoumanis, N., & Duda, J. (2006). A test of self-determination theory in the exercise domain. *Journal of Applied Social Psychology, 36*, 2240–2265.

Estabrooks, P., & Carron, A. (1999). Group cohesion in older adult exercisers: Prediction and intervention effects. *Journal of Behavioral Medicine, 22*, 575–588.

Estabrooks, P., & Carron, A. (2000). The physical activity group environment questionnaire: An instrument for the assessment of cohesion in exercise classes. *Group Dynamics: Theory, Research, and Practice, 4*, 230.

Kahn, E. B., Ramsey, L. T, Brownson, R. C., Health, G. W., Howze, E. H., Powell, K. E., Stone, E. J., Rajab, M. W., & Corso, P. (2002). The effectiveness of interventions to increase physical activity: A systematic review. *American Journal of Preventive Medicine, 22*, 73–107.

Loughead, T., Colman, M., & Carron, A. (2001). Investigating the mediational relationship of leadership, class cohesion, and adherence in an exercise setting. *Small Group Research, 32*, 558–575.

McGran, K. (2012). Los Angeles Kings win first Stanley Cup, *The Toronto Star*.

Prapavessis, H., Carron, A. A., & Spink, K. S. (1996). Team building in sport. *International Journal of Sport Psychology, 27*, 269–285.

Shapcott, K., Carron, A., Burke, S., Bradshaw, M., & Estabrooks, P. (2006). Member diversity and cohesion and performance in walking groups. *Small Group Research, 37*, 701–720.

Spink, K. S., & Carron, A. V. (1993). The effects of team building on the adherence patterns of female exercise participants. *Journal of Sport & Exercise Psychology, 15*.

Van der Bij, A., Laurant, M., & Wensing, M. (2002). Effectiveness of physical activity interventions for older adults: A review. *American Journal of Preventive Medicine, 22*, 120–133.

Chapter 12

Fear of Re-Injury

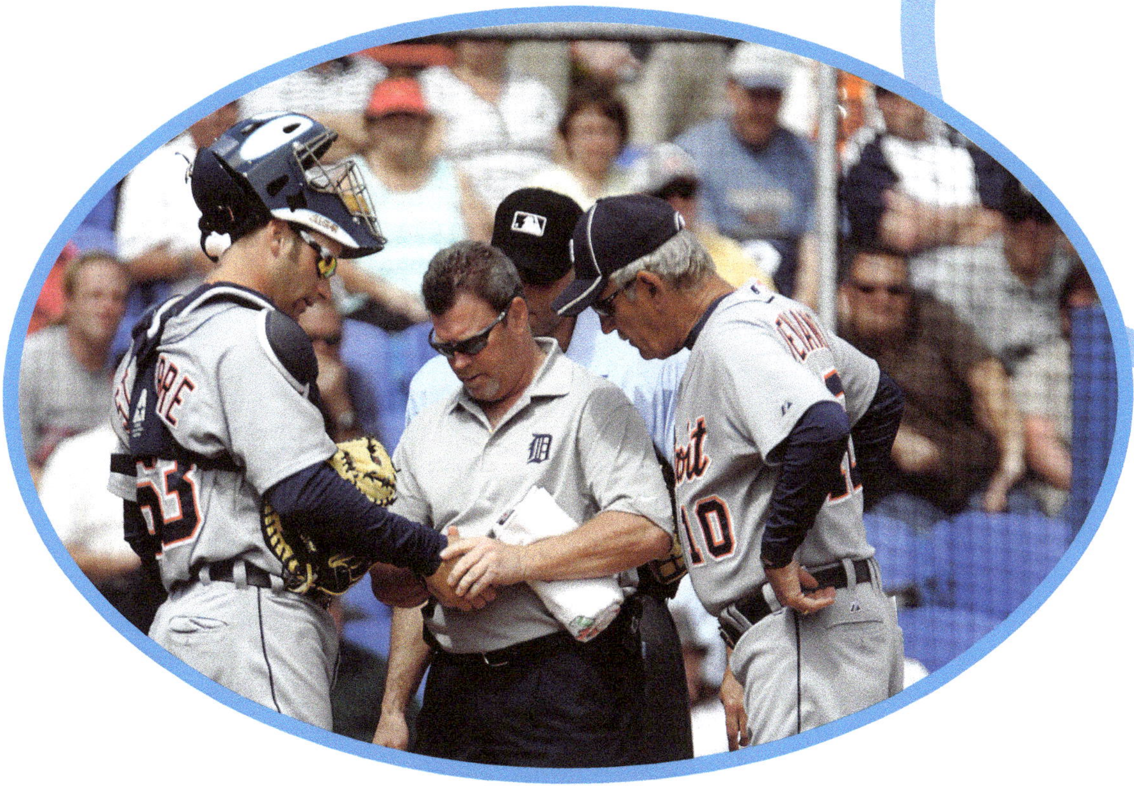

Introduction

Anecdotally, we have all encountered situations in which we choose not to engage in a specific behavior because we are afraid of either injuring ourselves, or running the risk of aggravating an old injury. Athletes and exercisers can encounter similar difficulties during rehabilitation and return to activity following a sport or recreation-related injury. Rehabilitation is a period of time often characterized by the unknown, with individuals potentially uncertain about their health, their status on their team, and even their ability to continue participating in their chosen activity. It is therefore not surprising that fear is a common emotional response following injury (Andersen, 2001; Brewer, 2001; Bianco, Malo, & Orlick, 1999; Johnston & Carroll, 1998; May & Sieb, 1987; Podlog & Eklund, 2006; Rotella, 1985; Wiese-Bjornstal, Smith, Shaffer, & Morrey, 1998).

The two most common fears associated with injury have been identified as a fear of re-injury, and a fear of being unable to perform at pre-injury levels upon return to play (Podlog & Eklund, 2004; Podlog & Eklund, 2005). Other sources of fear may include anxiety about missing practice, losing fitness, and the projected length of recovery time (Tracey, 2003). In a qualitative study involving adolescent gymnasts, Chase, Magyar, and Drake (2005) found that athletes were most fearful of injuries occurring because of the difficulty in returning from them and being unable to participate in practices and competitions while recovering.

Injury-related fear is common in rehabilitation settings, regardless of the population or type of injury being treated. Not only is it distressing to the individual, it can also present a barrier to recovery or return to activity. Although there has been relatively little research into fear in the context of sport and exercise, strong theoretical arguments and evidence from clinical research indicate the importance of its consideration in the management of sport or recreational injury. In the rest of this chapter, we will review the existing literature in this area and provide recommendations for intervention design in treatment settings.

Kinesiophobia

A specific type of injury-related fear is kinesiophobia, or a fear of movement. This is defined as "an excessive, irrational, and debilitating fear of physical movement and activity resulting from a feeling of vulnerability to painful injury or re-injury" (Kori, Miller, & Todd, 1990). Kinesiophobia is commonly an issue in chronic pain populations, but does occur following acute sport/recreation injury as well.

Most of the research on kinesiophobia has occurred in clinical contexts with low back pain patients. These studies have shown that fear of movement is not always related to pain intensity (Swinkels-Meewisse, Roelofs, Verbeek, Oostendorp, & Vlaeyen, 2003; Vlaeyen, Kole-Snijders, Boeren, & van Eek, 1995a), but may arise from a fear of anticipated pain (Vlaeyen, Kole-Snijders, Rotteveel, Ruesink, & Heuts, 1995b). Individuals who report high levels of pain-related fear tend to avoid situations that might cause discomfort, which might actually decrease pain tolerance or heighten sensitivity to pain over time (Vlaeyen et al., 1995b). Avoiders tend to report more frequent pain, pain of longer duration, and more pain- and injury-related fear than those who do not suffer from kinesiophobia (Crombez, 1994). There is also some indication that pain-related fear might perpetuate pain through symptom-specific muscle reactivity under fear-inducing conditions (Vlaeyen, Seelen, Peters, de Jong, Aretz, Beisiegel et al., 1999), although this has not been investigated thoroughly.

Kinesiophobia has also been strongly linked to catastrophizing and depression (Vlaeyen et al., 1995a; Vlaeyen et al., 1995b). Catastrophizing refers to a bias toward negative aspects of a situation and an exaggeration of their importance or influence in relation to the outcome (Vlaeyen et al., 1995b). Catastrophizing can be focused on the present (e.g., dwelling on one's own inability to cope and imagining the worst possible result of current circumstances, even though they may be only temporary) or future-oriented (e.g., anticipating all of the things that might go wrong in the future, and creating a reality to match those thoughts) (see Figure 12–1; Vlaeyen et al., 1995b). This type of negative thought process can be linked to hopelessness or depression, and can result in a sort of "self-fulfilling prophecy" (e.g., the individual behaves in such a way that the imagined worst-case scenario actually happens).

Although catastrophizing is typically related to personal beliefs that a situation is worse than it really is, it can be influenced by external factors, such as the interaction a patient has with his or her therapist. Caregivers and others in social support roles may verbally or non-verbally convey messages that lead an athlete or exerciser to believe that the prognosis of an injury is insurmountable (Vlaeyen & Crombez, 1999). It is therefore important to consider how the environment may be affecting fear and fear-related behaviors in rehabilitation settings.

Lethem, Slade, Troup, and Bentley (1983) introduced a "fear-avoidance" model to better articulate the relationship between pain, fear, and behavior. In this model, "confrontation" and "avoidance" are given as the two extreme responses to fear. Confrontation is believed to reduce fear over time, whereas avoidance is presumed to maintain or exacerbate fear (Vlaeyen & Crombez, 1999). After injury, those who exhibit high levels of fear-related avoidance are therefore postulated to experience decreased physical activity and a reduction of activity-related social interaction, which ultimately leads to greater disability and, potentially, chronic pain.

FIGURE 12–1 Cognitive-Behavioral Model of Fear of Movement/(Re)injury

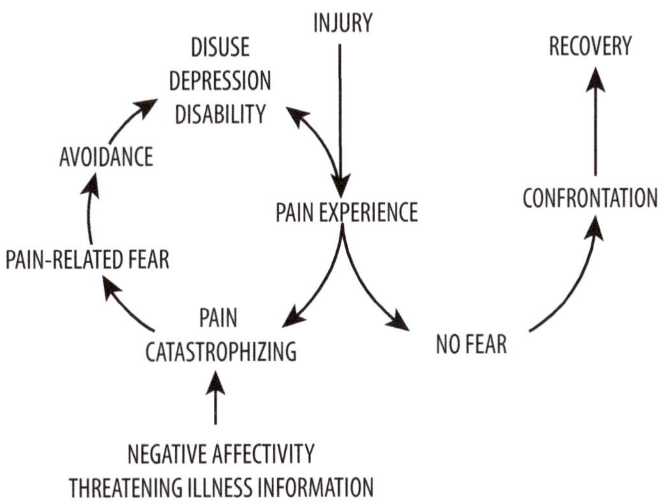

Vlaeyen et al., 1995b

It has been empirically demonstrated that fear of movement may manifest as early as the first treatment appointment following injury, and baseline fear may be predictive of future activity participation or disability (Swinkels-Meewisse, Roelofs, Schouten, Verbeek, Oostendorp, & Vlaeyen, 2006). This has prompted researchers to recommend identifying fearful patients and classifying them as "avoiders" or "confronters" in order to facilitate interventions that reduce pain-related fear in the acute stage of injury (Swinkels-Meewisse et al., 2003; Swinkels-Meewisse et al., 2006). Yet, in a review of the evidence in support of the "fear-avoidance" model, Pincus and colleagues concluded that, because of the paucity of research literature and the limited accuracy of current measurement techniques, it may be premature to promote fear reduction as a central component of treatment until we better understand the relationship between pain, fear, and avoidance behavior (Pincus, Smeets, Simmonds, & Sullivan, 2010).

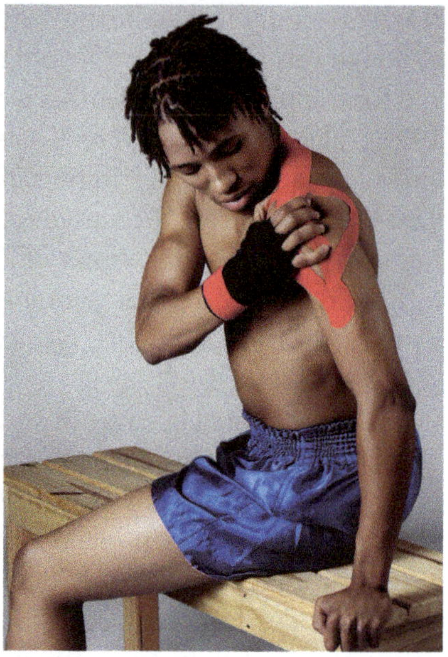

Return to Play

Returning to sport or exercise after rehabilitation can be perceived as threatening because of the many "unknowns" that characterize this period. Individuals often express concerns about whether or not the injured body part is properly healed, or how performance may be affected after time away. They might also express concern about putting themselves in a situation similar to the one in which their initial injury occurred. Feelings of fear during this time are often centered on concerns over re-injury and worry about not being able to reach performance goals.

Re-injury fear can be particularly important when considering the outcomes of surgical interventions. For example, in one study of 64 patients who were followed up a minimum of five years post-ACL reconstruction, the researchers found that nine individuals (14%) had not returned to their previous level of sport participation because they were afraid of re-injury (Yee, Karim, & Chang, 2008). This finding is consistent with a number of other ACL reconstruction studies that also found re-injury fear to be a strong predictor of return to activity (Ardern, Webster, Taylor, & Feller, 2011a; Ardern, Webster, Taylor, & Feller, 2011b; Kvist, Ek, Sporrstedt, & Good, 2005; Tripp, Stanish, Ebel-Lam, Brewer, & Birchard, 2007).

In a review and meta-analysis of 30 ACL reconstruction studies, Ardern et al. (2011b) found that 63% of patients returned to their pre-injury sport level after surgery, and 44% had returned to competitive sport. The 12 studies that examined the reasons why participants did not return to their previous sport level indicated that fear of re-injury accounted for 19% of decisions not to return, with social reasons (18%), knee function problems (13%), and fear of job loss with re-injury (11%) being the next most common responses. These results suggest that re-injury fear is a common and somewhat debilitating issue that arises with injuries that are severe in nature and/or require extensive rehabilitation. Moreover,

Grimmer, Jones, and Williams (2000) reported that up to 8% of youth athletes drop out of sport each year because of either an actual injury or a fear of injury. These results suggest that injury-related anxiety is not simply a matter of personal concern for athletes undergoing rehabilitation, but might actually have a cascade effect that contributes to declining physical activity levels in a number of populations.

For those who do ultimately return to activity, the onset of re-injury fears can be associated with a number of factors. For example, those who have never been injured before tend to experience heightened re-injury fear, as do those whose injuries are chronic in nature (Podlog & Eklund, 2006). Additionally, it has been suggested that strong identification with the athlete role or being externally motivated can be associated with negative outcomes, such as reduced confidence and greater fear (Podlog & Eklund, 2005). Consistent findings indicate that the sport context into which the individual is returning (e.g., highly competitive or contact sports) can prompt increased competitive anxiety or greater focus on the injured area (Bianco et al., 1999; Gould, Udry, Bridges, & Beck, 1997; Podlog & Eklund, 2005). Furthermore, although kinesiophobia has been shown to decrease over time during rehabilitation, it often remains a salient concern at return to play (Chmielewski, Jones, Day, Tillman, Lentz, & George, 2008).

According to Johnston and Carroll (1998), fear of injury can manifest in many ways upon return to activity, including being hesitant, holding back, not giving maximal effort, or being cautious of injury-provoking situations (especially those similar to the context of the injury occurrence). These behaviors have the potential to dramatically impair performance, and as such warrant further research attention.

Fear and Injury Risk

Whereas a number of researchers have focused on fear and stress management during rehabilitation in order to help athletes and exercisers return to activity successfully, others have looked at the likelihood of injury-related fear actually increasing injury risk. Andersen and Williams (1988) proposed in their initial stress-injury model that a history of stressors, such as major life events, daily hassles, or previous injury, could increase the risk of an athlete becoming injured. Aside from the obvious risk of re-injury associated with playing before a first injury is healed, the authors suggested that re-injury fear could also be a risk factor because it would lead to a significant stress response, which has been shown to increase the risk of injury (Williams & Andersen, 1998). The idea of a "self-fulfilling prophecy" has also been considered in this context (Podlog & Eklund, 2005; Rotella, 1985; Williams & Andersen, 1998), but has not been empirically supported (McKay, Campbell, Meeuwisse, & Emery, 2013).

Previous injury is consistently reported as one of the most robust predictors of sustaining another, but few researchers have examined the specific relationship between previous injury stress and re-injury, and these studies have yielded inconclusive results. For example, Hanson, McCullagh, and Tonymon (1992) found that time since previous injury was not related to frequency or severity of re-injury occurrence; conversely, Lysens et al. (1984) found that students with a history of injury were at high risk of recurrence. Although the nature of the association between fear and injury risk has not been thoroughly examined since it was first proposed, it is recommended that sport psychology consultants help individuals to develop strong coping skills to offset potential stress arising from re-injury fear.

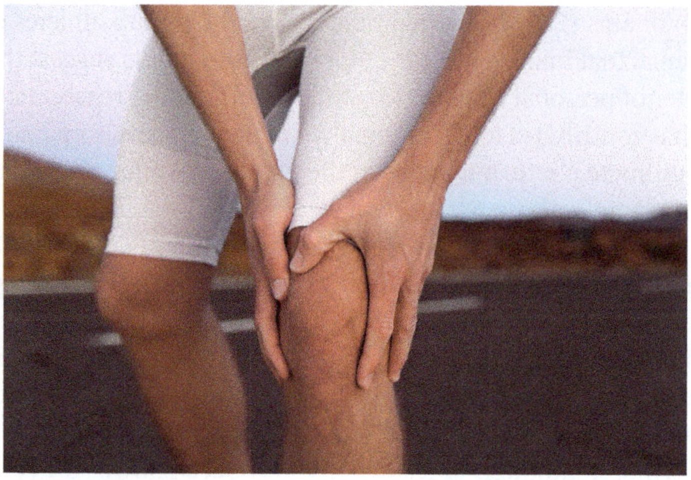

Interventions for Re-Injury Anxiety

Relaxation and Imagery

One potential avenue for reducing injury-related fear is to take a stress management approach. In rehabilitation contexts, helping patients relax and reframe their treatment expectations can reduce anxiety and facilitate more successful recovery. Using this strategy, and as earlier mentioned in our discussion of imagery interventions, Cupal and Brewer (2001) recruited 30 athletes following ACL surgery to engage in a study of relaxation and guided imagery. Participants were athletes from recreational and competitive sports who were block randomized into one of three groups: treatment, placebo, or control. The treatment condition consisted of 10 individual sessions of relaxation and guided imagery over a six-month period, using videos of the surgery as a visual baseline for imagery of rehabilitation goals. The placebo group was given equal attention time and encouragement, and the control group received no additional attention. The results demonstrated that between 2 and 24 weeks post-operatively, all three groups had a reduction in injury-related anxiety, but the treatment group had a significantly greater decrease, alongside greater measures of strength and less reported pain.

Despite somewhat promising results, there has been relatively little additional research effort in extending these findings through replication or trials in other populations. Yet, given the body of literature supporting the use of relaxation and imagery techniques, it remains a viable intervention strategy for addressing re-injury fear.

Stress Inoculation

Stress inoculation training (SIT) is another possible intervention alternative. This cognitive-behavioral therapy is based on principles from clinical psychology, and entails the three-step development of progressive relaxation and coping techniques that are applied through graded exposure to stressors (Meichenbaum & Deffenbacher, 1988). Step one, or the *conceptualization* phase, involves the development of a collaborative relationship between the athlete and counselor, and reconceptualization of the individual's stress response into a series of short-term, intermediate, and long-term coping goals. The *skills acquisition and rehearsal* phase is when the athlete learns and practices coping skills in the clinic or other training setting with gradual in vivo exposure to specific stressors (e.g., rehabilitation). In the final *application and follow through* stage, athletes are encouraged to apply their personal coping approach to increasing levels of stressors in real world situations, with the opportunity for "booster sessions" to maintain the effectiveness of the intervention (Meichenbaum, 1996).

SIT alongside physical therapy has been investigated following meniscus injury and has been shown to decrease post-surgical pain and anxiety, with patients requiring fewer days to return to criterion physical functioning than controls (Ross & Berger, 1996). There is also some support for SIT in reducing pain-related fear in low back pain patients (de Jong, Vlaeyen, Onghena, Goossens, Geilen, & Mulder, 2005; Vlaeyen, de Jong, Geilen, Heuts, van Breukelen, 2002), but these studies have been conducted with small convenience samples, and larger studies will be required to draw broader inferences about the efficacy of SIT as a treatment modality.

How It Is Measured

The most common method of assessing injury-related fear is the Tampa Scale for Kinesiophobia (TSK), a 17-item instrument originally developed to measure fear of movement/(re)injury in chronic pain patients (Clark et al., 1996). It is a psychometrically sound tool that demonstrates convergent validity with measures of fear-avoidance beliefs, pain catastrophizing, pain-related disability, and general negative affect (French, France, Vigneau, French, & Evans, 2007). Ratings on the scale are summed to yield a total score, where higher values indicate greater fear of re-injury.

Although the TSK has been used across many populations in research and clinical applications, there is some debate as to its interpretation. Confirmatory factor analysis has yielded both two-factor (Swinkels-Meewisse et al., 2003; Roelofs, Sluiter, Frings-Dresen, Goossens, Thibault, Boersma et al., 2007) and three-factor (French et al., 2007) models of fit, suggesting that additional research is needed to fully articulate the latent constructs that are tapped by the scale. Moreover, the TSK specifically addresses kinesiophobia, and as such is not appropriate for addressing other injury-related fears. These are often measured using single items or study-specific surveys, which have been inconsistent and potentially subject to misclassification bias in previous studies (McKay et al., 2013; Chase et al., 2005; Podlog & Eklund, 2005; Tracey, 2003).

Some General Recommendations

Threat appraisals have been associated with adherence to physiotherapy treatment. In a prospective study of 62 sport medicine clinic patients, Taylor and May (1996) found that injury severity and perceptions of susceptibility to slow recovery at the first treatment appointment were related to subsequent non-adherent behavior. The results suggested that injury severity was the strongest threat appraisal predictor of adherence to prescribed therapy modalities, but those with higher perceptions of susceptibility to re-injury or slow recovery were more likely to follow advice to rest. Clinicians should therefore be aware that there could be differential adherence to their recommendations, depending on whether or not their patients exhibit avoidance behavior related to kinesiophobia, or re-injury fear.

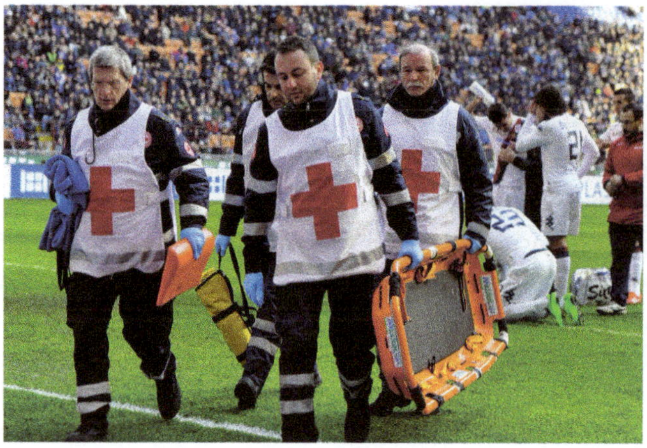

Image © Paolo Bona, 2014. Used under license from Shutterstock, Inc.

Additional recommendations for addressing fear in rehabilitation include:

- Many athletes report that actually testing the injured body part in a sport scenario is the only way to alleviate their fear (Podlog & Eklund, 2005). It is therefore important that enough physical challenges are presented during rehabilitation to give athletes confidence that their injury has healed and the body part can withstand the rigors of sport participation.
- Open discussion of return to activity fears can dispel myths associated with recovery and prevent irrational beliefs from undermining the individual's confidence (Podlog & Eklund, 2004).
- Psychological techniques used for other issues in rehabilitation, such as goal setting, imagery, and self-talk, can be used to alleviate re-injury fears. Initiating these interventions early in rehabilitation and continuing to use them through the return to activity phase can help reduce the impact of re-injury fear on performance.

CHAPTER SUMMARY

Fear, anxiety, and worry are common emotions following injury. These can arise in response to concerns about re-injury, lost training time, or the individual's ability to reach performance goals. Although there has been little research into the impact of these emotions on re-injury risk or performance, there is considerable theoretical and anecdotal support to suggest that fear is a salient issue for athletes and exercisers during rehabilitation.

Psychological interventions have been used to address fear, particularly kinesiophobia. Cognitive techniques, such as relaxation and imagery, have shown promise but much more research is needed to determine how beneficial they might be. Stress inoculation training also appears to be a useful method of mitigating fear, but its application has been limited to date. In practice, there are most likely many intervention strategies that will yield positive outcomes for athletes and exercisers who are struggling with re-injury fear, but current approaches are limited by a paucity of empirical evidence. Despite this, fear remains a pertinent issue in the sport injury domain, and practitioners should be aware of its potential effects on recovery and return to activity.

REVIEW QUESTIONS

1. What are the two most common fears associated with injury?
2. Define catastrophizing and discuss how it can affect injury recovery.
3. Select one intervention technique that can be used to reduce fear in rehabilitation, and describe how it could be implemented.

SUGGESTED READINGS

Kvist, J., Ek, A., Sporrstedt, K., & Good, L. (2005). Fear of re-injury: a hindrance for returning to sports after anterior cruciate ligament reconstruction. *Knee Surgery, Sports Traumatology, Arthroscopy, 13*, 393–397.

Podlog, L., & Eklund, R. C. (2005). Return to sport after serious injury: A retrospective examination of motivation and psychological outcomes. *Journal of Sport Rehabilitation, 14*, 20–34.

Tripp, D. A., Stanish, W., Ebel-Lam, A., Brewer, B. W., & Birchard, J. (2007). Fear of re-injury, negative affect, and catastrophizing predicting return to sport in recreational athletes with anterior cruciate ligament injuries at 1 year post-surgery. *Rehabilitation Psychology, 52*, 74–81.

REFERENCES

Andersen, M. (2001). Returning to action and the prevention of future injury. In J. Crossman (Ed.), *Coping with sports injuries: Psychological strategies for rehabilitation* (pp. 162–173). New York: Oxford University Press.

Andersen, M. B., & Williams, J. M. (1988). A model of stress and athletic injury: Prediction and prevention. *Journal of Sport & Exercise Psychology, 10*, 294–306.

Ardern, C. L., Webster, K. E., Taylor, N. F., & Feller, J. A. (2011a). Return to the pre-injury level of competitive sport after anterior cruciate ligament reconstruction surgery: Two-thirds of patients have not returned by 12 months after surgery. *American Journal of Sports Medicine, 39*, 538–543.

Ardern, C. L., Webster, K. E., Taylor, N. F., & Feller, J. A. (2011b). Return to sport following anterior cruciate ligament reconstruction surgery: a systematic review and meta-analysis of the state of play. *British Journal of Sports Medicine, 45*, 596–606.

Bianco, T., Malo, S., & Orlick, T. (1999). Sport injury and illness: Elite skiers describe their experiences. *Research Quarterly for Exercise and Sport, 157*, 157–169.

Brewer, B. (2001). Psychology of sport rehabilitation. In R. Singer, H. Hausenblas, & C. Janelle (Eds.), *Handbook of sport psychology* (2nd ed.) (pp. 787–803). New York: John Wiley & Sons, Inc.

Chase, M. A., Magyar, T. M., & Drake, B. M. (2005). Fear of injury in gymnastics: Self-efficacy and psychological strategies to keep on tumbling. *Journal of Sports Sciences, 23*, 465–475.

Chmielewski, T. L., Jones, D., Day, T., Tillman, S. M., Lentz, T. A., & George, S. Z. (2008). The association of pain and fear of movement/re-injury with function during anterior cruciate ligament reconstruction rehabilitation. *Journal of Orthopaedic & Sports Physical Therapy, 38*, 746–753.

Clark, M. E., Kori, S. H., & Brockel, J. (1996, September). Kinesiophobia and chronic pain: psychometric characteristics and factor analysis of the Tampa Scale. In *American Pain Society Abstracts* (Vol. 15, p. 77).

Crombez, G. (1994). *Pijnmodulatie door anticipatie (Pain modulation through anticipation).* (Doctoral dissertation), University of Leuven, Belgium.

Cupal, D. D., & Brewer, B. W. (2001). Effects of relaxation and guided imagery on knee strength, re-injury anxiety, and pain following anterior cruciate ligament reconstruction. *Rehabilitation Psychology, 46*, 28–43.

de Jong, J. R., Vlaeyen, J. W. S., Onghena, P., Goossens, M. E. J. B., Geilen, M., & Mulder, H. (2005). Fear of movement/(re)injury in chronic low back pain. Education or exposure in vivo as mediator to fear reduction? *Clinical Journal of Pain, 21*, 9–17.

French, D. J., France, C. R., Vigneau, F., French, J. A., & Evans, R. T. (2007). Fear of movement/(re)injury in chronic pain: A psychometric assessment of the original English version of the Tampa scale for kinesiophobia (TSK). *Pain, 127*, 42–51.

Gould, D., Udry, E., Bridges, D., & Beck, D. (1997). Stress sources encountered when rehabilitating from season-ending ski injuries. *Journal of Sport Psychology, 11*, 361–378.

Grimmer, K., Jones, D., & Williams, J. (2000). Prevalence of adolescent injury from recreational exercise: An Australian perspective. *Journal of Adolescent Health, 27*, 266–272.

Hanson, S. J., McCullagh, P., & Tonymon, P. (1992). The relationship of personality characteristics, life stress, and coping resources to athletic injury. *Journal of Sport & Exercise Psychology, 14*, 262–272.

Johnston, L., & Carroll, D. (1998). The context of emotional responses to athletic injury: A qualitative analysis. *Journal of Sport Rehabilitation, 7*, 206–220.

Kori, S. H., Miller, R. P., & Todd, D. D. (1990). Kinesiophobia: a new view of chronic pain behavior. *Pain Management, 3*, 35–43.

Kvist, J., Ek, A., Sporrstedt, K., & Good, L. (2005). Fear of re-injury: a hindrance for returning to sports after anterior cruciate ligament reconstruction. *Knee Surgery, Sports Traumatology, Arthroscopy, 13*, 393–397.

Lethem, J., Slade, P. D., Troup, J. D., & Bentley, G. (1983). Outline of a fear-avoidance model of exaggerated pain perception. *Behaviour Research and Therapy, 21*, 401–408.

Lysens, R., Stevrrlynck, A., Vanden Auwrele, Y., Lefevre, J., Renson, L., Claessens, A., & Ostyn, M. (1984). The predictability of sports injuries. *Sports Medicine, 1*, 6–10.

May, J., & Sieb, G. (1987). Athletic Injuries: Psychosocial factors in the onset, sequelae, rehabilitation, and prevention. In J. May & M. Asken (Eds.), *Sport psychology: The psychological health of the athlete* (pp. 157–185). New York: PMA Publishing Corp.

McKay, C., Campbell, T., Meeuwisse, W., & Emery, C. (2013). The role of psychosocial risk factors for injury in elite youth ice hockey. *Clinical Journal of Sport Medicine, 23*, 216–221.

Meichenbaum, D. (1996). Stress inoculation training for coping with stressors. *The Clinical Psychologist, 49*, 4–7.

Meichenbaum, D. H. & Deffenbacher, J. L. (1988). Stress inoculation training. *The Counseling Psychologist, 16*, 69–90.

Pincus, T., Smeets, R. J. E. M., Simmonds, M. J., & Sullivan, M. J. L. (2010). The fear avoidance model disentangled: Improving the clinical utility of the fear avoidance model. *Clinical Journal of Pain, 26*, 739–746.

Podlog, L., & Eklund, R. C. (2004). Assisting injured athletes with the return to sport transition. *Clinical Journal of Sport Medicine, 14*, 257–259.

Podlog, L., & Eklund, R. C. (2005). Return to sport after serious injury: A retrospective examination of motivation and psychological outcomes. *Journal of Sport Rehabilitation, 14*, 20–34.

Podlog, L., & Eklund, R. C. (2006). A longitudinal investigation of competitive athletes' return to sport following serious injury. *Journal of Applied Sport Psychology, 18*, 44–68.

Roelofs, J., Sluiter, J. K., Frings-Dresen, M. H. W., Goossens, M., Thibault, P., Boersma, K., & Vlaeyen, J. W. S. (2007). Fear of movement and (re)injury in chronic musculoskeletal pain: Evidence for an invariant two-factor model of the Tampa Scale for Kinesiophobia across pain diagnoses and Dutch, Swedish, and Canadian samples. *Pain, 131*, 181–190.

Ross, M. J., & Berger, R. S. (1996). Effects of stress inoculation training on athletes' postsurgical pain and rehabilitation after orthopedic injury. *Journal of Consulting and Clinical Psychology, 64*, 406–410.

Rotella, B. (1985). The psychological care of the injured athlete. In L. Bunker, R., Rotella, & A. Reilly (Eds.), *Sport psychology: Psychological consideration in maximizing sport performance* (pp. 273–287). Ann Arbor: McNaughton & Gunn, Inc.

Swinkels-Meewisse, I. E. J., Roelofs, J., Schouten, E. G. W., Verbeek, A. L. M., Oostendorp, R. A. B., & Vlaeyen, J. W. S. (2006). Fear of movement/(re)injury predicting chronic disabling low back pain: A prospective inception cohort study. *Spine, 31*, 658–664.

Swinkels-Meewisse, I. E. J., Roelofs, J., Verbeek, A. L. M., Oostendorp, R. A. B., & Vlaeyen, J. W. S. (2003). Fear of movement/(re)injury, disability and participation in acute low back pain. *Pain, 105*, 371–379.

Taylor, A. H., & May, S. (1996). Threat and coping appraisal as determinants of compliance with sports injury rehabilitation: An application of Protection Motivation Theory. *Journal of Sports Sciences, 14*, 471–482.

Tracey, J. (2003). The emotional response to the injury and rehabilitation process. *Journal of Applied Sports Psychology, 15*, 279–293.

Tripp, D. A., Stanish, W., Ebel-Lam, A., Brewer, B. W., & Birchard, J. (2007). Fear of re-injury, negative affect, and catastrophizing predicting return to sport in recreational athletes with anterior cruciate ligament injuries at 1 year post-surgery. *Rehabilitation Psychology, 52*, 74–81.

Vlaeyen, J. W. S., & Crombez, G. (1999). Fear of movement/(re)injury, avoidance and pain disability in chronic low back pain patients. *Manual Therapy, 4*, 187–195.

Vlaeyen, J. W. S., de Jong, J., Geilen, M., Heuts, P. H. T. G., & van Breukelen, G. (2002). The treatment of fear of movement/(re)injury in chronic low back pain: Further evidence on the effectiveness of exposure in vivo. *The Clinical Journal of Pain, 18*, 251–261.

Vlaeyen, J. W. S., Kole-Snijders, A. M. J., Boeren, R. G. B., & van Eek, H. (1995a). Fear of movement/(re)injury in chronic low back pain and its relation to behavioural performance. *Pain, 62*, 363–372.

Vlaeyen, J. W. S., Kole-Snijders, A. M. J., Rotteveel, A. M., Ruesink, R., & Heuts, P. H. T. G. (1995b). The role of fear of movement/(re)injury in pain disability. *Journal of Occupational Rehabilitation, 5*, 235–252.

Vlaeyen, J. W. S., Seelen, H. A. M., Peters, M., de Jong, P., Aretz, E., Beisiegel, E., & Weber, W. E. J. (1999). Fear of movement/(re)injury and muscular reactivity in chronic low back pain patients: an experimental investigation. *Pain, 82*, 297–304.

Wiese-Bjornstal, D. M., Smith, A. M., Shaffer, S. M., & Morrey, M. A. (1998). An integrated model of response to sport injury: Psychological and sociological dynamics. *Journal of Applied Sport Psychology, 10*, 46–69.

Williams, J. M., & Andersen, M. B. (1998). Psychosocial antecedents of sport injury: Review and critique of the stress and injury model. *Journal of Applied Sport Psychology, 10*, 5–25.

Yee, D. Y. H., Karim, S. A., & Chang, H. C. (2008). Return to sports after anterior cruciate ligament reconstruction–A review of patients with minimum 5-year follow-up. *Annals Academy of Medicine Singapore, 37*, 273–278.

Index

C

D

E

K

L

M

R

S

www.ingramcontent.com/pod-product-compliance
Ingram Content Group UK Ltd.
Pitfield, Milton Keynes, MK11 3LW, UK
UKHW052008041026
15590UKWH00008B/2214

9 781465 268952